# Building the Future of Food Safety Technology

# Building the Future of Food Safety Technology

## Blockchain and Beyond

**Darin Detwiler, LP.D**

*Assistant Dean and Associate Teaching Professor*
*Northeastern University*
*Founder and CEO of Detwiler Consulting Group*
*Boston, MA, United States*

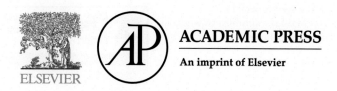

ELSEVIER

**ACADEMIC PRESS**
An imprint of Elsevier

Academic Press is an imprint of Elsevier
125 London Wall, London EC2Y 5AS, United Kingdom
525 B Street, Suite 1650, San Diego, CA 92101, United States
50 Hampshire Street, 5th Floor, Cambridge, MA 02139, United States
The Boulevard, Langford Lane, Kidlington, Oxford OX5 1GB, United Kingdom

**Notices**
Knowledge and best practice in this field are constantly changing. As new research and experience broaden our understanding, changes in research methods, professional practices, or medical treatment may become necessary.

Practitioners and researchers must always rely on their own experience and knowledge in evaluating and using any information, methods, compounds, or experiments described herein. In using such information or methods they should be mindful of their own safety and the safety of others, including parties for whom they have a professional responsibility.

To the fullest extent of the law, neither the Publisher nor the authors, contributors, or editors, assume any liability for any injury and/or damage to persons or property as a matter of products liability, negligence or otherwise, or from any use or operation of any methods, products, instructions, or ideas contained in the material herein.

**Library of Congress Cataloging-in-Publication Data**
A catalog record for this book is available from the Library of Congress

**British Library Cataloguing-in-Publication Data**
A catalogue record for this book is available from the British Library

ISBN: 978-0-12-818956-6

For information on all Academic Press publications visit our website at
https://www.elsevier.com/books-and-journals

*Publisher:* Charlotte Cockle
*Acquisitions Editor:* Patricia Osborn
*Editorial Project Manager:* Emerald Li
*Production Project Manager:* Kiruthika Govindaraju
*Cover Designer:* Alan Studholme

Typeset by TNQ Technologies

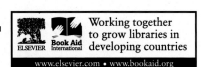

Working together
to grow libraries in
developing countries

www.elsevier.com • www.bookaid.org

# Contents

## SECTION 1    Defining blockchain and regulatory technology

## SECTION 7 Data and food supply chain

## SECTION 8 IT Data security

# Contributors

**Jason P. Bashura, MPH, RS**
Food Defense Subject Matter Expert, New York, United States

**Jennifer Crandall**
Founder and CEO, Safe Food En Route, LLC., Independence, KY, United States

**Kevin Dean, MBA**
Technology Strategist, Dolphin Data Development Ltd., Toronto, ON, Canada

**Darin Detwiler, LP.D**
Assistant Dean and Associate Teaching Professor, Northeastern University, Founder and CEO of Detwiler Consulting Group, LLC., Boston, MA, United States

**Laurette Dube, PhD**
Professor, McGill University, Montreal, QC, Canada

**Adam Friedlander, MS**
Manager, Food Safety and Technical Services, FMI, Washington, D.C., United States

**Karen J. Hand, PhD**
Director, Research Data Strategy, Food for Thought, University of Guelph, Guelph, ON, Canada

**David Hatch**
Chief Strategy and Growth Officer, Corvium, Boston, MA, United States

**Karen Jensen, MBA, RD**
Senior Manager of Regulatory & Sustainability, Reily Foods Company, Knoxville, TN, United States

**John G. Keogh, MBA, MSc**
Doctoral researcher, Henley Business School, University of Reading

**Nida Khan**
Doctoral researcher in blockchain and data analytics for traceability in finance, The Interdisciplinary Centre for Security, Reliability and Trust, University of Luxembourg, Luxembourg City, Luxembourg

**Thodoris Kontogiannis**
Researcher and Author, AgroKnow, Marousi, Attica, Greece

**Bobby Krishna, MSc**
Senior Specialist for Food Permits and Applied Nutrition Section, Dubai Municipality, Dubai, United Arab Emirates

**Vijay Laxmi, LPD, MSc**
Security, Architecture & Engineering Director, Information Technology, Iron Mountain, Inc., Boston, MA, United States

**Wendy Maduff, PhD**
Vice President of Corporate Food Safety and Quality, The Wonderful Company, Los Angeles, CA, United States

**David Mahoney, JD**
Senior Corporate Counsel, Indigo Ag, Inc., Boston, MA, United States

**Abderahman Rejeb**
Doctoral Researcher, School of Regional Sciences and Business Administration, The Széchenyi István University, Győr, Hungary

**Mira Rodgers, MS**
Enologist at Courtside Cellars, LLC., San Luis Obispo, California, United States

**Brian Ronholm, MS**
Director of Food Policy, Consumer Reports, Washington, D.C., United States

**David Shelep**
Microbiologist and Consultant, Paramount Sciences, Los Angeles, CA, United States

**Steven Sklare**
President, Food Safety Academy, Chicago, IL, United States

**Giannis Stoitsis**
CEO/Founder/Owner at FOODAKAI, Marousi, Attica, Greece

**Bridget Sweet, LPD, MS, REHS/RS, CP-FS**
Executive Director of Food Safety at Johnson & Wales University, President and CEO of Sweet Safe, LLC., Providence, RI, United States

**Gary M. Weber, PhD**
Senior Director Food Safety and Contamination Prevention, Worldaware, Washington, D.C., United States

**Ed Wogan, MS**
Vice President, Brand Development-Retail Expansion, Catalina USA, Gloucester, MA, United States

**Jeremy Zenlea, MBA**
Head of Food Safety for EG America, Westborough, MA, United States

**Gennette Zimmer, MBA, MSc**
Data Analytics, Boston University, Boston, MA, United States

# Author biography

**Darin Detwiler, LP.D., M.A.Ed.** is the Assistant Dean at Northeastern University's College of Professional Studies and the Lead Faculty of the MS: Regulatory Affairs of Food and Food Industries. As a professor of food regulatory policy, he has specialized in food safety, global economics of food and agriculture, blockchain, and food authenticity.

An internationally recognized and respected food policy and technology expert with over 25 years' experience in shaping federal food policy, consulting with corporations, and contributing thought leadership to industry events and publications. Detwiler advises industry, NGOs, and government agencies, addressing food safety and authenticity issues in the United States and abroad. In 2018, Detwiler received the International Association for Food Protection (IAFP) Distinguished Service Award (sponsored by *Food Safety Magazine*).

Over the past 25 years, Detwiler has consulted with the US Department of Agriculture in strengthening food safety policies, particularly in the areas of consumer education, product labeling, and their pathogen reduction program. In addition to serving in various educational and advisory capacities, his committee work includes appointments to two terms as a member of the National Advisory Committee on Meat and Poultry Inspection (NACMPI) for the USDA, where his work improved standards and policies related to risk-based sampling. Detwiler's collaboration with the Food and Drug Administration (FDA) includes stakeholder advisory groups, FSMA preimplementation, and on the "New Era of Smarter Food Safety." He also speaks at FDA events and training sessions.

Detwiler holds degrees in history, social studies, and education from Western Washington University, a Master of Arts and Education from the University of Phoenix, and a Doctorate in Law and Policy from Northeastern University's College of Professional Studies.

Detwiler is the author of *Food Safety: Past, Present, and Predictions* (Elsevier Academic Press, 2020)

# Contributor biographies

**Jason Bashura, MPH, RS:** Food Defense Subject Matter Expert. He previously served as the Senior Food Defense Analyst for the US Food and Drug Administration's Center for Food Safety and Applied Nutrition (CFSAN)—Food Defense and Emergency Coordination Staff. Bashura is a former Public Health Preparedness Coordinator and a Senior Environmental Sanitarian. He holds a master's degree in Public Health from the University of Connecticut and a BSc in Public Health from Southern Connecticut State University.

**Jennifer Crandall:** Food Safety Consultant with over 22 years of experience. She has a strong background in supplier management and compliance. Her experience includes 8 years in food manufacturing in various roles such as Quality Assurance Manager, Product Development Manager, Sanitation Supervisor, and Production Supervisor. She gained 12 years corporate experience with the Kroger Company, managing private label suppliers and produce, seafood and meat products with food safety and quality compliance. In 2018, Jennifer founded Safe Food En Route, LLC, where she and her team provide Supplier Compliance Management services including verification services for importers in accordance with FSMA's Foreign Supplier Verification Program Rule. They also provide QA/Food Safety services including specification management, FDA label review services, prevetting food safety of suppliers, GFSI audit gap analysis and consulting, general food safety consulting, and monitoring supplier compliance management and assistance with HACCP, Food Safety Plans, and Produce Safety Rule management. Jennifer holds a BS in Food Science from Purdue University.

**Kevin Dean, MBA:** Toronto-based technology strategist and a licensed engineer. He has been working as a consultant in manufacturing, logistics and supply chain industries for 25 years. Kevin holds a BASc and an MBA from Queen's University.

**Laurette Dube, PhD:** Full Professor at the Desautels Faculty of Management, McGill University. Her research focuses on the study of affects, behavioral economics, and neurobehavioral processes underlying consumption, lifestyle, and health behavior. Her translational research examines how such knowledge can inspire effective interventions. She is also the founder and scientific director of The McGill Centre for the Convergence of Health and Economics, a unique initiative to push the boundaries of science to tackle societal and economic challenges and foster individual and collective health and wealth. Initially trained as a nutritionist, she also holds degrees in finances (MBA), marketing (MPS), and behavioral decision-making/consumer psychology (PhD).

**Adam E. Friedlander, MS:** Food safety scientist at FMI, the food industry association. He is an advocate for food safety and agricultural industries working to advance food safety programs for retailers and product suppliers throughout the country. He is a member of the International Association for Food Protection, Institute of Food Technologists, Conference for Food Protection, Partnership for Food Safety Education, and Association of Food and Drug Officials. Friedlander graduated from Cornell University with a Bachelor of Science in Food Science and Operations Management and a minor in Music. He received his Master of Science in Regulatory Affairs of Food and Food Industries from Northeastern University's College of Professional Studies. He is the coeditor of the textbook *Food System Transparency* (A volume in the Advances in Agroecology series) (Taylor & Francis Group, 2020).

**Karen Hand, PhD:** Involved in numerous research and industry projects involving the analysis and management of Canadian agri-food data. Dr. Hand is keenly interested in the establishment of a comprehensive digital transformation strategy for Canadian Agri-Food to ensure our position as leaders in the global marketplace and for a global sustainable food system. Dr. Karen Hand received her PhD in biostatistics from the University of Guelph.

**David Hatch**: Chief Strategy and Growth Officer at Corvium, a food safety and risk-reducing software company in Boston, MA. David has over 30 years of technology marketing, sales, and customer success leadership experience. He is the founder of CMO in Residence, a marketing and business development consulting firm. Formerly, David was CMO at IANS, an information security services firm, and was the EVP/GM of Harte Hanks Technology Market Solutions and Aberdeen Group, a Boston-based market research firm.

**Karen Jensen, MBA, RD:** Senior Manager of Regulatory and Sustainability at Reily Foods Company, leading all regulatory compliance across Reily Foods' portfolio and managing new label reform and bioengineering. Her experience in the industry includes having served as Associate Principal Scientist at PEPSICO and as the Regulatory Affairs Nutrition Labeling Specialist at Nestlé, USA. A Registered Dietitian, Jensen holds an MBA in Marketing from Northern Illinois University—College of Business and a BS in Dietetics from University of Wisconsin-Stout.

**John G Keogh, MBA, MSc:** President and principal advisor at Toronto-based, niche advisory and research firm Shantalla Inc. He has held executive leadership roles in IT, Technology Consulting, Industry Standards, and Supply Chain Management. A frequent keynote speaker and media analyst, he is currently a doctoral researcher on transparency and trust in food chains at the Henley Business School, University of Reading.

**Nida Khan:** Doctoral researcher in blockchain and data analytics for traceability in finance from the Interdisciplinary Centre for Security, Reliability and Trust (SnT), University of Luxembourg. The research proposal by her won the prestigious

FNR grant, given by the government of Luxembourg for innovative industrial projects. She has worked on decentralized app development for financial contracts, blockchain-based micropayments, blockchain governance, privacy-preserving blockchains, and management of smart contracts. Her research interests include blockchain, artificial intelligence, and cryptography.

**Thodoris Kontogiannis:** Researcher and Author at AgroKnow.

**Bobby Krishna, MSc:** Senior Specialist for Food Permits and Applied Nutrition Section at Dubai Municipality. Krishna has organized and managed several food safety conferences, workshops, scientific meetings, exhibitions, and trainings in Dubai, including the annual Dubai International Food Safety Conference. He is a visiting faculty member at the Canadian University in Dubai. Krishna holds a BSc in Agricultural Sciences from Agra University and an MSc Food Science and Technology—focus on Food Science, QA from the University of New South Wales.

**Vijay Laxmi, LPD, MSc,** is the Security, Architecture and Engineering Director, Information Technology at Iron Mountain Inc, an American enterprise information management services company. Her previous experience includes that of Principal Architect, Cybersecurity and Strategic IT at Biogen, an American multinational biotechnology company, as Senior Global Architect at Schneider Electric, a French multinational corporation providing energy and automation digital solutions for efficiency and sustainability, Senior Technical Lead at Intuit, an American business and financial software company, Senior Architect and Senior Program Manager at Microsoft, and Lead Software Engineer at webMethods focusing on application integration, business process integration, and B2B partner integration. Laxmi has also worked in Software Engineering and IT Consulting for clients including the Union Bank of Switzerland. Laxmi holds a BSc in Mathematics (Hons) from Delhi University, an MSc in Computer Applications from Devi Ahilya Vishwavidyalaya State University of Madhya Pradesh, India, an MSc in Applied Mathematics from The University of Washington, and a Doctor of Law and Policy from Northeastern University's College of Professional Studies.

**Wendy Maduff, PhD:** Vice President of Corporate Food Safety and Quality at The Wonderful Company, responsible for food safety and quality systems, corporate incident management team, and centralizing functions of the four separate business units. While as the Global Food Safety Officer for Subway Restaurants, she supervised all food safety, regulatory, food tracking, quality assurance of the food products and equipment, regulatory, packaging, and nutrition used throughout Subway's nearly 44,900 stores in 112 countries. Dr. Maduff has helped previous positions as the Principal Microbiologist with ConAgra Foods and the Director of Technical Services and Manager of Technical Services for Food Safety Net Services. She received a BA from Virginia Polytechnic Institute and State University, a master's degree from Clemson University, and a Doctorate in Food Safety from the University of California, Davis.

**David Mahoney, JD:** Senior Corporate Counsel at Indigo Ag, Inc., drafting and negotiating agreements on licensing, services, compliance, and joint research. Mahoney has been practicing law since 2002, focusing on intellectual property, corporate and regulatory law in the pharmaceutical, biotechnology, scientific device, and agricultural industries. David's prior positions have included serving as US General Counsel for Lion Bioscience, Inc. (later renamed Sygnis Pharma) as well as US General Counsel for Febit, Inc., an international biotechnology and scientific device company. His professional experience also includes serving as legal counsel for other innovative companies as well as the Massachusetts Institute of Technology, in the Office of the General Counsel. He teaches in Boston and online. He is an assistant teaching professor in Northeastern University College of Professional Studies' Master of Science in the Regulatory Affairs of Drugs, Biologics, and Medical Devices program. He has been teaching at Northeastern since 2012. David holds a Bachelor of Science from Cornell University and a JD, with Distinction, from Suffolk University Law School.

**Abderahman Rejeb:** Student at the Doctoral School of Regional Sciences and Business Administration, The Széchenyi István University, Győr, Hungary. His research interests are Supply Chain Management, Information Management, and Technology Applications.

**Mira Rodgers, MS:** Enologist at Courtside Cellars, LLC., where she has previously served as a Quality Technician and a Grape Evaluation Intern. She was a Quality Compliance Specialist and an Analytical Technologist at Bolthouse Farms as well as a Researcher at Cal Poly State University. Mira earned degrees in biology, anatomy, and physiology at Cal Poly, San Luis Obispo, winemaking certification at UC Davis, and a Master of Science in Regulatory Affairs of Food and Food Industries at Northeastern University's College of Professional Studies.

**Brian Ronholm, MS:** Director of Food Policy at Consumer Reports. Ronholm's background includes serving as the Senior Director of Regulatory Policy at two DC area law firms. Prior to that, Ronholm served as the US Department of Agriculture's Deputy Under Secretary, Food Safety from 2011 to 2017. He also served as the Agriculture Appropriations Associate for the US House of Representatives, in the office of Representative Rosa L. DeLauro (D-CT3). Ronholm holds a BS in Finance from Cal State University:East Bay and an MS in Public Policy Management from The George Washington University.

**David Shelep:** Microbiologist and Consultant at Paramount Sciences. His previous experience includes Director of Sales at AEMTEK, focusing on Environmental

Monitoring for food manufacturing and food Safety, Business Development for Eurofins Lancaster Laboratories, focusing on analytical testing laboratory, primarily for pharmaceutical and biotechnology companies, Senior Account Manager and Director of Sales for Accugenix, Inc., specializing in microbial identifications primarily for the pharmaceutical market, as well as other positions within the bioscience arena. He additionally has experience in clinical microbiology and began his career with Deibel Laboratories performing microbiological analyses. He has previously authored and presented on Microbial Identifications, Business strategy in Outsourcing, and Contamination Control. David holds degrees in Microbiology and Chemistry from Bowling Green State University.

**Steven Sklare:** President of the Food Safety Academy. He previously served as the Director, Customer Engagement:Foods Program (Food Fraud Mitigation/Food Safety Solutions) at US Pharmacopeia, the Strategic Business Development Executive at UL Everclean, and as a Food Safety Consultant at Zep Industries (Food Division). Sklare holds a BA in Economics from The University of Wisconsin-Madison.

**Giannis Stoitsis:** CEO/Founder/Owner at FOODAKAI (an enterprise software platform that collects, translates, and enriches global food safety data in order to extract tailor-made insights for the global supply chain). He is also a Partner and Innovation Advisor at Agroknow.

**Bridget Sweet, LPD, MS, REHS/RS, CP-FS:** Executive Director of Food Safety at Johnson & Wales University (JWU). She is the President and CEO of Sweet Safe, LLC. In addition to practical experience, she serves as an Adjunct Professor and Lead Course Developer for the JWU College of Culinary Arts, lecturing and developing material for food safety programs at the undergraduate and graduate levels. She previously served as a Global Food Safety Specialist for Whole Foods, an Environmental Public Health Officer at Harvard University, and as a local Director of Public Health for a city in Massachusetts. Sweet is a technical expert on food safety matters and her list of professional credentials includes the following: Massachusetts Registered Sanitarian (RS), Registered Environmental Health Specialist/Registered Sanitarian (REHS/RS), Certified Professional-Food Safety (CP-FS), Certified HACCP Manager, FSPCA Preventive Controls for Human Food Lead Instructor, and Managing Retail Food Safety Certified Trainer. She serves as a member of the Conference for Food Protection and the Rhode Island Food Policy Council. She is an elected member of the Board of Health in her hometown and currently serves as Chairman of the Board. Sweet holds a Doctorate in Law and Policy from Northeastern University's College of Professional Studies, an MS in Food Safety from Michigan State University, and a BS in Marine Safety and Environmental Protection from Massachusetts Maritime Academy.

**Gary M. Weber, PhD:** Senior Director Food Safety and Contamination Prevention at WorldAware, a global integrated risk management firm. Dr. Weber's career spans nearly four decades. He grew up in a farming community in Indiana and worked on a family dairy and swine, and crop farm. He received his BS and MS degrees from Purdue University and Doctorate degree from Michigan State University. There he served as an Adjunct Assistant Professor of Animal Science and Area Livestock Agent. He then accepted an appointment as the National Program Leader for Animal Science with the US Department of Agriculture in Washington, DC. Following this assignment, he became the Executive Director of Scientific and Regulatory Affairs for the cattle industry in Washington, DC. During that time, he provided leadership to preventing the introduction or spread of Bovine Spongiform Encephalopathy (BSE) and he served on the National Advisory Committee on Meat and Poultry Inspection (NACMPI) which advises the Secretary of Agriculture on matters affecting federal and state inspection program activities. He served as the President of Bioniche Food Safety, United States, and Prevention Manager for the Food and Drug Administration's Coordinated Outbreak Response and Evaluation Network. The opinions shared here are his own.

**Ed Wogan:** A marketing services professional with an extensive background in retail, supply chain, and emerging technologies serving the industry. Wogan holds graduate degrees from Northeastern University's D'Amore McKim School, Harvard University, as well as a Bachelor of Science Degree from Utica College of Syracuse University. Wogan is an active member in industry associations like the National Association of Convenience Stores and FMI, has presented at the Path to Purchase Institute, and is an advisor/mentor to early stage start-ups via Northeastern's Venture Mentoring Network organization.

**Jeremy Zenlea, MBA:** Head of Food Safety for EG America, a nationwide chain of food service focused convenience store brands. In this role, he oversees all aspects of food safety, including international and domestic regulatory compliance, retail and commissary food safety/QA operations, and supply chain integrity. Jeremy has worked with a variety of different product categories, including refrigerated, high-risk ready-to-eat foods (meat, poultry, pork, and fresh-cut produce), chocolate, and confectioneries. He is an expert in constructing, implementing, and managing complex food safety, food fraud, and food defense systems for large domestic and international food companies. Jeremy is also a lecturer at Northeastern University College of Professional Studies' Master of Science in Regulatory Affairs of Food and Food Industries program. He is an active member of the International Association for Food Protection and the Partnership for Food Safety Education. Jeremy holds a BSc from the University of Massachusetts-Amherst and an MBA from Northeastern University.

**Gennette Zimmer, MBA, MSc:** Data Analytics Facilitator at Boston University who brings a rich background of experience from her career, having previously served as a Senior IT Knowledge and Learning Specialist at Tufts University, a Risk Management Specialist and Trainer at the law firm of Wiley Rein LLP in Washington, DC, and as a Computer Applications Instructor at The Art Institute of Los Angeles. Zimmer earned an MBA from the University of Phoenix and a Master of Science in Computer Information Systems (Data Analytics) from Boston University.

# Foreword

When Darin Detwiler asked me to write a preface to this book, it was very early in 2020, before the coronavirus upended the world. The final writing of this preface has coincided with the realization of how the pandemic would affect all people and business. The size and scope of the potential disruption became increasingly apparent as the COVID-19 crisis, and its impacts on society, has unfolded. Darin requested that I write from my perspective as a Chief Strategy Officer. This is my current role at CORVIUM: a company that develops and markets food safety technology that is integrated within several testing, sanitation, audit, and diagnostic solutions.

As the head of strategy, it is my responsibility to understand the world as it exists and how both direct and indirect pressures will impact and manifest themselves among our customers, partners, stakeholders, and our own company as a whole. My work experiences have been a privilege. I thought I had lived through a majority of the challenges the world could throw at me. I was wrong. We are now living in an unprecedented time when all businesses, organizations, and the people who work and interact with them will reevaluate their strategies in light of the coronavirus crisis and its aftermath of a "new normal." This is just as true in the food industry, and for food safety professionals, as it is for any other profession, with the caveat that food is, indeed, an essential industry and staple. With the beginnings of this new understanding, it is indeed a privilege to write this preface to a book that helps point us in the direction of how food safety, through the use of technology, can and will change over time.

"Strategist" is not something I majored in at university or a profession that is listed in the typical online form pull-down menu we encounter when subscribing to content. Becoming a strategist is the result of over 30 years of work across a variety of organizations within several industries. My experiences have included executive and ownership roles managing market research, technology advisory, and consulting organizations, as well as many years of prior stints as a technology developer, user, marketer, and executive. I have studied the digital transformations that have occurred in financial services, healthcare, manufacturing, publishing, and most recently, the very nascent advances being made in the food industry.

In school, I majored in none of the above. I am a graduate of the University of Massachusetts School of Social and Behavioral Sciences, with a BA in Communication. My academic training focused on how to clearly articulate thoughts and ideas, and my career has allowed me to leverage that training and apply it to the challenges of technology adoption across a multitude of industry challenges.

All of the years and decades in business have helped me to accumulate a well-rounded view into why organizations invest in technology, the intended purposes and objectives that technology is tasked to address, and the efficacy of technology's impact on organizations. Therefore, I write this preface in the voice of a strategist, as I now focus my attention on the evolving use of technology within food safety environments.

After the flush of flattery that Darin's request evoked had worn off, and through the new lens that the coronavirus crisis has provided, I realized three things:

**First**-*This book is very much needed.* The food industry, and "food safety" in particular, is startlingly behind the curve when it comes to the use of data technology. Even in today's digitized world, many food safety teams (even at some of the largest food suppliers in the world) operate within an environment of paper-based reporting, and at best, a manually administered spreadsheet. This must change.

**Second**-*Technology evokes fear and risk.* While the industry continues to "talk the talk" regarding modernization and digitization of food safety, few have begun to "walk the walk." We hear a lot about Blockchain, for example, but see few if any meaningful applications of it in the food industry. This is not due to any fundamental disagreement with the concept or its potential value in preventing real public health issues-but rather the fear of the unknown-the fear of what *could* happen in an increasingly transparent industry. A disturbingly significant percentage of food suppliers express an aversion to allowing their food safety data to be transformed into digital records. This fear is founded on the risk of those records being exposed to an audience of consumers who are uneducated in the complexities of pathogen, allergen, and other food safety testing programs. The fear of liability, in other words, is blocking the very clear path to alleviating liability risks.

**Third**-*The Coronavirus Crisis changes everything.* Mere months before the pandemic became a reality, a senior food company executive said to me "I don't think we'll see digital transformation really take hold in our industry for at least a decade." He was putting up an objection to considering the digitization of his food safety data. Today, that same organization is prioritizing a project with the objective of enabling their food safety teams to monitor their sanitation controls and FSQA programs remotely through use of digital, web-based technology. There is nothing like a life-changing crisis to put a spotlight on a pent-up need. The food industry has seen a particular vulnerability emerge via the pandemic impact: *human safety.* Now, in addition to the risks that foodborne pathogens represent, the threat to facility workers adds a new layer of risks to be managed. This is driving increased demand for testing, monitoring, and "workplace distancing"-the likes of which we have not encountered before. Technology definitely has a role to play in all of this.

As with anything involving fear and overcaution regarding the unknown, the answer lies in education. That which we understand, we adopt and embrace. That which we do not understand, we fear and avoid.

Slow technology adoption was illustrated perfectly through the advent of online banking. The industry and consumers alike rebelled against this concept for many years, touting fear of online fraud and the potential for customer churn. Over time, however, the idea of NOT offering online banking, purchasing, and financial services has now become ludicrous. Why? Because the benefits of offering digital services far outweighed the danger and risks. Today, online banking risks are mitigated to an acceptable level. Is it perfect? No. Is it tolerable? Apparently so.

The same can be said about our healthcare system, and the push for migration to a system based on electronic health records, which is now known simply by its acronym: "EHR." (If it has an acronym, you KNOW it has been adopted!) While there is a fear of access to our digitized personal health information, the benefits of having an EHR system far outweigh the risks. Healthcare providers can now share information, coordinate treatment plans, alleviate known drug interaction risks, and practice far safer medicine as a result of the transparency that an EHR-based system provides. Gone are the days of shelves filled with color-coded folders for each patient, full of manually created, human error-prone data.

And yet today, when an auditor or inspector visits a food production plant, they face the unfortunate "norm"-a massive vault of paper-based reports and logs. The lack of automation extends throughout the food supply chain, from upstream farms and raw goods suppliers all the way to the restaurants and grocers where we purchase and consume food. It is no wonder, therefore, that our food supply chain continues to experience an ever-increasing number of food safety issues and recalls.

The CDC now estimates that over one-sixth of the US population (48 million people!) will suffer a foodborne illness and 3000 people die each year as a result of ingesting contaminated food (CDC, 2018). Added to that now will be an estimate and set of guidelines to deal with human-borne pathogens that could, if left unchecked, pose a serious threat to the food supply chain if processing plant workers are not able to safely operate their production lines.

Traditional methods must give way to digital transformation. "Digital transformation" enables the correlation of data pertaining to a variety of food safety activities-such as how sanitation effectiveness is related to allergen and pathogen testing or how weather fluctuations impact food production environmental cleanliness, the analysis of which a manual paper-based approach makes impossible. The current manual error-prone means by which food safety programs are being managed is clearly not working, and the increasing complexities of the global food supply chain are making it impossible to track and manage food safety adherence using traditional methods.

This book is an essential read for the industry. As a community, *we must get past our fear of digitizing food safety data.* Perhaps the pandemic and its aftereffects will accelerate this movement. Regardless, it is the only path to gaining control, analyzing, and managing food safety performance in a world that requires us to do so or fail at the peril of thousands. As dramatic as that sounds, it is where we are, and given the lessons of adjacent industries, proper use of technology and data is the answer.

**David Hatch**
*Chief Strategy and Growth Officer*
*Corvium, Boston, MA, United States*

## Reference

CDC. (2018, November 15). *CDC and food safety*. Retrieved from https://www.cdc.gov/foodsafety/cdc-and-food-safety.html.

# Introduction to building the future of food safety technology

One of the hottest topics at food industry events is technology. Today's stakeholders across the entire spectrum of seed to fork live in a world where technology-in a variety of forms-is all around them. Those in the industry may see it in the form of software, robotics, satellite imagery, and even virtual reality. Consumers may see advances in food technology in the way they gain information about food, share feedback, order food, and even in how they pay for food.

In a way, technology has always been part of how humans as consumers have been defined over time. When we talk about the transition from hunter/gatherers to agriculture, from hand tools to steam or electric engines, from analog to digital platforms, and even from horse-drawn carriages to unmanned drones for delivery, we are characterizing the advancement of industrialization at the same time we are describing the evolution of society (see Table 1.1).

With these changes in technologies, significant transformations impacted the geography of food supply (distances for import/export) and of consumers (eating outside the home and, now, ordering delivery over the smartphone.) They impacted the economics of farmers, producers, and consumers-such as efficiency and new markets. They resulted in the demand for changes in policies and in laws-mostly related to protecting public health. Finally, they forced radical changes in our social behavior as workers, consumers, and even as families.

## Blockchain: The Buzz Word

Any modern discussion of the food industry and technology will inevitably include a focus on data collection and analysis related to compliance and reputation. Some new technologies, or "RegTech," are promised as key optimization tools not only for the future of the industry but also for consumers as they "can now expect to see the entire histories of the products they buy, and hence make more informed decisions" (Rivers, 2019). The most talked about and written about of all technologies today is Blockchain. Some in the food industry describe Blockchain using words such as transparency, traceability, network, partnership, and big data. Some retail giants use words such as "required."

Walmart describes itself as "...the world's largest retailer" due to having become "the masters of supply chain management." The retail giant has "endeavored to become a leader in the area of implementing supply chain technologies to achieve the kind of operational efficiency that make these cost savings possible" (West, n.d). In a September 24, 2018, press release, Walmart and Sam's Club (a chain of membership-only retail warehouse clubs owned and operated by Walmart Inc.)

**Table 1.1** Comparing changes in Industrial Revolutions to changes in Societies.

| Description | Industrial revolutions | Societies | Description |
|---|---|---|---|
| | | Society 0.1 (30,000 to 70,000 years ago) | Cognitive Revolution: *Toolmaking* |
| | | Society 1.0 (circa 10,000BC) | Agricultural Revolution: *Domestication* |
| Steam engine machines/ urbanization | First Industrial Revolution (18th to 19th centuries) | Society 2.0 (1760–1960s) | Industrial Revolution: *Urbanization* |
| Internal combustion engine/ urbanization/ imperialism/ immigration | Second Industrial Revolution (between 1870 and pre-World War I) | | |
| "Digital Revolution"/the Internet | Third Industrial Revolution (1980s–today) | Society 3.0 (1950–today) | Information Revolution: *Digitalization* |
| Robotics/artificial intelligence (AI)/ nanotechnology/ quantum computing/ Blockchain/ biotech/the Internet of things (IoT)/autonomous vehicles | Fourth Industrial Revolution (2010s and beyond) | Society 4.0 (2010–2090) | Egregore Revolution: *Convergence* |
| | | Society 5.0 (circa 2100) | Transapience Revolution: *Transcendence* |

*Table 1.1 Created by author, based on information from Schwab, K. (2017). The Fourth Industrial Revolution. New York: Crown Business and Haupt, M. (2018, January 21). The Evolutionary Journey to Society 4.0. Medium. Retrieved from https://medium.com/society4/evolution-of-societies-93a5f0f9b31*

announced that they will require real-time, end-to-end food traceability from their suppliers of leafy green vegetables by September 2019. Specifically, their suppliers must use IBM Blockchain technology (Walmart, 2018).

According to Walmart,

> *Blockchain is a way to digitize data and share information in a complex network in a secure and trusted way. For food safety, this helps to more accurately pinpoint*

*issues in the food chain and further protect customers against foodborne ill-nesses.... For more than a year, Walmart, working with IBM and 11 other food companies, has successfully developed a Blockchain-enabled food traceability network built on open-source technology. In an initial pilot conducted by Walmart and IBM, the amount of time it took the retailer to trace an item from store to farm was reduced from seven days to just 2.2 seconds (Walmart, 2018).*

According to IBM,

*Blockchain offers complete visibility of the data behind the many stages of product creation. Manufacturers, farmers, wholesalers, suppliers, delivery services and stores each input information that details and verifies their roles in the process — creating a log that provides irrefutable evidence of a product's provenance (Rivers, 2019).*

With all this hype over Blockchain, exhibitor halls at food safety conferences are full of booths displaying everything from sanitation devices to sensors to software. This more complete view of the ecosystem of technologies includes the work horses of data collection, storage, packaging, analysis, and beyond. To fully understand the future of food safety technology, one needs to aim far beyond simply a look at Blockchain.

## Digitalization: A Critical Next Step

One critical concern to explore is the shift to the digitization of information within the food industry. Most regulations or other advances in data tied to food safety have been paper-based. The advent of bar codes in 1974, the 1989 GS1-128 bar codes, and the 2011 Produce Traceability Initiative were all paper-based (Libbey, 2018). Even with the **FDA Food Safety Modernization Act ("FSMA") of 2011** (Pub.L. 111−353, 124 STAT 3885) that had effective implementation dates of 2016−2018, paper was the standard for records. Only recently has the industry seen a change in the government's stance on digitization of records.

Only 2 days before Thanksgiving, 2018, the Centers for Disease Control and Prevention (CDC) issued a press release (CDC, 2018b) and a Food Safety Alert (CDC, 2019) regarding an outbreak of *Escherichia coli* tied to romaine lettuce that ultimately resulted in 62 reported cases across 16 states (and in Canada) with 25 hospitalizations (no deaths) and the triggering of an FDA recall (unlike a few previous outbreaks tied to leafy greens when the FDA did not issue a recall.) The CDC, along with (then) FDA Commissioner Scott Gottlieb, urged consumers to dispose of all romaine lettuce (Gottlieb, 2018b). Later that month, Commissioner Gottlieb issued a statement in which he declared that "Complicating this already large-scale investigation, the majority of the records collected in this investigation were either paper or handwritten" (Gottlieb, 2018a). Thus, the FDA's emphasis on industry work to standardize record-keeping and adopt traceability best practices now includes the use of state-of-the-art technologies. But this was only a suggestion from the US government. Unfortunately, a repeat of an outbreak tied to romaine lettuce from Salinas, CA, took place almost 1 year to the date, thus sparking another Thanksgiving recall in 2019—resulting in 167 reported cases across 27 states with 85 hospitalizations (no deaths) and the triggering of an FDA recall (CDC, 2020; FDA, 2020).

## Canada's position on Digitalization

In Canada, the Safe Food for Canadians Act (SFCA) (S.C. 2012, c. 24) and the Safe Food for Canadians Regulations (SFCR) (SOR/2018-108) came into effect in January 2019. SFCA and SFCR cover imported, exported, interprovincially and, in some cases, intraprovincially traded food products.

> As risks to food, animal health and plants have changed considerably and continue to change rapidly, the Agency must continue to adapt and be more efficient and responsive while supporting Canada's ability to compete in the global market (Canadian Food Inspection Agency, 2018).

What makes Canada's SFCA stand out is that it was the first widespread regulation in North America to suggest that "standard commercial software" is acceptable for record-keeping (Canadian Food Inspection Agency, 2019).

## So where does the FDA stand on Blockchain?

In the opening session for the 2017 Dubai International Food Safety Conference, Frank Yiannas, then Walmart's vice president in charge of food safety, delivered his thoughts on "Why Should Technology Trend in Food Safety: Exploring Blockchain." Yiannas shared his observation of weaknesses in the food industry when it comes to traceability and how he was once a major skeptic of Blockchain. Having become a believer that Blockchain can be a digital solution, he showed the international audience a video in which he highlighted his work at Walmart with IBM and nine other major food brands including Dole, Nestle, Tyson, and Unilever to pilot Blockchain technology. In December of 2018, Frank Yiannas took office as the FDA's Deputy Commissioner for Food Policy and Response.

On April 30, 2019, Yiannas and Acting FDA Commissioner Ned Sharpless, MD, released a statement on a **"New Era of Smarter Food Safety"** (Sharpless and Yiannas, 2019). Previously, the FDA's FSMA set forth new definitions and rules. Yiannas had initially added to FSMA through his support for the development of a food safety culture (as defined in his 2008 book titled "*Food Safety Culture*"). This 2019 statement initiated an advancement in the FDA's approach to food safety in that the administration now calls for industry support through incorporating the use of new and emerging technologies throughout the global supply chain.

As of June 2019, the FDA, authorized under the 2013 US Drug Supply Chain Security Act (Pub.L. 113−54), has embarked on a pilot program with Walmart, IBM, and Merck that will explore using Blockchain. The goals of this real-time monitoring test of the pharmaceutical supply chain include improving the security of prescription drug supply and distribution as well as increasing regulatory oversight of counterfeit, stolen, contaminated, or otherwise harmful drugs (Mathias, 2019). While large retailers have increased the use of digital solutions within the food industry over the past 50 years, one can see how success with this pilot will impact the FDA's initial steps towards a more proactive position on digital solutions for the food industry's future.

On October 21, 2019, Yiannas facilitated an FDA public meeting for the industry to hear about this "New Era of Smarter Food Safety," to participate in breakout sessions and to contribute statements on the Era's four pillars (FDA, 2019):

- Tech-Enabled Traceability and Foodborne Outbreak Response (reactive use of technologies, data streams, and processes to trace back and respond to public health risks).
- Smarter Tools and Approaches for Prevention (proactive use of new knowledge, new data analysis tools, and predictive analytics to mitigate potential food safety risks within the preventive controls framework established by FSMA).
- Adapting to New Business Models and Retail Food Safety Modernization (consideration of new business models, e-commerce, modern delivery methods).
- Food Safety Culture (promoting commitment in the industry and consumer education).

Of note with this public meeting on the FDA's "New Era of Smarter Food Safety" is the fact that none of the FDA's supporting documents mention "Blockchain" by name, opting instead to discuss transparency and traceability technologies. Presentations and breakout sessions also avoided deliberately focusing on "Blockchain" as a specific item.

## The Future of Food Safety Technology: Getting it Right

Blockchain (and other data collection technology) is often described as being able to improve food safety. These messages typically include how it would improve traceability and speed up a recall. While this increased reactive focus on data collection has a definite place in response to failures in food safety, this takes place after incidents or crises have occurred; when real people have been harmed; and consumers have become victims, hospital patients, and worse.

Much like a car's airbag, Blockchain definitely may be part of the solution, but deployment after an incident has already happened, regardless of its efficiency, forces consumers to accept that harm already has occurred. Over time, after-the-fact responses reduce a company's options to identify, stop, and correct a failure, while the liabilities of that company continue to increase. History shows where hindsight usually includes lawsuits, court trials, and sometimes even changes in legislation.

This is where, according to a 2012 study, many companies will experience a sharp drop in their NYSE stock value over an entire quarter of trading, then a return to preincident values that requires at least three additional quarters of stock trading (Seo et al., 2013).

Consumers are aware that new technologies and food safety practices come with a price tag that increases the grocery bill. But consumers will question what they are paying for if these steps fall short of protecting them. Consider, also, that while companies frequently recover (or at least survive) after these incidents, those consumers and their families most impacted by a foodborne illness or food allergen crisis never fully recover.

No large corporation is immune to failures that happen before, during, or after their involvement with a product. Since 1993, Americans have seen the seemingly uninterrupted cycle of crisis-and-reform through headline after headline of multistate outbreaks and huge recalls involving major labels and national retail or restaurant chains. While early food safety concerns focused on meat and poultry, more recent recalls and outbreaks have been tied to cantaloupe, leafy greens, sprouts, caramel apples, ice cream, peanut butter, and other produce. Ready-to-eat and commercially packaged goods such as cereals and salads also found their way onto lists of contaminated products.

Many times, even the efforts of those companies and leaders who did everything they could to protect their consumers would be thwarted by improper handling, inadequate cooking, or some other action down the line.

American economist George Stigler, PhD, received the 1982 Nobel Prize in Economic Sciences for his "seminal studies of industrial structures, functioning of markets and causes and effects of public regulation" (George, n.d.). Stigler's contributions, through his work in the economic theory of utility maximizing behavior-involving the concept that people in a market will alter their behavior to maximize their utility, meaning to increase their satisfaction (Posner, 2010)-are considered to be influential and responsible for its existence in modern economic thinking (Rosen, 1993).

Stigler's Nobel lecture included a discussion of a lack of serious professional attempts to measure the impact of public regulation; Stigler stated that while policymakers and traders differ by the "rules and constraints" of how they operate in markets, the theory of utility-maximizing behavior can still be used to analyze their behaviors. Stigler noted how economists believe that voters are "myopic and forgetful" of the causes of certain policy concerns while our elected officials (perhaps through design or perversion of our political institutions) are able to pursue their own interests (Mäler, 1992).

"Myopic and forgetful" could be used to explain how utility and concern (as in the case of food) sit on opposite ends of a spectrum. Some recent events serve as a reminder of how consumers and policymakers fit into this spectrum.

In her 2019 Eater article about "The Ice Cream Licker"-whose viral video (Today, 2019) angered so many across the nation that summer-Jenny Zhang went well beyond the facts behind both the behavior of the young woman in the video and the 2010-2015 *Listeria* outbreak (and subsequent recall) tied to Blue Bell Creameries' ice cream. The video demonstrates how technology can divide public opinion. Conversely, technicians in a food lab first detected the *Listeria* outbreak while testing new equipment and protocols, whereas technologies on hand in the ice cream production facilities did not mitigate the pathogen's presence. Thus, the use of technology, much like public opinion, can become a "double-edged sword."

Zhang's analysis of the polarized public perception of the two events should be mandatory reading for students of all disciplines. In Zhang's words,

> *It's a strange quirk of the human psyche that we are so often more preoccupied with the actions of individuals, rather than the actions of the larger corporations, institutions, and systems that have a lot more say in how the world works….When a teenage girl faces more hostility and calls for jail time for a prank than a multi-million-dollar company that failed to protect its consumers, that's when you really have to stop and consider who gets assigned blame, and who gets exoneration, in the eyes of the public (Zhang, 2019).*

The FDA's desire for public trust policy around food safety transparency and culture can also be a "double-edged sword" in the hands of federal regulators.

In 2018, (then) FDA Commissioner Scott Gottlieb's hesitancy to inform the public early about outbreaks and recalls-or even to declare a recall-has been characterized by what he called the agency's "culture of caution-a fear that putting out a false alarm about an *E .coli* outbreak could damage public trust in the FDA-and needlessly alarm consumers" (Haughney, 2020). Sure, the FDA wants to be absolutely certain they have found the correct source before going public with information. A year later, the FDA held their October 21, 2019 public meeting on their "New Era of Smarter Food Safety," (FDA, 2019) with significant messages of commitment, transparency, and consumer education.

However, on October 31, 2019, just 10 days after the FDA's public meeting, the FDA announced an *E. coli* outbreak and recall that would later carry-on throughout the Thanksgiving season and result in 167 reported cases across 27 states with 85 hospitalizations (no deaths) and the triggering of an FDA recall (CDC, 2020; FDA, 2020). That same day, the internationally respected food safety lawyer William "Bill" Marler penned a blog post:

> *I call Bullshit on the FDA, CDC and Health Departments of Arizona, California, Florida, Georgia, Illinois, Maryland, North Carolina, Nevada, New York, Oregon, Pennsylvania and South Carolina (Marler, 2019).*

Marler called out stakeholders (in the know about the outbreak) who "… all chose to hide it until late this evening," adding "so much for 'transparency' and so much for 'food safety culture.'" (Marler, 2019). His words about their actions speak volumes for the hope and hype around Blockchain and other forms of RegTech, in that all the collection of data and all the facts, or actionable information we can extract through analysis, are meaningless if we fail to act on them.

> *We will not have a safe food supply when facts are hidden from consumers. We will not have a safe food supply until there really is honesty and transparency by those in government, industry (growers, shippers, processors and retailers— grocery stores and restaurants) and academia charged with consumer food safety (Marler, 2019).*

The next day, Consumer Reports posted a statement online (Loria, 2019) indicating that they believe the FDA waited too long to alert consumers, listing a domino chain of separate outbreaks of *E. coli* O157:H7 tied to Romaine lettuce-December 2017, spring 2018, and fall 2018. Consumer Reports characterized the spring 2018 outbreak as "the largest and most deadly *E. coli* outbreak in the U.S. in decades" (Loria, 2019) and indicated that this pattern should have prompted the FDA to release information to the public earlier.

Again, insight from Consumer Reports' statement applies to the future of food safety technology. All of the data and all of the technology are meaningless to those who are harmed unless those in industry and government go beyond the data and consider the patterns to mitigate as much as possible. This FDA "culture of caution" (Haughney, 2020) with a fear of needlessly alarming consumers must not be prioritized subsequent to any fear on the part of the FDA of needlessly harming industry.

Food safety for all consumers, as well as an integrated food safety partnership and a true food safety culture, can and should be measured by elements of honesty, transparency, and speed of communication when it comes to critical information. The relationship between the industry and state/federal regulators is critical in this recipe. However, some experts point out that policy or politics may not be solely at fault for such delays.

Gary M. Weber, PhD, who wrote earlier in the chapter on "Food Safety," is the Senior Director Food Safety and Contamination Prevention at WorldAware. He shares his hope that the CDC will step up and achieve the promises they made in 2010 to improve illness and illness cluster analysis faster.

> *They take too long to provide actionable information for the FDA. It's disappointing when people attack FDA for being slow when they are more often than not waiting on CDC and the States to do their work. The CDC has been pushing the traceability issue on FDA while seemingly ignoring the real rate-limiting step in all this that sits in the hands of the CDC and the state labs. Too many people get sick and die because of a slow process of identifying suspect and implicated food vehicles. WGS should be making this much faster Gary Weber, Personal Communication, 2020*

The future of food safety technology is nowhere near as simple as any single "silver bullet" technology solution. In order for effective and sustainable use of any new RegTech-with results that benefit both industry and consumers-advancement will need to be coordinated and evaluated along with policy and the culture of those many technology stakeholders. The journey of data will, in many ways, parallel the journey of food from source to end user. Respecting the quality, safety, defense, security, and authenticity of data should be treated as critical as doing the same for food. Without this respect, the futures of food safety technology and of consumers are both at increased risk.

The CDC estimates that each year 48 million Americans become ill from foodborne pathogens, 128,000 are hospitalized, and 3000 die (CDC, 2018a). Since the landmark 1993 *E. coli* outbreak, the math shows that over 80,000 American consumers have died from foodborne illnesses, a large portion of which could have been prevented (Mead et al., 1999). The frequency and quantity of recalls, along with the number of outbreaks, illnesses, and deaths tied to foodborne pathogens, indicate that problems still exist somewhere between the farm and the table.

Industry use of Blockchain must include a parallel focus on its use to predict and prevent failures before they become crises that harm consumers. This approach brings an increase of options while minimizing (if not eliminating) liabilities. The impact on consumer safety adds great value to technology used in the most proactive sense.

Not all failures can be identified and stopped before it is too late. Predictive analytics should be driven by a balance of data literacy, technology literacy, and human literacy (Aoun, 2017). At the heart of human literacy should be found an understanding of the true burden of disease. With this, our use of data and technology can be transformed by asking the right questions, looking beyond simple cost-benefit analysis, and prioritizing consumers' safety. If industry leaders fail to develop practices or even a culture that embraces this balance, then consumers will ultimately pay for new technologies that protect industry more than they protect families.

This book brings together academic research with the first-hand perspectives of 25 diverse and seasoned experts in the food industry, data, technology, law, and beyond to explore the many dimensions of concern when faced with the future of food safety technology.

**Darin Detwiler, LP.D**
*Assistant Dean and Associate Teaching Professor*
*Northeastern University*
*Founder and CEO of Detwiler Consulting Group, LLC.*
*Boston, MA, United States*

# References

Aoun, J. (2017). *Robot-proof: Higher education in the age of artificial intelligence*. Cambridge: MIT Press.

Canadian Food Inspection Agency. (2019, June 12). *Safe food for Canadians regulations tool kit for food businesses fact sheet: traceability*. Retrieved from https://www.inspection.gc.ca/food/toolkit-for-food-businesses/traceability/eng/1427310329573/1427310330167.

Canadian Food Inspection Agency. (2018). *Understanding the safe food for Canadians regulations a handbook for food businesses* (CFIA publication no. P0965E-18 catalogue no.: A104-142/2018E-PDF), ISBN 978-0-660-26985-6. Retrieved from https://www.inspection.gc.ca/DAM/DAM-aboutcfia-sujetacia/STAGING/text-texte/regs_safe_food_regulations_handbook_business_1531429195095_eng.pdf.

CDC. (2018a). *Estimates of foodborne illness in the United States*. Retrieved from https://www.cdc.gov/foodborneburden/index.html.

CDC. (2018b). *Food safety alert:* E. coli *outbreak linked to romaine lettuce* [Press Release]. Retrieved from https://www.cdc.gov/media/releases/2018/s1120-ecoli-romain-lettuce.html.

CDC. (2019, January 9). *Food safety alert: Outbreak of* E. coli *infections linked to romaine lettuce* [Final update]. Retrieved from https://www.cdc.gov/ecoli/2018/o157h7-11-18/index.html.

CDC. (2020, January 15). *Outbreak of* E. coli *infections linked to romaine lettuce* [Final Update]. Retrieved from https://www.cdc.gov/ecoli/2019/o157h7-11-19/index.html.

FDA Food Safety Modernization Act ("FSMA") of 2011 (Pub.L. 111−353, 124 STAT 3885).

FDA. (2019, November 25). *Public meeting on a new era of smarter food safety: October 21, 2019* [Updated Press Release]. Retrieved from https://www.fda.gov/food/workshops-meetings-webinars-food-and-dietary-supplements/public-meeting-new-era-smarter-food-safety-10212019-10212019.

FDA. (2020, January 27). *Outbreak Investigation of* E. coli*: romaine from salinas, California (November 2019)*. Retrieved from https://www.fda.gov/food/outbreaks-foodborne-illness/outbreak-investigation-e-coli-romaine-salinas-california-november-2019.

George J. Stigler − Facts. (n.d.). Nobelprize.org. Retrieved from http://www.nobelprize.org/nobel_prizes/economic-sciences/laureates/1982/stigler-facts.html.

Gottlieb, S. (2018a). *Statement from FDA Commissioner Scott Gottlieb, M.D., on findings from the romaine lettuce* E. coli *O157:H7 outbreak investigation and FDA's efforts to prevent future outbreaks* [Press Release]. Retrieved from https://www.fda.gov/news-events/press-announcements/statement-fda-commissioner-scott-gottlieb-md-findings-romaine-lettuce-e-coli-o157h7-outbreak.

Gottlieb, S. (2018b). *Statement from FDA Commissioner Scott Gottlieb, M.D., on the current romaine lettuce* E. coli *O157:H7 outbreak investigation*. Retrieved from https://www.fda.gov/news-events/press-announcements/statement-fda-commissioner-scott-gottlieb-md-current-romaine-lettuce-e-coli-o157h7-outbreak.

Haughney, C. (2020, January 23). Is the FDA ready for the next *E. coli* outbreak? *The Boston Globe*. Retrieved from https://www.bostonglobe.com/2020/01/23/metro/is-fda-ready-next-e-coli-outbreak/.

Haupt, M. (2018, January 21). *The evolutionary journey to Society 4.0*. Medium. Retrieved from https://medium.com/society4/evolution-of-societies-93a5f0f9b31.

Libbey, N. (2018, November 15). *Presentation on evolution of food traceability*. Schaumburg, IL: Food Safety Consortium.

Loria, K. (2019, November 1). *FDA discloses new* E. Coli *romaine outbreak after it ends: CR believes the agency waited too long to alert consumers.* Retrieved from https://www.consumerreports.org/e-coli/fda-discloses-new-e-coli-romaine-outbreak-after-it-ends/.

Mäler, K. (1992). *Nobel lectures, Economics 1981−1990.* Singapore: World Scientific Publishing, Co.

Marler, B. (2019, October 31). *I call bullshit on the FDA, CDC and Health Departments of Arizona, California, Florida, Georgia, Illinois, Maryland, North Carolina, Nevada, New York, Oregon, Pennsylvania and South Carolina.* Marler Blog. Retrieved from https://www.marlerblog.com/legal-cases/i-call-bullshit-on-the-fda-cdc-and-health-departments-of-arizona-california-florida-georgia-illinois-maryland-north-carolina-nevada-new-york-oregon-pennsylvania-and-south-carolina/.

Mead, P., Slutsker, L., Dietz, V., McCaig, L., Bresee, J., Shapiro, C., et al. (1999). *Food-related illness and death in the United States.* Centers for Disease Control and Prevention. Available from http://wwwnc.cdc.gov/eid/article/5/5/99-0502.

Mathias, T. (2019, June 13). *IBM, Walmart, Merck in blockchain collaboration with FDA.* Reuters New Service. Retrieved from https://www.reuters.com/article/us-fda-block-chain/ibm-walmart-merck-in-blockchain-collaboration-with-fda-idUSKCN1TE1SA.

Posner, R. (2010). *Economic Analysis of Law.* New York: Aspen Pub.

Rivers, S. (2019, April 22). Win customers' hearts with a transparent supply chain. In *IBM food trust's blockchain pulse: IBM blockchain blog.* Retrieved from https://www.ibm.com/blogs/Blockchain/2019/04/win-customers-hearts-with-a-transparent-supply-chain/.

Rosen, S. (1993). George J. Stigler and the industrial organization of economic thought. *The Journal of Political Economy, 101*, 51.

(SFCA) 2012   Safe Food for Canadians Act (SFCA) (S.C. 2012, c. 24).

(SFCR) 2018   Safe Food for Canadians Regulations (SFCR) (SOR/2018-108).

Schwab, K. (2017). *The fourth industrial revolution.* New York: Crown Business.

Seo, S., et al. (2013, June). The impact of food safety events on the value of food-related firms: An event study approach. *International Journal of Hospitality Management, 33*. Retrieved from https://www.sciencedirect.com/science/article/abs/pii/S0278431912000989.

Sharpless, N., & Yiannas, F. (2019). *FDA Statement: Statement from Acting FDA Commissioner Ned Sharpless, M.D., and Deputy Commissioner Frank Yiannas on steps to usher the U.S. into a new era of smarter food safety* [Press Release]. FDA. Retrieved from https://www.fda.gov/news-events/press-announcements/statement-acting-fda-commissioner-ned-sharpless-md-and-deputy-commissioner-frank-yiannas-steps-usher.

The Today Show. (2019, July 6). *Blue bell ice cream licker identified by police.* NBC News. YouTube. Retrieved from https://www.youtube.com/watch?v=N7u37pCIwz8&fbclid=IwAR1xJmjGJnJj6cM_0jjspT_l7-3zc42JESC-bFW26tQNdZ0_j9KI6k0XIME.

*U.S. Drug Supply Chain Security Act (Pub.L. 113−54).*(2013).

Walmart. (2018, September 24). *Walmart and Sam's Club to require real-time, end-to-end food traceability with blockchain* [Press release]. Retrieved from https://corporate.walmart.com/media-library/document/leafy-greens-on-Blockchain-press-release/_proxyDocument?id=00000166-0c4c-d96e-a3ff-8f7c09b50001.

West. C. et al. (n.d.) "RFID Technology." Walmart supply chain. Retrieved from https://walmartsupplychain.weebly.com/rfid-technology.html.

Yiannas, F. (2008). *Food safety culture: Creating a behavior-based food safety management system.* New York: Springer.

Zhang, J. (2019, July 12). *Why there's more outrage over the ice cream licker than a listeria outbreak.* Eater. Retrieved from https://www.eater.com/2019/7/12/20691669/blue-bell-ice-cream-licker-corporation-listeria-accountability.

# Building the future of food safety technology

## Introduction

When Walmart conducted its test on the use of Blockchain technology in 2018 and was able to trace a package of sliced mangoes from the store shelf back to the exact source in 2.2 seconds, it served as an emphatic announcement on the potential of technology's role in food traceability (Corkery and Popper, 2018). Under traditional methods, the tracing of this product typically would have taken almost a week to complete. The difference between 1 week and 2 seconds is, of course, very significant; when applied to food safety, specifically traceability and outbreak containment, the difference is several lifetimes.

Think of how quickly potentially contaminated products can be identified and removed from store shelves; think of how quickly the source of the contamination can be identified and corrective measures implemented; think of how many potential problems could be identified even before a product reaches the consumer.

Stakeholders in the food policy arena had been aware of the emerging concept and promise of Blockchain for a few years but were waiting to see if that promise eventually would translate into successful implementation. The test Walmart conducted, combined with their subsequent announcement that it would require its leafy green suppliers to trace their products using Walmart's Blockchain system, served notice that the concept had emerged and held significant promise (Walmart, 2018).

The impact that a fully realized, developed, and implemented technology like this could have in reducing, and even preventing, foodborne illness is immense. It may have transformed many skeptics into believers. And, to think, Blockchain is not the only technology related to traceability that offers this promise.

## Edible DNA

Imagine an edible, inactive DNA-based bar code that is invisible, tasteless, and designed to trace a particular food product back to its source within a few minutes. On immediate consideration of this technology, this would appear to address concerns about Blockchain in terms of reducing potential errors by reducing the number of data input variables throughout the process.

A company called SafeTraces*, based in Pleasanton, California, has developed this technology-short DNA tracers-and sells it to food producers and other companies throughout the food supply chain. While the concept may seem like it originated from science fiction, the tracers it created can identify the origin of a commodity, intermediate handlers, processors, and final disposition for retail.

The process is fascinating. The DNA-based material can be incorporated into a product through a powder or liquid formulation, in a wash step, or included in coatings in produce items. Using apples as an example, after harvest, most produce is washed and coated with natural waxes to reduce moisture loss, extend shelf life, and improve its appearance. The tracer product is integrated with the washing and coating process and is added to the wax or other coating.

According to information on the company's website, to trace the product, sampling is performed with a swab or a rinse, and analysis of the short DNA sequences is a rapid step that can be performed at a customer site. Through the use of a special device that can read the DNA bar code, the sequence information can then be mapped to a database with the detailed traceability information. Obviously, food that has been consumed cannot be traced, but the technology offers food producers an opportunity to limit the scope of a recall once they learn of a problem.

This was such a notable technology that The Wall Street Journal included it on a list of six inventions that are part of a technological revolution involving the food industry (Gasparro & Newman, 2018).

In case you were wondering about the identity of the other five technologies outlined in the article, they include 3D printed foods; algae farming for use in foods; the use of organic agricultural by-products like grape skins to develop an ultrathin edible coating that can be applied to the surface of fruit to maintain its freshness longer; facial recognition technology to help track behavior of dairy cows; and a food computer that helps set up a controlled environment that can mimic climates around the world. As these other examples demonstrate, technology is not limited to traceability goals.

## The regulatory dynamic

It is the regulatory aspect that can often be the most intriguing and vexing component of developing a new technology. When start-up companies reach the conclusion of a product's development process and are prepared to enter the marketplace, they may have the impression that the most difficult part is over. In fact, navigating the regulatory process also can impose some barriers to the process, and sometimes, a company can find itself proceeding down the wrong path. This is how many consulting firms are able to stay in business.

Once companies figure out how they intend to navigate the regulatory path, they often have the misconception that the officials they are meeting with can provide an endorsement of the company or product. I encountered this frequently during my time as a regulator, and as a congressional staff member.

While government officials may be intrigued by a particular technology, ethics rules prohibit them from providing any type of endorsement. They may refer companies to meet with other relevant officials as a way of notifying others of a developing technology, but they are not able to provide a formal endorsement that the company can use in promotional material.

Depending on the product or technology, once companies determine the relevant agencies they need to interact with, the regulatory process can truly begin. The short DNA tracers offer a good example of the regulatory process that a company can encounter with new technology.

After obtaining generally recognized as safe status from the Food and Drug Administration (FDA) in 2014, one of the goals SafeTraces tried to pursue was filing a petition with the National Organic Standards Board (NOSB) to include short DNA tracers on a list of allowed substances that could be used on organic products. Formally called the National List of Allowed and Prohibited Substances, this list identifies the synthetic substances that may be used and the natural substances that may not be used in organic crop and livestock production. The list also identifies a limited number of nonorganic substances that may be used in or on processed organic products.

Changes to the National List can be accomplished through a petition that can be initiated by anyone. In its petition submission, SafeTraces asserted that the short DNA tracers would be used in food production as inactive ingredients with no technical effect. They also noted that the tracers are not classified as inert substances of toxicological concern and are not recombinant or GMO materials. The company explained that the manufacturing of short DNA tracers starts with a naturally occurring material, which is DNA purified from an edible plant or fungus, and uses naturally occurring enzymes and nucleotides to copy a short section of the starting DNA.

SafeTraces argued that the addition of short DNA tracers to the National List would offer important advantages to the organic community. They added that the material is naturally derived, is safe for the environment, and offers traceability advantages that cannot be achieved through other means.

While I used to work for a firm that represented SafeTraces, I coincidentally now work for an organization that filed comments urging the NOSB to reject the petition. In its comments submitted in March 2017, Consumer Reports argued that the petition should be rejected because short DNA tracers were created using excluded methods. The groups also contended that the tracers do not meet the criteria outlined in the Organic Food Production Act because they are not essential for raising environmental and human health concerns. Although Consumer Reports did not necessarily express an objection to the technology itself, the group did oppose the use of short DNA tracers within the context of organic production.

Ultimately, the NOSB followed the recommendation of its subcommittee panel and rejected the SafeTraces petition, and short DNA tracers were not recommended for the National List.

## Be careful what you wish for

One technology rumored to be currently in use by large food companies is a mobile testing kit that tests for antibiotic residue in livestock at very sensitive levels. If this technology becomes widely available, not only would it have a significant impact on market behavior and producer accountability, but it would impact regulatory policy as well.

With the current public health goal of limiting the use of antibiotics in food-producing animals, a mobile testing kit that could provide immediate information on residue levels would have important public policy implications. If meat and poultry companies are currently using this technology to hold their producers accountable, there would be considerable demand from consumers to make this information widely available to serve as a guide for product purchases. Regulators also could use this to verify that products are free of antibiotics.

If the rumors of this technology prove to be true, the regulatory dynamic this would create will be interesting to observe.

Difficult politics have always surrounded regulations of feedlots. The primary reason for this is a strong, independent sentiment that rejects any hint of outside intrusions, whether from big food companies or the government. This mindset permeates the industry and prevents meaningful food safety proposals from being implemented at these establishments. The US Department of Agriculture's Food Safety and Inspection Service cannot regulate these feedlots because their jurisdiction begins only when livestock enters the slaughterhouse.

The FDA is unable to investigate feedlots either. During an FDA investigation into a romaine lettuce outbreak in 2019, the agency never could identify the source of the contamination. They did find the strain of *Escherichia coli* that made people sick in sediment from a water reservoir on one of the California farms that grew contaminated lettuce. When the FDA sought to take samples from a nearby feedlot to see if there was a match, they were denied entry (FDA, 2019).

Introducing better technology into the system does provide a slight change to the dynamic. Because food companies are their customers, producers often have no choice but to allow these companies to access their facilities and monitor operations to ensure contractual standards and obligations are being met. However, similar entreaties by a government agency to monitor regulatory compliance would be met with much skepticism and, in worst case scenarios, hostility.

It is widely recognized in the food policy arena that, in order to make significant progress in reducing foodborne illness rates-and have a true, prevention-based food safety system-there needs to be additional regulations on the farm part of the "farm-to-fork" spectrum. While policies such as food safety modernization, stricter performance standards, and enhanced traceability measures can have an impact, these efforts are not able to directly impact behavior at the source of food production.

Technology will continue to bring us one step closer to the ideal prevention-based food safety system. The following chapters help chart this course.

## Disclosure

I worked for a firm that represented SafeTraces on regulatory issues, and that is how I became aware of their product. While I participated in some calls with the client with other members of the firm, I did not perform any substantive work and did not have any financial interest in the company; I also have no financial interest in the firm.

**Brian Ronholm, MS**

*Director of Food Policy, Consumer Reports*
*Washington, D.C., United States*

## References

Corkery, M., & Popper, N. (2018, September 24). *From farm to Blockchain: Walmart tracks its lettuce (The giant retailer will begin requiring lettuce and spinach suppliers to contribute to a Blockchain database that can rapidly pinpoint contamination).* The New York Times. Retrieved from https://www.nytimes.com/2018/09/24/business/walmart-Blockchain-lettuce.html.

FDA. (2019, October 31). *FDA, CDC and other health partners investigated outbreak of E. coli O157:H7 possibly linked to romaine lettuce, outbreak appears to be over* [Press Release]. Retrieved from https://www.fda.gov/news-events/fda-brief/fda-cdc-and-other-health-partners-investigated-outbreak-e-coli-o157h7-possibly-linked-romaine.

Gasparro, A., & Newman, J. (2018, October 2). *Six technologies that could shake the food world.* The Wall Street Journal. Retrieved from https://www.wsj.com/articles/six-technologies-that-could-shake-the-food-world-1538532480.

Walmart. (2018, September 24). *Walmart and Sam's club to require real-time, end-to-end food traceability with Blockchain* [Press release]. Retrieved from https://corporate.walmart.com/media-library/document/leafy-greens-on-Blockchain-press-release/_proxyDocument?id=00000166-0c4c-d96e-a3ff-8f7c09b50001.

# Defining blockchain and regulatory technology

1

# Defining Terms

1

**Gennette Zimmer, MBA, MSc**

*Data Analytics, Boston University, Boston, MA, United States*

With so many technology terms bandied about today, there is not always a clear understanding of what these terms actually mean. For example, whenever the term Blockchain is brought into a conversation, it inevitably includes the question "Is it like (throw in a technology buzzword)?" And often that technology buzzword thrown in has very little to do with Blockchain. So rather than leave the reader to their own devices and hope they know about the technology described in this book, this section is designed to provide a very basic understanding of these and other terms the reader will encounter later in this book or in discussions on this topic.

One of the most common technology buzzwords associated with **Blockchain** is Bitcoin. And while it has its roots in this form of cryptocurrency, Blockchain has taken on a life of its own and is now being applied to myriad industries including food. Also known as an immutable distributed ledger, Blockchain is the process used to simultaneously store digital information on multiple databases. Each transaction or set of transactions becomes a block. The first recorded transaction is known as the genesis block. When a new block is created, it contains a time stamp and information linking it to the previous block. Because duplicate copies of the database exist on multiple computers, these computers all need to agree on the blocks as they are recorded. The purpose is to track each step so that it is impossible to modify, manipulate, or fake the transactions once they are recorded in a block.

Blockchain was born out of the creation of **cryptocurrency**. Just like the dollar is an asset used to exchange for an item, cryptocurrency is a digital asset as a means for exchange. This digital payment system uses cryptography to create secure financial transactions that would be difficult to fake by translating readable data into illegible and unbreakable codes. Individual transactions for cryptocurrency are recorded and managed on the Blockchain.

Transactions are managed by **miners**. These miners are individuals, or more likely a company, who use specialized computers to solve computational puzzles in order to add the next block in the chain. The goal is securing the network and confirming transactions. Miners are rewarded with new cryptocurrency (e.g., Bitcoin or Ethereum) either for solving the puzzle or based on the amount of time spent mining.

**Bitcoin**, created in 2009, is the first form of cryptocurrency to be introduced to the general public. Since its inception, it has had very dramatic financial growth.

**Building the Future of Food Safety Technology.** https://doi.org/10.1016/B978-0-12-818956-6.00001-4

When it was first introduced to the marketplace in 2010, it was valued $0.0003 per Bitcoin (BTC) and grew from there. Bitcoin trading did not really start to take off until 2013 (Edwards, 2019). At the beginning of that year, Bitcoin was valued at about $13.50 per BTC. And by the end of 2017, just 5 years later, Bitcoin had risen to nearly $20,000 per BTC before taking a dramatic downturn in November 2018 to just $3500 per BTC (Edwards, 2019). The value of a BTC has demonstrated fluctuating growth ever since.

With the success of Bitcoin came cryptocurrency competitors. Often known as altcoin, because it is an alternative to Bitcoin, there are several thousand variations available today. But the most successful alternative to Bitcoin is **Ethereum**. Ethereum does not just provide its own form of cryptocurrency known as **Ether** (ETH), but unlike Bitcoin (which focuses solely on cryptocurrency) Ethereum has also created a programmable Blockchain framework for **smart contracts**. Developers use Ethereum's smart contracts to build their own decentralized applications (Buterin, 2020).

Smart contracts are automated agreements used to enable transactions between parties. These agreements, which comprise lines of code on a Blockchain, define the terms and conditions agreed upon by all parties, as well as any penalties for not adhering to them. Once created, rules are automatically executed when a condition is met without the need of an intermediary. Because of its structured nature, smart contracts create a transparency that helps mitigate mistrust between parties, thus supporting reputations, and since they are stored on the Blockchain, there is also a transactional lineage for each smart contract. A simple example of how smart contracts can be used extrapolated from an IBM scenario (Gopie, 2018) is as follows:

> Store X *wants to purchase a product from* Food 4 U—*a food manufacturer that ships their product through* Shipping Inc. Food 4 U *and* Store X *can create a smart contract whereby* Store X *puts money in escrow to be released upon delivery of the product ordered.* Food 4 U *and* Shipping Inc *create their own smart contract whereby* Food 4 U *puts money into escrow for* Shipping Inc *to pick up said product and deliver it to* Store X. *Beyond just moving the product from point A to point B, additional rules set forth could be delivery times, temperature requirements, testing, and audit results. All of these agreements are programmed into the smart contract and stored on the Blockchain. Once* Store X *has received the product, provided all rules were adhered to, the money from their escrow is now released to* Food 4 U *and the money from* Food 4 U's *escrow is released to* Shipping Inc. *If for any reason* Shipping Inc *does not deliver the product to* Store X *or the additional conditions are not met, then based on the agreed upon parameters in the smart contract, the money in escrow is returned to the original parties.*

Another prominent Blockchain framework is **Hyperledger Fabric**. Hyperledger Fabric is a distributed ledger software product from **Hyperledger**. Hyperledger was launched in 2016 and is hosted by the Linux Foundation. Hyperledger Fabric's framework differs from Bitcoin or Ethereum in that it is not dependent on cryptocurrency to operate. Companies like IBM and Walmart use this framework for their Blockchain platform as early as 2016 when they partnered with Tsinghua University in China to use Hyperledger to improve food safety by tracking the Chinese pork market. On March 3, 2020, it was announced that Walmart has taken its involvement a step further and joined Hyperledger's open-source Blockchain consortium (Haig, 2020).

Blockchain technology and smart contracts are currently in exploration mode and its future is undecided. Similar to the volatile nature of Bitcoin, another way to look at how Blockchain's value is perceived can be seen in how 2019 started off with food and beverage industry conversations centered on Blockchain being imperative to the future of food safety. In February 2019, Commissioner Scott Gottlieb, MD, announced that the FDA will be testing new technologies to enhance industry track-and-trace systems for the drug supply chain.

> *We're also focused on making improvements across the other products we regulate, especially related to food and our ability to address foodborne outbreaks. We're invested in exploring new ways to improve traceability, in some cases using the same technologies that can enhance drug supply chain security, like the use of blockchain*
>
> **FDA, 2019.**

During the middle of the same year, some industry groups had reported pulling out of pilot testing or downplaying investment in Blockchain, at this time (Detwiler, 2020). And by the end of 2019, the FDA's public event on the "New Era of Smarter Food Safety" barely mentioned Blockchain by name. This is not to say Blockchain is out of consideration as a useable tool; however, the recent conversations have revealed an understanding of how complicated the modern food supply and distribution chains impact the ease of adoption. Further, there is a growing awareness of the timeline for ROI, from an earlier perception of 5 years to a more realistic estimate of 25 years before it could be successfully implemented (Detwiler, 2020).

One potential alternative to traditional Blockchain is a distributed ledger from the ITOA Foundation called **Tangle**. Tangle is similar to Blockchain in that transactions are distributed and stored across a decentralized network of participants. But it distinguishes itself because, as opposed to Blockchain, it "… does not consist of transactions grouped into blocks and stored in sequential chains, but as a stream of individual transactions entangled together" ("What is IOTA?", 2020). The goal is to use Internet of things (IoT) and Web 3.0 to enhance distributed ledger technology to address what the IOTA Foundation sees as issues plaguing the current Blockchain technology.

Just as Facebook or Instagram are examples of social media, Blockchain is a part of an ecosystem of technologies that at its core is still just data. Although, many of the terms in this next section can be applied to any industry, they also have their place in understanding the future of food safety technology.

While data are just individual units of information, there is an incredible amount of it collected and analyzed every day. Data are referred to as **structured**, **unstructured**, or **semistructured**. Structured data are clearly defined with specified fields and easily searchable and easily stored in a relational database. An example of structured data would be the information stored in each block of a Blockchain. Unstructured data are disorganized data that do not contain specified fields making it more difficult to search. Videos, audio recordings, blog posts, text messages, etc., are considered unstructured. As the name implies, semistructured data are somewhere in between the former two data types. Semistructured data are not easily organized but do have some properties, such as metadata, that make analysis easier (Robb, 2017; "Structured Data vs. Semi Structured Data", 2020).

The term **big data** refers to data that demonstrate volume (how much data are collected), velocity (how fast they are being collected), and variety (what kind of data are being collected) that cannot be stored in a traditional relational database. Unfortunately, there is ambiguity in this definition. Given the speed and quantity with which data are collected today are not the same as what were being collected even a few years ago. Another feature of big data is that data can be stored in their originating format, meaning it is not necessary to impose a structure onto a set of unstructured data (Coronel and Morris, 2019).

In November 2018, the International Data Corporation (IDC) predicted that the amount of data stored in the Global Datasphere will grow from 33 zetabytes to 175 zetabytes in 2025. For context, one zetabyte is approximately one trillion gigabytes (Reinsel, Gantz, & Rydning, 2018). So where are all of these data coming from? So much of these data are propagated by people interacting with computers or mobile devices. But another way data are generated is by devices interacting with other devices. **IoT** are devices that are either connected to the Internet or devices that are connected to each other. This includes sensors or some other technology built into the device that has automated functions to generate and collect data for a specific objective.

With the existence of so much information, where is it being stored? Data are stored in myriad locations. The devices people use, such as a smartphone, or companies servers store a vast amount of information. But a growing amount of data are being stored in what is known as the cloud. **Cloud computing** is defined by the National Institute of Standards and Technology as

> *… a model for enabling convenient, on-demand network access to a shared pool of configurable computing resources (e.g., networks, servers, storage, applications, and services) that can be rapidly provisioned and released with minimal management effort or service provider interaction.*
>
> **"NIST Cloud Computing Program", 2019.**

Some of the prominent providers of cloud computing services include but are not limited to Amazon Web Services, Google Cloud Platform, Microsoft Azure, VMWare, and IBM Cloud.

**Table 1** Four different types of cloud services.

| | |
|---|---|
| Public cloud | Built and managed by a third party that offers services via the Internet to the public. |
| Private cloud | Services offered over the Internet or over a private internal network built by a company that may have large geographically dispersed locations that need flexibility in accessing information. |
| Hybrid cloud | A combination of both public and private that host applications that need more security on a private server and other applications on a more public server. |
| Community cloud | Built by and for a specific group that has similar needs or goals and can only be accessed by members of said community. |

*Table 1 by author, based on information from Coronel, C., & Morris, S. (2019). Database systems: Design, implementation, & management. 13th ed. Boston: Cengage.*

The four types of cloud services are public, private, hybrid, and community (see Table 1)

There are currently three types of cloud computing platforms. **Software as a Service** provides software that can be accessed via an Internet connection rather than having it installed directly on a device. **Platform as a Service** provides a cloud-based environment for building applications and hosts servers, networks, storage, operating system software, and databases at its data center. **Infrastructure as a Service** provides servers, networking, storage, and data center space ("Cloud Computing Overview," N.D.). IDC predicts that, by 2025, 49% of the world's stored data will reside in public cloud environments (Reinsel et al., 2018).

Beyond looking at simply where data are stored comes consideration of how data move from one location to another. When data stay at one place, they are classified as being in the *at-rest* stage. Interstakeholder or intrastakeholder movement of data classifies it as being in the *in-transit* stage. Finally, data can be classified as being in an *in-use* stage when the information system packages and analyzes the data. In all three stages, protecting the security of the data is essential.

Some technologies are used to collect, store, package, and analyze data, while other technologies are used to remove the element of human error, such as robotics in packaging and pelleting operations. Some technologies are used to simplify areas of work, such as the scanning of bar codes, while others are used to increase speed and/or reduce costs, such as unmanned delivery drones on land or in the air. All of these technologies use data and data science methods to improve performance.

**Data science** is a field of study that applies scientific methods to data in order to extract knowledge and insights. But within data science contains other terms that are sometimes used synonymously, but are actually different pieces of the whole pie. **Data mining**, often referred to as knowledge discovery in databases, uses machine learning and statistics to find patterns within a dataset. For example, a grocery store finding a relationship between product A and product B. **Data analysis** is a term that covers the methods used for extracting data, organizing it, then making decisions based on the conclusions drawn. **Data analytics** organizes the data and applies statistical methods in order to develop models based on the results. These methods take information and reveal stories from the data that may help inform the present or future. For example, the grocery store has a loyalty card that contains the shopping habits of its customers. By analyzing the shopping habits of all customers they can find purchasing patterns and send an email to a customer stating "Because you purchased product A, you may be interested in product B."

**Predictive analytics** uses data to predict future trends. Machine learning and artificial intelligence (AI) are methods associated with predictive analytics. As opposed to statistical modeling, which is based on proven mathematical theories that analyze data that meet certain assumptions, **machine learning** uses computers to look for patterns in the data to create theories based on what it learned. These computers continue to learn without having to be expressly programmed. Based on the idea of making computers that think more like humans, machine learning is a key part of **AI,** but there is more to AI overall. AI is able to correctly interpret external data, learn from it, and then use what it has learned to achieve specific goals and tasks through flexible adaptation (Kaplan and Haenlein, 2019). AI is how tools like Siri and Alexa not only answer questions but also improve upon the quality of its answers as it learns from the questions its users ask.

One thing to consider is that while there may be zetabytes of data at rest, there is only a small fraction of that data that can be classified as in-use. While there has been exponential growth of data collection, only about 0.5% of data are currently analyzed (Guess, 2015). And even though companies are talking about the importance of big data and finding tools to capture more information, between 60% and 73% of all data within an enterprise go unused for analytics (Barrett, 2018). So while companies are talking about and working toward improvement in the amount of collected data being analyzed, there is still a long way to go. Especially as more RegTech, such as Blockchain, is created for the food industry. It is not just important to collect information, but analysis of it, be it predictive or otherwise, may be the key to keeping our food safe.

## References

Barrett, J. (2018, April 12). *Up to 73 percent of company data goes unused for analytics. Here's how to put it to work.* Inc.. Retrieved from https://www.inc.com/jeff-barrett/misusing-data-could-be-costing-your-business-heres-how.html.

Buterin, V. (2020, February 10). *What is Ethereum?.* Ethereum.com. Retrieved from https://ethereum.org/what-is-ethereum/.

Cloud Computing Overview. (n.d.) *IBM.* Retrieved from https://www.ibm.com/cloud/learn/cloud-computing.

Coronel, C., & Morris, S. (2019). *Database systems: Design, implementation, & management* (13th ed.). Boston: Cengage.

Edwards, J. (2019, November 3). *Bitcoins price history.* Investopedia. Retrieved from https://www.investopedia.com/articles/forex/121815/bitcoins-price-history.asp.

Food and Drug Administration. (2019, February 7). *FDA takes new steps to adopt more modern technologies for improving the security of the drug supply chain through innovations that improve tracking and tracing of medicines* [Press Release]. Retrieved from https://www.fda.gov/news-events/press-announcements/fda-takes-new-steps-adopt-more-modern-technologies-improving-security-drug-supply-chain-through.

Guess, A. (2015, June 10). *Only 0.5% of all data is currently analyzed.* Dataversity. Retrieved from https://www.dataversity.net/only-0-5-of-all-data-is-currently-analyzed/.

Haig, S. (2020, March). *Walmart joins hyperledger alongside 7 other companies.* Retrieved from https://cointelegraph.com/news/walmart-joins-hyperledger-alongside-7-other-companies.

Kaplan, A., & Haenlein, M. (2019, January). Siri, Siri, in my hand: Who's the fairest in the land? On the interpretations, illustrations, and implications of artificial intelligence. *Business Horizons, 62*(1), 15—25. Retrieved from https://www.sciencedirect.com/science/article/pii/S0007681318301393.

NIST Cloud Computing Program. (2019, July 9). *The National Institute of Standards and Technology.* Retrieved from https://www.nist.gov/programs-projects/nist-cloud-computing-program-nccp.

Reinsel, D., Gantz, J., & Rydning, J. (2018, November). *The digitization of the world: From edge to core.* Retrieved from https://www.seagate.com/files/www-content/our-story/trends/files/idc-seagate-dataage-whitepaper.pdf.

Structured Data vs Semi Structured Data. (2020). *Tealium learning center.* Retrieved from https://community.tealiumiq.com/t5/Customer-Data-Hub/Structured-Data-vs-Semi-Structured-Data/ta-p/15617.

*What is IOTA?.*(2020). Retrieved from https://www.iota.org/get-started/what-is-iota.

# The future food chain: digitization as an enabler of Society 5.0

**John G. Keogh, MBA, MSc [1], Laurette Dube, PhD [2], Abderahman Rejeb[3], Karen J. Hand, PhD [4], Nida Khan[5], Kevin Dean, MBA [6]**

[1]*Doctoral researcher, Henley Business School, University of Reading;* [2]*Professor, McGill University, Montreal, QC, Canada;* [3]*Doctoral Researcher, School of Regional Sciences and Business Administration, The Széchenyi István University, Győr, Hungary;* [4]*Director, Research Data Strategy, Food for Thought, University of Guelph, Guelph, ON, Canada;* [5]*Doctoral researcher in blockchain and data analytics for traceability in finance, The Interdisciplinary Centre for Security, Reliability and Trust, University of Luxembourg, Luxembourg City, Luxembourg;* [6]*Technology Strategist, Dolphin Data Development Ltd., Toronto, ON, Canada*

## Introduction

Academic literature on Society 5.0 is in the nascent stage of development. However, its evolution may have a considerable impact on how we conceive and architect our future food systems and food supply chains (FSCs). Considering the current rapid evolution of technology and the digitization of FSCs, it is necessary to investigate the conceptual Society 5.0 paradigm and the proposed creation of more sustainable food ecosystems. Therefore, this chapter draws mainly on secondary sources to conduct a narrative literature review to summarize prior studies on food chain digitization from a Society 5.0 perspective. The concept of Society 5.0 is not yet clearly defined (Džbánková & Sirůček, 2018), with an insignificant number of papers published in academic journals, which constrains a systematic literature review. In order to investigate the latest development in the field and extract valuable insights for industry practitioners and policymakers, we chose to incorporate gray literature from several sources in our analysis. Various scientific databases queried in January 2020 included Scopus, Web of Science, EBSCO Business Source Premier, IEEE Xplore, ScienceDirect, and Google Scholar. This writing includes information from conference papers and screened the references of publications to obtain additional relevant materials or pertinent references not captured during our initial search. The following search string was applied: "Society 5.0" AND food*, and the authors screened each paper for relevance.

The overarching and newly emerging research theme of **convergent innovation** (CI) is described by Dubé et al. (2017) as a solution-oriented paradigm at the interface of public and private sector value creation, which provides the construct to interweave the complexity of food systems digitalization and Society 5.0. In this chapter, the authors draw on their findings to unravel the different components and drivers of Society 5.0. and to illustrate how the CI paradigm powered by digital technology and human creativity can inform the next iteration in the evolution of our food systems and society (Dubé, Pingali, & Webb, 2012, Dubé et al., 2018, Dubé, Jha, et al., 2014).

## Society 5.0

The concept of **Society 5.0**, first conceived in Japan to establish a supersmart, high-tech enabled society (Hamid, 2018), is defined as a new societal ecosystem that involves several strategic changes based on the continued penetration of digital technologies into all spheres of human existence (Bryndin, 2018). According to Fukuyama (2018, p. 48), Society 5.0 is "an information society built upon Society 4.0 aiming for a prosperous human-centered society." As such, Society 5.0 is an era of increasing digitization and modernization of industrial and societal infrastructures (Fukuda, 2019). The concept of Society 5.0 shares certain similarities and parallels with the Industrial Revolution phase of "Industry 4.0" which started in Germany, the "Industrial Internet" in the United States, "Made in China 2025," and "Smart Cities" efforts globally. However, Society 5.0 has a more comprehensive vision that looks beyond the idea of a purely technology-driven phase (Industry 4.0) to one which is human-centric and considers the whole of society (Keidanren, 2016). As Fukuda (2019) highlights, the Society 5.0 vision recognizes global trends, considers the rapid pace of technology-driven change, the unprecedented explosion in data generation, and acknowledges a society that struggles to keep pace. Fig. 1 below (not to timescale) overlays and distinguishes the societal evolution phases from the industrial revolution phases.

The UN 2030 agenda, with SDGs (see Fig. 2) as its core, aims to create inclusive socioeconomic transformations with an integrative vision of economic prosperity, environmental sustainability, and social reforms that include poverty eradication (Griggs et al., 2013). As with Japan's vision of Society 5.0, the UN developed the SDGs to enable a new world wherein *"all human beings can enjoy prosperous and fulfilling lives and that economic, social, and technological progress occurs in harmony with nature"* (UN, 2020).

Several of the SGDs are concerned with increasing and promoting more sustainable food production, enabling society to overcome specific food system challenges (e.g., food security, food safety, and food nutrition). While the total economic burden of unsafe food on society is unknown, a study by the World Bank (2018) estimated that foodborne illnesses cost US$ 110 Billion annually in low- and middle-income economies. Food is intimately connected to every aspect of our society, and Bildt-gÅrd (2008, p. 101) argued that culture, tradition, and location historically bound communities together and "regulated what to eat, when to eat it, how to prepare it." This intimacy presents societal risks, specifically those posed by foodborne diseases, exemplified throughout history as mild or severe illness and mortality in humans, food, and companion animals. While acknowledging significant

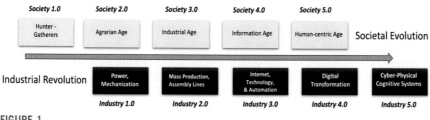

**FIGURE 1**

Societal evolution and Industrial Revolution.

*Created by author.*

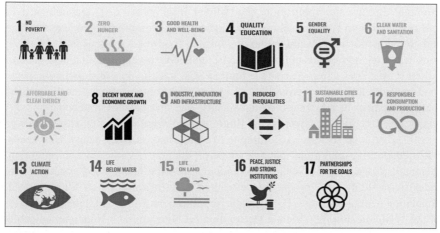

**FIGURE 2**

United Nations Sustainable Development Goals (SDGs) https://www.un.org/sustainabledevelopment/wp-content/uploads/2019/01/SDG_Guidelines_AUG_2019_Final.pdf.

underreporting of foodborne illnesses and deaths, the World Health Organization (WHO) highlighted in 2015 that 31 global hazards (i.e., foodborne diseases) resulted in 600 million foodborne disease illnesses and 420,000 deaths in 2010 (WHO, 2015a). Furthermore, recurring food safety outbreaks, food fraud scandals, and ethical lapses, amplified by social media (BildtgÅrd, 2008), combine to erode trust in our food systems (Edelman, 2020). Importantly, the food system significantly affects economic conditions and impacts upon our planetary health. To prepare for an uncertain future, nations must adopt an interdisciplinary approach to meet the SDG goals (Beer, 2007). A CI approach will enable appropriate digitization of FSCs and alignment with the vision of Society 5.0 and UN SDG goals-together, an agile future global food system to ensure food security, eradication of poverty, and planet sustainability.

Society 5.0 sets out to create a common societal infrastructure based on advanced service platforms (Onday, 2019). Driven to establish a resilient and agile food ecosystem, the Japanese National Agricultural and Food Research Organization (NRO) strives to achieve the vision of Society 5.0 by creating a "smart food chain" from breeding to cultivation, harvesting, storage, processing, distribution, consumption, and food waste reduction (SPHSIT, 2019). Smart food chains and their ecosystems (illustrated by the Japanese NRO) are conceptualized as agile and responsive, leveraging technological advancements to mitigate risks and meet the challenges facing today's FSCs including a fast-growing global population, rapid urbanization, an aging society, and uncertainties related to climate change (Pandey et al., 2016).

With the increasing globalization of FSCs, Society 5.0 offers several opportunities for food organizations to unlock the full potential of new technologies. For example, through the application of **artificial intelligence** (AI) technologies, it will be possible to combine and analyze increasingly complex heterogeneous data and extract actionable insights regarding critical food-related issues such as allergens, nutrition, ingredients of food products, retail store inventories, and market conditions (CAO, 2020). In preparing the future FSCs, stakeholders (e.g., policymakers, food industry, technology providers, nongovernment organizations) must consider the development of a human-centered society, one that balances the economic dimensions of the food ecosystem with future needs for human health, sustainability, nutrition, and food security. According to Makoto Yano (2019), Society 5.0 extends FSCs beyond the traditional boundaries of production (supply) and consumption (demand). Conceptually, Society 5.0 encompasses the entire food ecosystem in order to facilitate new product development and (re)formulation for improved population health outcomes. For example, the European Union (EU) member states of the WHO created the "Vienna Declaration on Nutrition and Noncommunicable Diseases" in 2013 to address the high burden of noncommunicable diseases linked to unhealthy diets (WHO, 2015). A vital component of the Vienna Declaration was the creation and adoption of a standard nutrient profile model across EU Member States.

## Technology in food supply chains

According to the World Economic Forum (WEF),

> *Food plays a central role in human societies and is essential to the well-being of people and the planet. But a fundamental transformation is needed to meet the aspirations of an inclusive, efficient, sustainable, nutritious and healthy food system*

**WEF, 2019, p. 6.**

Furthermore, WEF argues that the application of modern information technology (IT) is a critical enabler for FSC development, especially food traceability. As such, a digital transformation will have a significant impact on global agri-food sectors

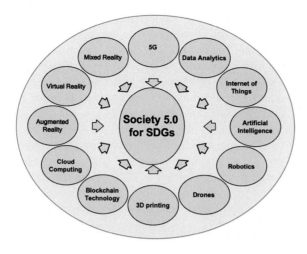

**FIGURE 3**

Technological enablers for Society 5.0 and SDGs.

*Image by author.*

and create new business opportunities. One can envision a future business-driven data architecture encompassing the entire agri-food ecosystem. In this scenario, a smallholder farmer is holding a digital device with information feeds and alerts from multiple on-farm technologies and cloud-based service providers (e.g., weather, market pricing, alerts to harvest before rain or frost). In essence, the small-holder has a handheld decision support system that acts to democratize technologies and makes it affordable and useable. From mobile devices to **Internet of things** (IoT) devices on equipment, vehicles, and farm animals, a broad spectrum of trans-formational and potentially disruptive technologies are deployed in FSCs. In Fig. 3 below and subsequent sections, we summarize 12 technologies (noninclusive list) that support the transition of FSCs toward the realization of the vision of Society 5.0 and the UN's SDGs.

## Data analytics

Data are generated at unprecedented rates by technology in FSCs and many other sectors of the economy (Sonka, 2014). The exponential growth of data lead to the generation of the **term "big data"** (BD), which Subudhi, Rout, & Ghosh (2019, p. 2) define as *"a conglomeration of the booming value of heterogeneous datasets, which is so huge and intricate that processing it becomes difficult, using the existing database management tools."* The process of collecting, structuring, and analyzing this data is known as **big data analytics**. Conceptually, Society 5.0 stresses the need for the creation of new value in FSCs through advanced analytical and predictive tools to analyze diverse data and information relating to meteorological conditions, crop growth, and marketing conditions along with food trends and needs (Hitachi,

2020). Furthermore, data can support the globalization of FSCs in adapting to market conditions by providing food producers with the capability to identify new and emerging markets and anticipate consumers' demands such as healthy and environmentally sustainable food products (Khanna, Swinton, & Messer, 2018). By implication, one can envision the use of technology to enable FSCs to be more responsive to consumers by offering food products tailored to their personal preferences in a prompt manner. Moreover, increased access to relevant data and information will allow food ecosystems to identify and address the issues of food waste and develop more efficient FSCs. The application of **predictive analytics** applied to integrated data systems will provide for optimization of food quality, food safety, and food security (Kamble, Gunasekaran, & Gawankar, 2019). As a result, the application of advanced analytics and predictive tools will be significant enablers of Society 5.0 and SGDs food goals and provide economic and societal value to all actors within the food ecosystem.

## Internet of Things

The IoT has become a critical sector within the global information and communication technology (ICT) industry (Park, Cho, Han, & Kwon, 2017). IoT represents a nascent communication paradigm where various devices share data within a single framework or behave as lone actors. At the factory level, IoT devices can help to visualize processes (Gružauskas, Baskutis, & Navickas, 2018) and operational performance of production lines as well as providing predictive, preventative maintenance alerts. At the farm level, precision agriculture, broadly conceptualized as the use of ICTs for improved control of crops, livestock, and physical resources to optimize economic, social, and environmental farm performance (Eastwood, Chapman, & Paine, 2012), utilizes numerous sensors and IoT devices. For example, IoT-enabled sensors implemented in farms monitor weather conditions, as well as the health and well-being of soil, crops, and livestock.

IoT can contribute to the development of more efficient, data-driven FSCs to improve food production and meet the increasing demand of the world population (Jeppesen, Ebeid, Jacobsen, & Toftegaard, 2018). The use of IoT helps to enhance supply chain visibility and decision-making by improving the real-time access to data, which aids communication, coordination, and cooperation between FSC actors (Ahumada & Villalobos, 2009). In order to balance global FSC demand and supply, IoT sensors and other ICTs can be leveraged to monitor food quality, food safety, and food security (Wang & Yue, 2017; Zhong, Xu, &Wang, 2017). Therefore, IoT has the potential to drive enhanced agility in FSCs, generating a plethora of data in real time that can be analyzed using advanced predictive analytics, allowing food organizations to identify supply chain weaknesses and introduce proactive measures (Verdouw, Wolfert, Beulens, & Rialland, 2016). As well, IoT can be applied in FSCs to preserve the quality of fresh produce and ensure the compliance to food safety standards, thereby reducing food waste and aiding food security (Ray, Harsh, Daniel, & Ray, 2019). Challenges remain at the farm level and across FSCs broadly to ensure the security, integration, and interoperability for IoT devices deployed across proprietary equipment, which must be addressed to ensure the full value of IoT is extracted. For example, a report from the WEF on food traceability (WEF, 2019) argues that food sensing technologies aimed at preserving food quality, food safety, and enabling traceability can reduce food waste by 5–7%. As a result, IoT devices can increase the global productivity of FSCs and accelerate the progress toward the realization of Society 5.0 and SDGs of global food security and sustainability.

## Artificial intelligence

In recent years, AI has advanced rapidly and has impacted several sectors, including FSCs. Mooney (2018) argued that AI has the potential for agri-food to be more efficient and resilient to climate uncertainty. For example, AI tools offer farmers the potential to grow different crops symbiotically, anticipate problems, and take appropriate preventative or corrective actions via robotics (Renda, 2019). AI has the potential to increase the efficiency of FSCs through process automation as well as intelligent and interoperable integration of food production operations (WEF, 2019). According to Atkinson and Ezell (2019, p. 8), *"The advent of AI will lead to a significant reorganization of tasks in the manufacturing environment,- displacing humans from repetitive and routine tasks, while creating new opportunities for them to focus on value-generating activities."*

Furthermore, AI supports agricultural activities relating to farming, land allocation (Pokhrel, Paudel, & Segarra, 2018), monitoring and control of irrigation processes (Ait-Mouheb et al., 2018; Mohanraj, Gokul, Ezhilarasie, & Umamakeswari, 2017), and robot guidance (Sheridan, 2016). Likewise, AI tools and techniques can improve the management of FSC activities by providing predictive capabilities using real-time data generated by sensors and by using machine learning algorithms. Defined as an application of AI, machine learning involves computers learning how to think and act like humans in an autonomous manner through data. One pertinent application area of machine learning is that it can help to optimize the route for each vehicle to bring down transportation costs, which is one of the foremost concerns of the FSC in recent times (Reuters, 2019). Machine learning can have diverse applications in FSCs, among which are its employment in anticipating the needs of the customer to enhance customer retention and predict product demand to manage supply. AI has the potential to be the gateway toward fulfillment of Society 5.0 by facilitating FSCs, to realize new value opportunities while empowering FSC actors to adapt to the dynamics of a sustainable global food system.

## Robotics

Robotics comprises a cluster of critical technologies that will enable new opportunities for automation within food ecosystems and underpin the transition toward

Society 5.0 and the realization of the SDGs. Within FSCs, robotics can perform both simultaneous and repetitive tasks and simplify the handling, labeling, movement, and tracking of food products throughout the manufacturing process, improving visibility and interventions to prevent food safety issues (Duckett et al., 2018). Moreover, the usage of collaborative robots or "cobots" aids human activities within FSCs, such as lifting or moving heavy totes or containers. Further introduction of this transformational technology into FSCs could optimize activities such as inspecting and monitoring of soil conditions, cultivation (feeding and weeding), automated harvesting using autonomous vehicles, and rapidly responding to changing conditions (Blackmore, 2009). Robotics combines with AI as enablers of higher levels of flexibility in FSCs, contributing to productivity gains and the automation of specific tasks that were previously dependent on humans (Atkinson & Ezell, 2019). Other possible productivity gains include the identification and removal of hazards in food manufacturing currently vulnerable to human error and qualitative and quantitative optimization of food production. Adoption of robotics and automation in the global food system will significantly increase efficiency and significantly contribute to the future needs of Society 5.0 and the fulfillment of the SDGs in terms of productivity, sustainability, and capacity for adaptation to climate change and extreme weather conditions (UN, 2020).

## Drone technology

Drone technology deployments in agriculture and fisheries are in a nascent stage yet moving at a fast pace according to the UNFAO (2018: V) who argue *"drones, and connected analytics has great potential to support and address some of the most pressing problems faced by agriculture in terms of access to actionable real-time quality data."* From a technical perspective, drones represent multiple classes of crewless robotic vehicles that are remotely controlled or autonomous and utilized on land (e.g., autonomous farm equipment), aerial (e.g., fixed-wing, multirotor or quadcopter), on water, or underwater (Companik, Gravier, & Farris, 2018; Fresco & Ferrari, 2018). FSCs could experiment with the technology to explore conceptual use cases such as the pickup of crop samples from remote farms for laboratory testing. Furthermore, drones have practical applications in FSCs from the monitoring of livestock movement on large acreage to operational efficiencies in distribution and retail. For example, Companik et al. (2018) noted that Walmart used drones to reduce its warehouse inventory count from 30 days to 1 day. As warehouse costs are 30% of total supply chain costs on average (AT Kearney, 2016), operational efficiencies can be significant. In the fisheries sectors, the UNFAO notes that several governments are using drones to monitor illegal fishing in protected waters while and at the farm level, drones provide an "eye in the sky for agriculture" (UNFAO, 2018, p. 1) enabling farmers to automatically collect data and monitor their crops in real time (van der Wal, Kooistra, & Poppe, 2015).

Similarly, land-based and aerial drones can effectively replace humans in time-consuming activities such as seeding and weeding operations and activities where human contact with fertilizer and chemical spraying may pose a health and safety risk. Remote data collection assists FSC actors in decision-making processes relating to disaster risk reduction (UNFAO, 2018), crop management, precision agriculture, yield forecasting, and environmental sustainability (Zhang & Kovacs, 2012). When FSC stakeholders have access to high-quality data in real time, it enables more effective policy decisions and practical interventions toward the achievement of Society 5.0 and SDGs (UNFAO, 2018).

## 3D printing

3D printing represents an advanced form of production automation, which consists of *"joining materials to make objects from 3D model data, usually layer upon layer, as opposed to subtractive manufacturing methodologies"* (ASTM, 2012, F2792-12a). Although this technology is not new, novel applications of the technology are relevant and will play a crucial role in the development of Society 5.0. The utility of 3D in research and development (R&D) and manufacturing facilitates creativity in product design, including shape, dimensions, internal structure, and taste, as well as personalized food formula (Ricci, Derossi, & Severini, 2019). As such, 3D printing offers the flexibility to design, premanufacture, and innovate foodstuffs that could be tailored to consumer requirements and preferences (Portanguen, Tournayre, Sicard, Astruc, & Mirade, 2019). The novel application of 3D technology intensifies the trend toward the personalization of food products through the fabrication of foods with complex dimensions and advanced textures, tailoring nutritional contents, and increasing consumer satisfaction (Godoi, Prakash, & Bhandari, 2016). Moreover, FSCs can rely on this technology to design attractive food packages while minimizing waste and reducing food product handling and possible contamination risks. The alignment of this technology with Society 5.0 and SDGs is rooted in the specific characteristics of 3D printing to encourage sustainable manufacturing, elimination of waste, reduced packaging, and increased worker safety.

## Blockchain technology

Treiblmaier (2018, p. 547) defines Blockchain as *"a digital, decentralized and distributed ledger in which transactions are logged and added in chronological order with the goal of creating permanent ad tamper-proof records."* Blockchain is considered a versatile technology that extends beyond its original technical underpinning of cryptocurrencies and considered both transformative and foundational in FSCs (WEF, 2019). Rejeb, Keogh, & Treiblmaier (2019), Rejeb, Sűle, & Keogh (2018) argued that a Blockchain could be considered a configuration of multiple technologies, tools, and methods that address a business problem or use case. Furthermore, the academic and industry literature views Blockchain as an indispensable technological innovation that enhances transparency and increases trust in FSCs (Lacity, 2018; Yiannas, 2018). Both transparency and trust are vital essential constructs in the envisioned Society 5.0. For example, trust is viewed as essential to the basic functioning of society and is described by Berg (2004, p. 22, citing Elster, 1989) as a "*social lubricant*" and vital during periods of social uncertainty such as a food-related crisis (BildtgÅrd, 2008; Luhmann, 2000). Hence, Blockchain can support enhanced transparency and trust building in FSCs by facilitating the seamless exchange of immutable data and information between trading partners.

Furthermore, retailers can manage the shelf life of food products in individual stores and apply additional safeguards and tools to ensure food authenticity (Galvez, Mejuto, & Simal-Gandara, 2018). The technology can also be used to enhance product traceability (Mattila, Seppälä, & Holmström, 2016) and improve the ability to identify and recall unsafe products rapidly. For example, Kamath (2017) notes that Walmart simulated a product safety recall for mango, which demonstrated advanced traceability and the potential to reduce the time to trace and recall from 7 days to 2.2 s.

The globalization of FSCs has posed several challenges for FCSs to secure and protect the movement of food and information throughout the entire supply chain. However, operating in a Blockchain environment, companies would be able to maintain real-time visibility over FSCs and to quickly identify the data origin and the physical path followed by food products (Kamilaris, Fonts, & Prenafeta-Boldú, 2019). The application of Blockchain, combined with other technologies (e.g., Smart Contracts, IoT, AI), methods (e.g., analytical science), and tools (e.g., covert, overt, and forensic security features in foods and packaging), allows FSCs a more significant opportunity to address FSC-related opportunism, sustainability, food quality, food safety, authenticity, provenance, and food fraud risks in an optimal and efficient manner (Fosso Wamba, Kamdjoug, Robert, Bawack, & G Keogh, 2020; Saberi, Kouhizadeh, Sarkis, & Shen, 2019).

The functional attributes of Blockchain technology, including disintermediation, high data security, and immutability, are essential enhancements for future global FSCs. Blockchain can reduce the complexity and costs of online transactions while reducing the risk of various forms of food-related crime, including product diversion and corruption. The adoption of Blockchain in global FSCs can help to achieve SDGs, especially those goals related to the proper functioning of commodity markets, the facilitation of timely access to market information, and the simplification of trade procedures (UN, 2020). Furthermore, the WEF suggests that Blockchain-enabled traceability can reduce food loss by 1−2% (WEF, 2019).

## Cloud computing

Cloud computing is a well-established technology that can help transfer, store, process, and share supply chain information more rapidly and more efficiently (Gnimpieba, Nait-Sidi-Moh, Durand, & Fortin, 2015). In the agri-food industry, cloud computing represents a driving force toward the development of more agile FSCs that can proactively respond to unpredictable variations in quality and quantity of food supply (Verdouw, Robbemond, Verwaart, Wolfert, & Beulens, 2018). Cloud computing offers several capabilities to FSC trading partners, such as parallel processing, virtualization of resources, data security, and high data storage capacity (Subudhi et al., 2019). Increasingly, the unique business environment of FSCs demands a virtual infrastructure based on cloud computing to integrate, monitoring devices, storage devices, analytics tools, visualization platforms, and client delivery (Armbrust et al., 2010). Li, Wang, & Chen (2012) note that cloud computing could enhance cold chain collaboration, enabling an increased cocontrol of product information such as in-transit temperature monitoring and enhanced efficiency in the delivery of perishable food products. Cloud computing can support the vision of Society 5.0 that aims to accelerate digitization and drive the interconnection of products, value chains, and business models by boosting various interoperability scenarios in the FSC, including real-time collaboration and interactions among FSC exchange partners. Moreover, cloud computing is a cost-effective tool as it enables food organizations to save costs associated with the investment in physical IT infrastructures.

## Augmented reality

Augmented reality (AR) is a technology wherein real and virtual environments are combined, interact in real time, and the images rendered in three dimensions (3D) (Azuma, 1997). While Society 5.0 promises to integrate the physical and digital worlds fully, the opportunities offered by AR could entice FSC actors to adopt this technology. In analyzing the possibilities of AR, Beck, Crandall, O'Bryan, & Shabatura (2016) argue that AR technology could enhance training procedures through maintaining more control of food processes, higher flexibility, and fast learning abilities. For example, the use of AR headsets in the food and beverage production and processing plants could provide assembly line workers with all necessary information to ensure proper food preparation or packaging. This finding is confirmed by Clark & Crandall (2019), who found AR-based smart glasses were 50% more efficient in on-the-job training of food service staff versus traditional classroom or video training methods. Regarding food consumers, Wang et al. (2019) posit that AR contains various pleasure-oriented features that could facilitate the creation of hedonic and interactive experience, allowing consumers to augment their senses while purchasing or eating food. The benefits of AR in the FSC also include the increasing visualization of food processes, the prevention of contamination risks, the facilitation of food training, the empowerment of food marketing, and the optimization of food logistics (e.g., warehousing activities) (Luque, Peralta, de las Heras, & Córdoba, 2017).

## Virtual reality

Different from AR, the focus of virtual reality (VR) is to create a simulated environment that immerses the user and gives the feeling of being present in that environment (Desai, Desai, Ajmera, & Mehta, 2014). Given that Society 5.0 demands sustainable development, food security, and food safety, VR can be a promising tool to drive behavioral change. In this regard, Ammann, Siegrist, & Hartmann (2019) point out that VR enables food researchers (and trainers) to augment the virtual environment with *disgust cues* (e.g., bacterial contamination on food preparation surfaces) that are invisible in the real world. The authors further note that VR acts as a catalyst for food training and hygiene-related behavioral change interventions. VR is an enabler for a plethora of applications in the FSC, particularly in food R&D. For example, a study by Crofton, Botinestean, Fenelon, & Gallagher (2019) revealed that VR systems offer an immersive and engaging tool for researchers to inspect and manipulate the internal structures of foods, resulting in new manufacturing practices, food products, and customer experiences.

Food packaging is another potential use case that benefits from VR (Vanderroost et al., 2017). In discussing visualization and immersive capabilities, Janssen, Nijenhuis-de Vries, Boer, & Kremer (2017) concluded that VR is a promising technology. The authors argue that VR could be useful in the future to understand the underlying behavioral drivers in consumer food waste patterns (i.e., a strong disgust cue could be an expired carton of milk whereas an expired bag of rice may be acceptable to consume due to a perceived lower risk).

## Mixed reality

In contrast to VR and AR, mixed reality (MR) engages the user in a space which consists of more profound experiences with both digital and real objects (Kim & Sohn, 2003). The application of MR to FSCs are similar to those outlined in the case of utilizing AR. However, Costanza, Kunz, & Fjeld (2009) illustrate that the mix of reality and virtuality could help consumers to browse food products, In this regard, MR is a more complex and multilayered rendering of virtual objects. An example is a consumer reaching out virtually and "picking up" a food package, turning it around, and reading the information on all sides of the packaging. In essence, it is a perfect digital twin to the physical product.

## 5G communication networks

The shift toward the development of Society 5.0 and the achievement of SDGs in FSCs requires a telecommunication network that spreads connectivity and blurs the boundaries between digital and physical space. The advent of 5G communication networks could bring the cost of connectivity into the reach of most FSC partners. 5G represents the next generation of wireless networks that will provide users—anyone or anything—access to information and the ability to share data anywhere, anytime (Dahlman et al., 2014). The deployment of 5G consolidates the existing communication infrastructure of the FSC and responds to the increasing requirements of FSCs in terms of high capacity, low latency, scalability, agility, and universal support for data and media applications and services (Borcoci, 2017). Besides, 5G is a foundational layer for several technologies used in the FSC, such as IoT (unprecedented data generation) and cyber-physical systems. Borcoci

(2017) argues that the adoption of 5G will facilitate and optimize the network management based on algorithms, advanced automation capabilities for optimization of complex business objectives, data analytics, and BD techniques. Hu (2016) suggests that 5G could respond to the requirements of immersive technologies such as AR, VR, and MR, which need to operate in an exceptionally high-speed network and within an efficient energy consumption environment.

Thanks to its high-speed throughput and low latency, 5G can also support machine-to-machine communications, as in the case of applying automatic guided vehicles for food logistics operations. The advanced technical capabilities of 5G networks will increase the degree of connectivity of FSCs since this emerging technology gives unprecedented options for data throughput (Faraci, Raciti, Rizzo, & Schembra, 2018). However, connectivity in rural areas connected to FSCs remains a technical challenge, also for 5G. Various stakeholders are engaged in research and experimentation. For example, the Department for Digital, Culture, Media and Sport in the United Kingdom is supporting a multistakeholder project called "5G Rural Integrated Testbed," see http://www.5grit.co.uk. Furthermore, Kota and Giambene (2019) and Völk et al. (2019) highlight research on drones and satellites in combination with 5G networks to extend coverage to underserved and remote areas as well as trains, vessels, aircraft, and terrestrial base stations.

Overall, the realization of Society 5.0 through the achievement of the UN's SDGs is a worthy pursuit and critical to our future as a healthy society and planet. New and emerging technologies are critical enablers for Society 5.0, which manifests in the characterization of the ongoing evolution of organizations through the increasingly interconnected nature of our society, business, and technology. It is delivering profound (and potentially disruptive) impacts by offering innovative business opportunities (products, distribution, supply chains, and ecosystems) and innovative solutions to societal challenges related to our environment, health, productivity, and resource allocation. Food convergence innovation (FCI) is a relevant framework to enable the full potential of digitization in FSCs where all actors need to engage and provide leadership to realize the UN's SDGs as we transition toward Society 5.0.

Before discussing FCI in detail, the following section elaborates the industry-driven, supply chain operations reference "SCOR" model and briefly discusses where relevant technologies are mapped to the various stages of the SCOR framework.

## Positioning technologies in the supply chain operations reference framework

### Food supply chain in Society 5.0

Digitization necessitates new strategic management approaches to supply chain management, which integrates the emerging technologies while accomplishing the goals of the SDGs that fall within the realm of the FSC. The SCOR model was developed by the supply chain council to address, improve, and communicate the strategic management decisions in the supply chain to critical entities like the suppliers and customers. Fig. 4 gives some of the technologies that would aid in the five areas of the supply chain, which are the focus of the SCOR framework. The SCOR model helps to analyze a supply chain and determine its level of advancement. The five categories of the SCOR methodology, under which all the processes of the supply chain can be grouped, are listed below with an indication of a few key technological advancements that can aid to leverage the designated process:

- **Plan**: This is a very crucial phase of the supply chain and helps to balance the supply and demand. It plans the communication methodology to be followed in the supply chain as well as outlines the business rules and improvements to enhance efficiency. Machine learning can help in forecasting demand, supply, and inventory through intelligent algorithms. Predictive analytics can be used in demand forecasting by analyzing supply chain data to find patterns to aid in the prediction of future sales (Blackburn, Lurz, Priese, Göb, & Darkow, 2015).
- **Source**: This phase of the supply chain deals with the acquisition of materials and the entire supplier infrastructure, including inventory and supplier network management. IoT devices can provide a more efficient system of managing inventories than humans alone can (Jayanth, Poorvi, & Sunil, 2017). AI can help in the identification of damaged products and delays in the supply chain through data collected from suppliers. 5G would help to increase the use of IoT devices through a reduction in their cost, increase in life, and a minimization of the power requirements. AR devices can aid in improved screening of raw materials for acquisition since they enable remote users to see what the wearer is seeing.
- **Make**: This phase focuses on manufacturing and production. AI can be used for predictive maintenance. IoT can aid in location tracking and identification of fault areas in the manufacturing unit. Robots and automation of repetitive tasks can help in the improvement of product quality. Drones can offer many utilities, among which is the transport of products. 3D printing lowers the production costs, ensures a shorter delivery time, and is more "eco-friendly" (Kubáč & Kodym, 2017). AR and VR can help to improve this phase from the design and prototyping to the final production and assembly.
- **Deliver**: This phase comprises order management, warehousing, and transportation. IoT can help to track and authenticate products and shipments, which enables the prediction of final delivery date. Drones can be used to transport products to distribution centers. Machine learning can be employed on data collected from the IoT sensors to help in pattern recognition for identification of mismanagement and improvement of maintenance of machinery, warehouse equipment, and transportation.
- **Return**: This phase deals with an essential aspect of supply chains, which deals with the return of a defective product, containers, and packaging. The phase is also important from the perspective of customer retention and achieving a green

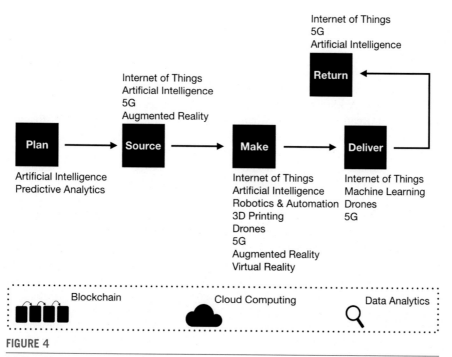

**FIGURE 4**

Digitization of an FSC in Society 5.0.

*Created by author.*

FSC in accordance with the SDG goals. Reverse logistics is an implausible step in the FSC, considering the perishable nature of food. However, one-third of the food produced globally is not consumed, and if food loss and waste were a "country," then it would rank as the third highest greenhouse gas emitter after the United States and China (Lott, 2013). A mechanism must be developed that will reduce food loss and waste by ensuring all stages of the FSCs (from seeding to cultivating, harvesting, post-harvest storage and distribution, production, distribution and logistics, retail, foodservice and household consumption) is optimized according to the products shelf life. AI can aid in this customization by raising alerts to indicate products that need a shorter delivery time to ensure their freshness. AI and IoT sensors can also optimize routings that minimizes the risk of the product becoming unfit for consumption.

FSCs will benefit from utilizing Blockchain functionality. In particular, a very positive consequence of implementing Blockchain is higher levels of data quality and improved integrity of the derived analytics.

The following section discusses in detail the concept of FCI, highlighting the need for a comprehensive framework that assists FSCs in achieving the expectations of Society 5.0 and the UN's SDGs.

## Food Convergence Innovation: accelerate industry 4.0 contribution to Society 5.0

The visionary features of Society 5.0 are (1) human-centered approach; (2) open, sustainable, and inclusive; and (3) experimentation-driven. These visionary features hold great promise for achieving the SDGs and rely on the embeddedness of digitization in everyday life of the citizen-consumer, organizations, systems, and society (as a whole). Realizing the SDGs demands not only a technological "fix" for our problems; they demand an encompassing societal change in human behaviors, choices, actions, interactions, and in the organization of society, including its policy. The ability to achieve individual and collective goals for integrative sustainable development hinges on the normative and adaptive quality of human behavior, be it at professional, organizational, institutional, system, or policy context (Cajaiba-Santana, 2014). Changes in everyday human behaviors in their personal lives are also an important prerequisite for societal-scale solutions (Pol & Ville, 2009; van der Have & Rubalcaba, 2016). To accelerate what Industry 4.0 can contribute to Society 5.0, we need to "innovate the way we innovate" to keep the human in the loop and set convergence targets within and across digital, physical, social, and economic systems in existence within and across jurisdictions around the world. The term CI has been coined for such integrative approach (Addy & Dubé, 2018; Buckeridge et al., 2012; Dubé et al., 2018, 2012; Dubé, Jha, et al., 2014; Hammond & Dubé, 2012; Lencucha et al., 2018).

Agri-food may be the sector of excellence whereby the interweaving of Industry 4.0 **digitization** to the aspirational features of Society 5.0 may accelerate the transformation of the structure and dynamics of traditional and modern systems needed for a full transition to Society 5.0, ensuring healthy diets from sustainable food systems for all. Food is a sturdy bridge between human biology and the agro-ecological, social, cultural, and economic contexts in which we live, be it in traditional or modern economies and societies. Digitalization linking biological, social, and commercial dimensions of agri-food systems offers the opportunity to develop an ecosystem of platforms that transcend the perspectives of individual actors that integrate ethical, social, environmental, and commercial concerns and that can legitimately aspire to do so at a societal level and scale. This section introduces the food convergence science and innovation (FCI) approach to sketch a powerful distributed alternative to the still prevailing vertically integrated model of agri-food systems. FCI aims to provide a framework to bridge or leapfrog the still prevailing socoeconomic divide structuring society (Dubé et al., 2018, 2012; Jha, Pinsonneault, & Dubé, 2016) while averting a potential digital divide (Bronson & Knezevic, 2019). CI targets not only the institutional transformation but also innovation at the level of technologies, communities, supply chains, markets, and other organizations and systems that form the economy and society.

The FCI framework places both general humanity and the human beings themselves at the center of transformation needed on supply and demand sides of the social and economic divide that has structured development since the onset of the first industrial revolution (Dubé et al., 2012; Jha et al., 2016). Large-scale data on human behavior in food, diet, lifestyle, and health domains are becoming available at an unprecedented level of contextual, spatial, and temporal granularity, opening new perspectives on bridging biological, social, and food environments. New digital methods of behavioral analytics integrate large-scale data on the diverse, dynamic, and oftentimes conflicting drivers of individual and household dietary behaviors. As such, AI and deep/machine learning and other methods aim to identify underlying behavioral patterns that were previously undetectable using traditional statistical analysis, along with their relationship to biological, social, and food systems (Dubé et al., 2018). In addition, the integration of consumer insights and behavioral economics may help to design and deploy interventions targeting lifelong nutrition, health, and wellness in a manner that is also economically, culturally, environmentally sustainable (Arora, Foley, Youtie, Shapira, & Wiek, 2014; Dubé, Addy, et al., 2014).

Broadly, CI further proposes to innovate the way we innovate by highlighting the fact that successful innovations with substantial economic and societal impacts tend to consist of a convergence of technological, business, social, and institutional innovations (see Fig. 5). In the agri-food space, examples of technological innovations

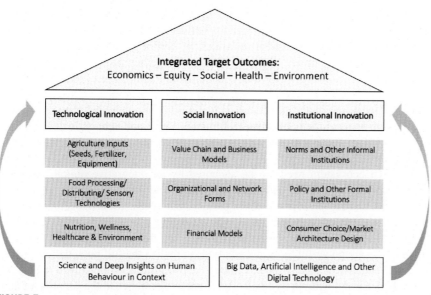

**FIGURE 5**

Convergent innovation framework.

*Adapted from Adapted from Dubé, L., Addy, N. A., Blouin, C., & Drager, N. (2014). From policy coherence to 21st century convergence: A whole-of-society paradigm of human and economic development. Annals of the New York Academy of Sciences, 1331(1), 201–215. https://doi.org/10.1111/nyas.12511. Created by author.*

include the use of agricultural inputs and applications, scientific or technical innovations in food processing and distribution, and even behavioral innovations (i.e., relating to nutritional intake, wellness, healthcare, and interactions with the environment). Adoption of technological innovations often requires the development of suitable business models to produce, deliver, and maintain the innovations, at times creating or disrupting entire value chains. This is the case when innovations are disruptive, as they tend to be accompanied by changes to social routines, networks, and, at times, even beliefs and attitudes (i.e., social innovations in the broad sense of the term).

## Discussion: challenges and further recommendations

The multistakeholder organizational form of FSCs (i.e., comprised of farmers, input suppliers, trusted advisors, for-profit, not-for-profit, associations, governmental, and academic institutions with competition at the local, regional, national, and global level) increases the complexity of the global food ecosystem. As a result, it is crucial to consider the diversity of actors involved and the scale at which either or both behavioral change and ecosystem transformation is necessary for integrative sustainable development. To account for the complexity and unique challenges of FSCs, CI proposes the creation of modular platforms and project portfolios in order to achieve a holistic transformation of agri-food, and indeed, Society 5.0. Modularity (Sanchez & Mahoney, 1996; Schilling, 2000) bridges the social and economic divide in a manner that supports individual and collective value creation. Modular projects cover the full spectrum of private, precompetitive, and public value creation targeting scopable and feasible solutions, regardless of their origin on one or the other side of the socioeconomic divide (Jha et al., 2016). Altogether, providing societal-scale solutions, while pursuing single and collaborative goals (Dubé et al., 2018, 2012; Dubé, Jha, et al., 2014), scientists and action partners from diverse disciplines and sectors at local, national, and global communities are assembled around targeted and feasible goals at the convergence of human, social and economic development with innovation, and intervention design being informed by deep understanding of individuals and contexts.

The FCI ecosystem needs to be anchored by an integrative digital backbone where technologies (digital and otherwise) are interwoven with data, human creativity, and social capital in portfolios of projects that, when stitched together, provide a societal-scale solution in focused domains (see Fig. 6).

Technologies (new and emerging) should not be regarded as an objective; instead, they are powerful tools and solutions to realize the full potential of Society 5.0 and sustainable FSCs. Of course, the move toward this oft perceived radical societal change is not without its challenges. A major hindrance to the adoption of new technologies in FCSs is implementation cost and the expected return on investment (OAFT, 2016).

For example, in a recent assessment concerning the adoption of precision dairy farming technology, producers indicated benefit-to-cost ratio as the most important

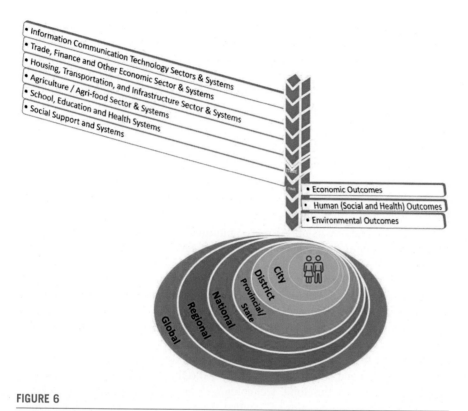

**FIGURE 6**

Convergent innovation framework.

*Adapted from Dubé, L., Addy, N. A., Blouin, C., & Drager, N. (2014). From policy coherence to 21st century convergence: A whole-of-society paradigm of human and economic development.* Annals of the New York Academy of Sciences, *1331(1), 201–215. https://doi.org/10.1111/nyas.12511. Created by author.*

consideration followed by total investment costs, simplicity of use, proven performance through independent research, and availability of local support (Borchers & Bewley, 2015). Moreover, the adoption factors of advanced technologies for a healthy environment and society should not be divorced from understanding the context and circumstances wherein FSCs operate. Such a lack of knowledge and uncertainty should be an impetus for FSC stakeholders to properly assess the societal, economic, and environmental benefits of technology adoption while considering any technology as fruitful and adoptable only if it is available at the right time and right place.

For agri-food, this is of utmost importance, as the accrual of economic and environmental benefits begins with on-farm technology adoption—the right technology on the right farm, and only then will we realize our SDGs. The complexity of FSCs also brings the challenge of data governance. For this reason, FCI takes a world perspective, bringing together relevant computer and data science and practices from industrialized and developing economies, illustrating how these perspectives can, in real time, support the design, delivery, and monitoring of targeted and effective innovation encapsulating behavioral change, product/program innovation, systems design, and data standards/policy. In other words, there is a need for an implementable governance framework designed by those who create (e.g., farmers), share (e.g., farmers), and consume the data. Although trust should be embedded (or enabled) as a foundational layer in technologies (Behnke & Janssen, 2019), adequate information policies should be established to empower and govern the trustworthiness of the data creators and data custodians. Blomqvist, Hurmelinna, & Seppänen (2005) argue that trust is of great importance in developing strong and productive collaborations. This implies that a trustworthy actor can help to simplify data governance, consent, and ownership. Also, a commitment from trustworthy organizations to establish strong linkages and integration between FSCs is also crucial for more sustainable FSC operations.

The agri-food sector needs to leverage trustworthy organizations, in addition to trusted technologies. An example in this context is the implementation of GS1 standards at the farm level and the leveraging of tools such as self-sovereign identity and digital farm wallets—certified by trustworthy farm organizations, which can enable confidence in data, ownership, access, and consent.

At present, IoT systems and on-farm technologies are isolated, siloed systems where integration and access to data are limited (Qiu et al., 2016). Broadly, siloed technologies and sensors limit technologies' ability to eliminate or eradicate endemic and or emerging crop and animal diseases. For example, a recent study on the use of precision dairy technologies concluded more work is required to improve disease detection by incorporating herd management software and recording of animal behaviors already known to producers as indicators of animal health (Eckelkamp & Bewley, 2020). It is therefore imperative that digitalization is based on shared standards and interoperability protocols in nonproprietary, multistakeholder digital architectures to overcome such problems.

Achieving the goals of Society 5.0 requires transdisciplinary collaboration to stimulate open science and equitable access to data and information. Moreover, sharing data, facilities, tools, and expertise enables breakthroughs in research, thereby supporting policy and innovation in the field of sustainable food, nutrition, and health (Musker, Tumeo, Schaap, & Parr, 2018) and potentially shaping public debate on the future of food.

An uncharted level of responsibility and collaboration by individuals, organizations, ecosystems, and institutions must occur in order to achieve and maintain best practices throughout the entire global food system. Leadership and a commitment to a more comprehensive, trustworthy digital agri-food strategy that accelerates our progression toward CI is demanded by the vision of Society 5.0 and required to achieve the SDG goals.

# References

Addy, N. A., & Dubé, L. (2018). Addressing complex societal problems: Enabling multiple dimensions of proximity to sustain partnerships for collective impact in quebec. *Sustainability, 10*(4), 980. https://doi.org/10.3390/su10040980.

Ahumada, O., & Villalobos, J. R. (2009). Application of planning models in the agri-food supply chain: A review. *European Journal of Operational Research, 196*(1), 1–20. https://doi.org/10.1016/j.ejor.2008.02.014.

Ait-Mouheb, et al. (2018). The reuse of reclaimed water for irrigation around the mediterranean rim: A step towards a more virtuous cycle? *Regional Environmental Change, 18*(3), 693–705. https://doi.org/10.1007/s10113-018-1292-z.

Ammann, J., Siegrist, M., & Hartmann, C. (2019). The influence of disgust sensitivity on self-reported food hygiene behaviour. *Food Control, 102*, 131–138. https://doi.org/10.1016/j.foodcont.2019.03.023.

Armbrust, et al. (2010). A view of cloud computing. *Communications of the ACM, 53*(4), 50. https://doi.org/10.1145/1721654.1721672.

Arora, S. K., Foley, R. W., Youtie, J., Shapira, P., & Wiek, A. (2014). Drivers of technology adoption—the case of nanomaterials in building construction. *Technological Forecasting and Social Change, 87*, 232–244. https://doi.org/10.1016/j.techfore.2013.12.017.

ASTM. (2012). Standard terminology for additive manufacturing technologies. *Astm International*. https://doi.org/10.1520/F2792–12A. Retrieved from www.astm.org.

AT Kearney. (2016). *Accelerating into uncertainty (CSCMP's 2017 annual state of logistics report.)*. Retrieved from https://www.kearney.com/transportation-travel/2017-state-of-logistics-report.

Atkinson, R. D., & Ezell, S. (2019). *The manufacturing evolution: How AI will transform manufacturing and the workforce of the future*. Information Technology and Innovation Foundation. Retrieved from https://itif.org/publications/2019/08/06/manufacturing-evolution-how-ai-will-transform-manufacturing-and-workforce. (Accessed 2 November 2020).

Azuma, R. T. (1997). A survey of augmented reality. *Presence: Teleoperators and Virtual Environments, 6*(4), 355–385. https://doi.org/10.1162/pres.1997.6.4.355.

Beck, D. E., Crandall, P. G., O'Bryan, C. A., & Shabatura, J. C. (2016). Taking food safety to the next level—an augmented reality solution. *Journal of Foodservice Business Research, 19*(4), 382–395. https://doi.org/10.1080/15378020.2016.1185872.

Beer, S. (2007). Food and society. In J. Eastham, L. Sharples, & S. Ball (Eds.), *Food supply chain management- issues for the hospitality and retail sectors* (pp. 21–36). Linacre House, Jordan Hill: Oxford OX2 8DP, Butterworth-Heinemann. Taylor & Francis.

Behnke, K., & Janssen, M. F. W. H. A. (2019). Boundary conditions for traceability in food supply chains using blockchain technology. *International Journal of Information Management*. https://doi.org/10.1016/j.ijinfomgt.2019.05.025, 101969.

Berg, L. (2004). Trust in food in the age of mad cow disease: A comparative study of consumers' evaluation of food safety in Belgium, Britain and Norway. *Appetite, 42*(1), 21–32. https://doi.org/10.1016/S0195-6663(03)00112-0.

Bildtgård, T. (2008). Trust in food in modern and late-modern societies. *Social Science Information, 47*(1), 99–128. https://doi.org/10.1177/0539018407085751.

Blackburn, R., Lurz, K., Priese, B., Göb, R., & Darkow, I.-L. (2015). A predictive analytics approach for demand forecasting in the process industry. *International Transactions in Operational Research, 22*(3), 407–428. https://doi.org/10.1111/itor.12122.

Blackmore, S. (2009). New concepts in agricultural automation. In *R&D conference "precision in arable farming: Current practice and future potential", Grantham, Lincolnshire, UK, 28th–29th October 2009* (pp. 127–137).

Blomqvist, K., Hurmelinna, P., & Seppänen, R. (2005). Playing the collaboration game right—balancing trust and contracting. *Technovation, 25*(5), 497–504. https://doi.org/10.1016/j.technovation.2004.09.001.

Borchers, M. R., & Bewley, J. M. (2015). An assessment of producer precision dairy farming technology use, prepurchase considerations, and usefulness. *Journal of Dairy Science, 98*(6), 4198–4205. https://doi.org/10.3168/jds.2014-8963.

Borcoci, E. (2017). Survey on software-defined networking and network functions virtualisation in 5G emerging mobile computing. *Cloud and Fog Computing in 5G Mobile Networks: Emerging Advances and Applications, 70*, 125.

Bronson, K., & Knezevic, I. (2019). The digital divide and how it matters for Canadian food system equity. *Canadian Journal of Communication, 44*(2). https://doi.org/10.22230/cjc.2019v44n2a3489.

Bryndin, E. (2018). System synergetic formation of society 5.0 for development of vital spaces on basis of ecological economic and social programs. *Annals of Ecology and Environmental Science, 2*(4), 12–19.

Buckeridge, D. L., Izadi, M., Shaban-Nejad, A., Mondor, L., Jauvin, C., Dube, L., et al. (2012). An infrastructure for real-time population health assessment and monitoring. *IBM Journal of Research and Development, 56*(5). https://doi.org/10.1147/JRD.2012.2197132, 2:1–2:11.

Cajaiba-Santana, G. (2014). Social innovation: Moving the field forward. A conceptual framework. *Technological Forecasting and Social Change, 82*, 42–51. https://doi.org/10.1016/j.techfore.2013.05.008.

CAO. (2020). *Examples of creating new value in the field of agriculture(Society 5.0)*. Retrieved from https://www8.cao.go.jp/cstp/english/society5_0/food_e.html. (Accessed 2 November 2020).

Clark, J., & Crandall, P. G. (2019). Educational affordances of Google glass as a new instructional platform for foodservice training. *Management & Education, 13*(1), 28–32.

Companik, E., Gravier, M., & Farris, M. (2018). Feasibility of warehouse drone adoption and implementation. *Journal of Transportation Management, 28*(2), 31–48. https://doi.org/10.22237/jotm/1541030640.

Costanza, E., Kunz, A., & Fjeld, M. (2009). Mixed reality: A survey. In D. Lalanne, & J. Kohlas (Eds.), *Human machine interaction: Research results of the MMI program* (pp. 47–68). Springer Berlin Heidelberg. https://doi.org/10.1007/978-3-642-00437-7_3.

Crofton, E. C., Botinestean, C., Fenelon, M., & Gallagher, E. (2019). Potential applications for virtual and augmented reality technologies in sensory science. *Innovative Food Science and Emerging Technologies, 56*. https://doi.org/10.1016/j.ifset.2019.102178.

Dahlman, E., Mildh, G., Parkvall, S., Peisa, J., Sachs, J., & Selén, Y. (2014). 5G radio access. *Ericsson Review (English Ed.), 91*(1), 42–47.

Desai, P. R., Desai, P. N., Ajmera, K. D., & Mehta, K. (2014). A review paper on oculus rift-A virtual reality headset. *ArXiv*, 1408.1173 [Cs]. Retrieved from http://arxiv.org/abs/1408.1173.

Detwiler, D. (2020). *Food safety: Past, present, and predictions* (1st ed.). Cambridge, MA: Elsevier Academic Press.

Dubé, L., Addy, N. A., Blouin, C., & Drager, N. (2014). From policy coherence to 21st century convergence: A whole-of-society paradigm of human and economic development. *Annals of the New York Academy of Sciences, 1331*(1), 201–215. https://doi.org/10.1111/nyas.12511.

Dubé, L., Du, P., McRae, C., Sharma, N., Jayaraman, S., & Nie, J.-Y. (2018). Convergent innovation in food through big data and artificial intelligence for societal-scale inclusive growth. *Technology Innovation Management Review, 8*(2), 49–65. https://doi.org/10.22215/timreview/1139.

Dubé, L., Jha, S., Faber, A., Struben, J., London, T., Mohapatra, A., et al. (2014). Convergent innovation for sustainable economic growth and affordable universal health care: Innovating the way we innovate. *Annals of the New York Academy of Sciences, 1*(1331), 119–141. https://doi.org/10.1111/nyas.12548.

Dubé, L., Pingali, P., & Webb, P. (2012). Paths of convergence for agriculture, health, and wealth. *Proceedings of the National Academy of Sciences, 109*(31), 12294–12301. https://doi.org/10.1073/pnas.0912951109.

Dubé, L., Subramanyam, R., Gold, R., Jha, S. K., Phelps, C., & Pinsonneault, A. (2017). Convergent Innovation: At the interface of private & public creation of economic & social value. *Academy of Management Proceedings, 2017*(1), 16859. https://doi.org/10.5465/AMBPP.2017.16859symposium.

Duckett, T., Pearson, S., Blackmore, S., Grieve, B., Chen, W.-H., Cielniak, G., et al. (2018). *Agricultural robotics: The future of robotic agriculture* [Whitepaper]. Retrieved from http://arxiv.org/abs/1806.06762.

Džbánková, Z., & Sirůček, P. (2018). Europe 4.0 vs Asia 4.0. *ICFE, 2018*, 313.

Eastwood, C. R., Chapman, D. F., & Paine, M. S. (2012). Networks of practice for co-construction of agricultural decision support systems: Case studies of precision dairy farms in Australia. *Agricultural Systems, 108*, 10–18. https://doi.org/10.1016/j.agsy.2011.12.005.

Eckelkamp, E. A., & Bewley, J. M. (2020). On-farm use of disease alerts generated by precision dairy technology. *Journal of Dairy Science, 103*(2), 1566–1582. https://doi.org/10.3168/jds.2019-16888.

Edelman. (2020). *Edelman trust barometer* [Global report]. 2/12/2020. Retrieved from https://www.edelman.com/trustbarometer.

Faraci, G., Raciti, A., Rizzo, S., & Schembra, G. (2018). A 5G platform for unmanned aerial monitoring in rural areas: Design and performance issues. In *2018 4th IEEE conference on network softwarization and workshops (NetSoft), 237–241. Montreal; QC; Canada.* IEEE. https://doi.org/10.1109/NETSOFT.2018.8459960.

Fosso Wamba, S., Kamdjoug, K., Robert, J., Bawack, R., & G Keogh, J. (2020). Bitcoin, Blockchain, and FinTech: A systematic review and case studies in the supply chain. *Production Planning and Control, 31*(2–3), 115–142.

Fresco, R., & Ferrari, G. (2018). Enhancing precision agriculture by internet of things and cyber physical systems. *Atti Soc. Tosc. Sci. Nat. Mem. Supplemento, 125*, 53–60.

Fukuda, K. (2019). Science, technology and innovation ecosystem transformation toward society 5.0. *International Journal of Production Economics*, 107460. https://doi.org/10.1016/j.ijpe.2019.07.033.

Fukuyama, M. (2018). Society 5.0: Aiming for a new human-centered society. *Japan Spotlight, 1*, 47–50.

Galvez, J. F., Mejuto, J. C., & Simal-Gandara, J. (2018). Future challenges on the use of blockchain for food traceability analysis. *Trends in Analytical Chemistry, 107*, 222–232. https://doi.org/10.1016/j.trac.2018.08.011.

Gnimpieba, Z. D. R., Nait-Sidi-Moh, A., Durand, D., & Fortin, J. (2015). Using internet of things technologies for a collaborative supply chain: Application to tracking of pallets and containers. *Procedia Computer Science, 56*, 550–557. https://doi.org/10.1016/j.procs.2015.07.251.

Godoi, F. C., Prakash, S., & Bhandari, B. R. (2016). 3d printing technologies applied for food design: Status and prospects. *Journal of Food Engineering, 179*, 44−54. https://doi.org/10.1016/j.jfoodeng.2016.01.025.

Gopie, N. (2018, July 2). *What are smart contracts on blockchain?* IBM Blockchain Blog. Retrieved from https://www.ibm.com/blogs/blockchain/2018/07/what-are-smart-contracts-on-blockchain/.

Griggs, D., Stafford-Smith, M., Gaffney, O., Rockström, J., Öhman, M. C., Shyamsundar, P., et al. (2013). Sustainable development goals for people and planet. *Nature, 495*(7441), 305−307. https://doi.org/10.1038/495305a.

Gružauskas, V., Baskutis, S., & Navickas, V. (2018). Minimizing the trade-off between sustainability and cost-effective performance by using autonomous vehicles. *Journal of Cleaner Production, 184*, 709−717. https://doi.org/10.1016/j.jclepro.2018.02.302.

Hamid, Z. A. (2018, October 15). *Japan's "Society 5.0*. NST. Retrieved from https://www.nst.com.my/opinion/columnists/2018/10/421551/japans-society-50. (Accessed 2 November 2020).

Hammond, R. A., & Dubé, L. (2012). A systems science perspective and transdisciplinary models for food and nutrition security. *Proceedings of the National Academy of Sciences, 109*(31), 12356−12363. https://doi.org/10.1073/pnas.0913003109.

van der Have, R. P., & Rubalcaba, L. (2016). Social innovation research: An emerging area of innovation studies? *Research Policy, 45*(9), 1923−1935. https://doi.org/10.1016/j.respol.2016.06.010.

Hitachi. (2020). *Our journey to evolution of society 5.0.* Retrieved from https://social-innovation.hitachi/en-in/knowledge-hub/viewpoint/society-5-0. (Accessed 2 November 2020).

Hu, F. (2016). *Opportunities in 5G networks: A research and development perspective.* CRC Press.

Janssen, A. M., Nijenhuis-de Vries, M. A., Boer, E. P. J., & Kremer, S. (2017). Fresh, frozen, or ambient food equivalents and their impact on food waste generation in Dutch households. *Waste Management, 67*, 298−307. https://doi.org/10.1016/j.wasman.2017.05.010.

Jayanth, S., Poorvi, M. B., & Sunil, M. P. (2017). Inventory management system using IOT. In S. C. Satapathy, V. K. Prasad, B. P. Rani, S. K. Udgata, & K. S. Raju (Eds.), *Proceedings of the first international conference on computational intelligence and informatics* (pp. 201−210). Springer. https://doi.org/10.1007/978-981-10-2471-9_20.

Jeppesen, J. H., Ebeid, E., Jacobsen, R. H., & Toftegaard, T. S. (2018). Open geospatial infrastructure for data management and analytics in interdisciplinary research. *Computers and Electronics in Agriculture, 145*, 130−141. https://doi.org/10.1016/j.compag.2017.12.026.

Jha, S. K., Pinsonneault, A., & Dubé, L. (2016). The evolution of an ICT platform-enabled ecosystem for poverty alleviation: The case of eKutir. *MIS Quarterly, 40*(2), 431−445. https://doi.org/10.25300/MISQ/2016/40.2.08.

Kamath, R. (2017). Food traceability on blockchain: Walmart's pork and mango pilots with IBM. *The Journal of the British Blockchain Association, 1*(1), 3712.

Kamble, S. S., Gunasekaran, A., & Gawankar, S. A. (2019). Achieving sustainable performance in a data-driven agriculture supply chain: A review for research and applications. *International Journal of Production Economics, 219*, 179−194. https://doi.org/10.1016/j.ijpe.2019.05.022.

Kamilaris, A., Fonts, A., & Prenafeta-Boldú, F. X. (2019). The rise of blockchain technology in agriculture and food supply chains. *Trends in Food Science & Technology, 91*, 640−652. https://doi.org/10.1016/j.tifs.2019.07.034.

Keidanren Policy & Action. (2016). *Toward realization of the new economy and society— reform of the economy and society by the deepening of "society 5.0".* https://www. keidanren.or.jp/en/policy/2016/029_outline.pdf. (Accessed 2 November 2020).

Khanna, M., Swinton, S. M., & Messer, K. D. (2018). Sustaining our natural resources in the face of increasing societal demands on agriculture: Directions for future research. *Applied Economic Perspectives and Policy, 40*(1), 38−59. https://doi.org/10.1093/aepp/ppx055.

Kim, H., & Sohn, K. (2003). Hierarchical depth estimation for image synthesis in mixed reality. *Stereoscopic Displays and Virtual Reality Systems X, 5006*, 544−553. https:// doi.org/10.1117/12.473879.

Kota, S., & Giambene, G. (2019). Satellite 5G: IoT use case for rural areas applications. In *Proceedings of the eleventh international conference on advances in satellite and space communications-SPACOMM. Valencia, Spain.*

Kubáč, L., & Kodym, O. (2017). The impact of 3D printing technology on supply chain. *MATEC Web of Conferences, 134*, 00027. https://doi.org/10.1051/matecconf/ 201713400027.

Lacity, M. C. (2018). Addressing key challenges to making enterprise blockchain applications a reality. *MIS Quarterly Executive, 17*(3), 201−222.

Lencucha, R., Dubé, L., Blouin, C., Hennis, A., Pardon, M., & Drager, N. (2018). Fostering the catalyst role of government in advancing healthy food environments. *International Journal of Health Policy and Management, 7*(6), 485−490. https://doi.org/10.15171/ ijhpm.2018.10.

Li, X., Wang, Y., & Chen, X. (2012). Cold chain logistics system based on cloud computing. *Concurrency and Computation: Practice and Experience, 24*(17), 2138−2150.

Lott, M. C. (2013). *UN says that if food waste was a country, it'd be the #3 global greenhouse gas emitter.* Scientific American Blog Network. Retrieved from https://blogs. scientificamerican.com/plugged-in/un-says-that-if-food-waste-was-a-country-ite28099d- be-the-3-global-greenhouse-gas-emitter/. (Accessed 2 November 2020).

Luhmann, N. (2000). Familiarity, confidence, trust: Problems and alternatives. In D. Gambetta (Ed.), *Trust: Making and breaking cooperative relations* (Vol. 6, pp. 94−107).

Luque, A., Peralta, M. E., de las Heras, A., & Córdoba, A. (2017). State of the industry 4.0 in the andalusian food sector. *Procedia Manufacturing, 13*, 1199−1205. https://doi.org/ 10.1016/j.promfg.2017.09.195.

Mattila, J., Seppälä, T., & Holmström, J. (2016). *Product-centric information management: A case study of a shared platform with blockchain technology.* Retrieved from https:// escholarship.org/uc/item/65s5s4b2.

Mohanraj, I., Gokul, V., Ezhilarasie, R., & Umamakeswari, A. (2017). Intelligent drip irriga- tion and fertigation using wireless sensor networks. In *2017 IEEE technological innova- tions in ICT for agriculture and rural development (TIAR)* (pp. 36−41). https://doi.org/ 10.1109/TIAR.2017.8273682.

Mooney, P. (2018). What's cooking for climate change? Techno-fixing dinner for 10 billion. *Bulletin of the Atomic Scientists, 74*(6), 390−396. https://doi.org/10.1080/ 00963402.2018.1533214.

Musker, R., Tumeo, J., Schaap, B., & Parr, M. (2018). *GODAN's impact 2014−2018 − improving agriculture, food and nutrition with open data* [Technical Report]. Retrieved from https://f1000research.com/documents/7-1328.

OAFT. (2016). *User needs assessment: Final report.* Ontario AgriFood Technologies. Retrieved from https://static1.squarespace.com/static/583f561af7e0ab824c0b77c8/t/

586ad4a23e00bec12e6c1ff7/1483396389489/User+Needs+Assessment.pdf. (Accessed 2 November 2020).

Onday, O. (2019). Japan's society 5.0: Going beyond industry 4.0. *Business and Economics Journal, 10*(389), 2.

Pandey, M. K., Roorkiwal, M., Singh, V. K., Ramalingam, A., Kudapa, H., Thudi, M., et al. (2016). Emerging genomic tools for legume breeding: Current status and future prospects. *Frontiers in Plant Science, 7*. https://doi.org/10.3389/fpls.2016.00455.

Park, E., Cho, Y., Han, J., & Kwon, S. J. (2017). Comprehensive approaches to user acceptance of internet of things in a smart home environment. *IEEE Internet of Things Journal, 4*(6), 2342–2350. https://doi.org/10.1109/JIOT.2017.2750765.

Pokhrel, B. K., Paudel, K. P., & Segarra, E. (2018). Factors affecting the choice, intensity, and allocation of irrigation technologies by U.S. Cotton farmers. *Water, 10*(6), 706. https://doi.org/10.3390/w10060706.

Pol, E., & Ville, S. (2009). Social innovation: Buzz word or enduring term? *The Journal of Socio-Economics, 38*(6), 878–885. https://doi.org/10.1016/j.socec.2009.02.011.

Portanguen, S., Tournayre, P., Sicard, J., Astruc, T., & Mirade, P.-S. (2019). Toward the design of functional foods and biobased products by 3D printing: A review. *Trends in Food Science & Technology, 86*, 188–198. https://doi.org/10.1016/j.tifs.2019.02.023.

Qiu, Z., Hu, N., Guo, Z., Qiu, L., Guo, S., & Wang, X. (2016). IoT sensing parameters adaptive matching algorithm. In Y. Wang, G. Yu, Y. Zhang, Z. Han, & G. Wang (Eds.), *Big data computing and communications* (pp. 198–211). Cham: Springer International Publishing.

Ray, P., Harsh, H. O., Daniel, A., & Ray, A. (2019). Incorporating block chain technology in food supply chain. *International Journal of Management Studies, 1*(5), 115–124.

Rejeb, A., Keogh, J. G., & Treiblmaier, H. (2019). Leveraging the internet of things and blockchain technology in supply chain management. *Future Internet, 11*(7), 161. https://doi.org/10.3390/fi11070161.

Rejeb, A., Süle, E., & Keogh, J. G. (2018). Exploring new technologies in procurement. *Transport & Logistics: The International Journal, 18*(45), 76–86.

Renda, A. (2019). The age of foodtech: Optimizing the agri-food chain with digital technologies. In R. Valentini, J. L. Sievenpiper, M. Antonelli, & K. Dembska (Eds.), *Achieving the sustainable development goals through sustainable food systems* (pp. 171–187). Cham: Springer International Publishing. https://doi.org/10.1007/978-3-030-23969-5_10.

Reuters. (2019). *Rising costs to challenge supply chain in 2019 | eft—supply chain & logistics business intelligence*. https://www.eft.com/supply-chain/rising-costs-challenge-supply-chain-2019. (Accessed 2 November 2020).

Ricci, I., Derossi, A., & Severini, C. (2019). Chapter 5—3D printed food from fruits and vegetables. In F. C. Godoi, B. R. Bhandari, S. Prakash, & M. Zhang (Eds.), *Fundamentals of 3D food printing and applications* (pp. 117–149). Academic Press. https://doi.org/10.1016/B978-0-12-814564-7.00005-5.

Robb, D. (2017, July 3). *Semi-structured data*. Datamation. Retrieved from https://www.datamation.com/big-data/semi-structured-data.html.

Saberi, S., Kouhizadeh, M., Sarkis, J., & Shen, L. (2019). Blockchain technology and its relationships to sustainable supply chain management. *International Journal of Production Research, 57*(7), 2117–2135. https://doi.org/10.1080/00207543.2018.1533261.

Sanchez, R., & Mahoney, J. T. (1996). Modularity, flexibility, and knowledge management in product and organization design. *Strategic Management Journal, 17*(S2), 63−76. https://doi.org/10.1002/smj.4250171107.

Schilling, M. A. (2000). Toward a general modular systems theory and its application to interfirm product modularity. *Academy of Management Review, 25*(2), 312−334. https://doi.org/10.5465/amr.2000.3312918.

Sheridan, T. B. (2016). Human−robot interaction: Status and challenges. *Human Factors, 58*(4), 525−532. https://doi.org/10.1177/0018720816644364.

Sonka, S. (2014). Big data and the Ag sector: More than lots of numbers. *International Food and Agribusiness Management Review, 17*(1), 1−20.

SPHSIT. (2019). Realization of society 5.0 by utilizing precision agriculture into smart agriculture in Naro, Japan. *International Workshop on ICTs for Precision Agriculture, 58.*

Subudhi, B. N., Rout, D. K., & Ghosh, A. (2019). Big data analytics for video surveillance. *Multimedia Tools and Applications, 78*(18), 26129−26162. https://doi.org/10.1007/s11042-019-07793-w.

Treiblmaier, H. (2018). The impact of the blockchain on the supply chain: A theory-based research framework and a call for action. *Supply Chain Management: An International Journal, 23*(6), 545−559. https://doi.org/10.1108/SCM-01-2018-0029.

UN. (2020). *Transforming our world: The 2030 agenda for sustainable development.* https://sustainabledevelopment.un.org/post2015/transformingourworld. (Accessed 2 November 2020).

UNFAO. (2018). *E-agriculture in action: Drones for agriculture.* Food and Agriculture Organization of the United Nations and International Telecommunication Union.

Vanderroost, et al. (2017). The digitization of a food package's life cycle: Existing and emerging computer systems in the logistics and post-logistics phase. *Computers in Industry, 87*, 15−30. https://doi.org/10.1016/j.compind.2017.01.004.

Verdouw, C. N., Robbemond, R. M., Verwaart, T., Wolfert, J., & Beulens, A. J. M. (2018). A reference architecture for IoT-based logistic information systems in agri-food supply chains. *Enterprise Information Systems, 12*(7), 755−779. https://doi.org/10.1080/17517575.2015.1072643.

Verdouw, C. N., Wolfert, J., Beulens, A. J. M., & Rialland, A. (2016). Virtualization of food supply chains with the internet of things. *Journal of Food Engineering, 176*, 128−136. https://doi.org/10.1016/j.jfoodeng.2015.11.009.

Völk, et al. (2019). Satellite integration into 5G: Accent on first over-the-air tests of an edge node concept with integrated satellite backhaul. *Future Internet, 11*(9), 193. https://doi.org/10.3390/fi11090193.

van der Wal, T., Kooistra, L., & Poppe, K. J. (2015). The role of new data sources in Greening Growth: The case of Drones. In *2015 OECD green growth and sustainable development Forum.*

Wang, Q. J., Mielby, L. A., Thybo, A. K., Bertelsen, A. S., Kidmose, U., Spence, C., et al. (2019). Sweeter together? Assessing the combined influence of product-related and contextual factors on perceived sweetness of fruit beverages. *Journal of Sensory Studies, 34*(3), e12492. https://doi.org/10.1111/joss.12492.

Wang, J., & Yue, H. (2017). Food safety pre-warning system based on data mining for a sustainable food supply chain. *Food Control, 73*, 223−229. https://doi.org/10.1016/j.foodcont.2016.09.048.

WEF. (2019). *Innovation with a purpose: Improving traceability in food value chains through technology innovations.* World Economic Forum. Retrieved from http://www3.weforum.

org/docs/WEF_Traceability_in_food_value_chains_Digital.pdf. (Accessed 2 November 2020).

WHO. (2015). *WHO estimates of the global burden of foodborne diseases*. Foodborne Disease Burden Epidemiology Reference Group 2007–2015.

WHO. (2015). *WHO Regional Office for Europe nutrient profile model (2015)*. Retrieved from http://www.euro.who.int/en/health-topics/disease-prevention/nutrition/publications/2015/who-regional-office-for-europe-nutrient-profile-model-2015. (Accessed 2 November 2020).

Yano, M. (2019). *Blockchain and the IoT*. RIETI special seminar. *RIETI-ANU-ERIA symposium: Asia's response to the trade war*. Retrieved from https://www.rieti.go.jp/jp/about/Highlight_73/Highlight_73.pdf. (Accessed 2 November 2020).

Yiannas, F. (2018). A new era of food transparency powered by blockchain. *Innovations: Technology, Governance, Globalization, 12*(1–2), 46–56. https://doi.org/10.1162/inov_a_00266.

Zhang, C., & Kovacs, J. M. (2012). The application of small unmanned aerial systems for precision agriculture: A review. *Precision Agriculture, 13*(6), 693–712. https://doi.org/10.1007/s11119-012-9274-5.

Zhong, R., Xu, X., & Wang, L. (2017). Food supply chain management: Systems, implementations, and future research. *Industrial Management & Data Systems, 117*(9), 2085–2114. https://doi.org/10.1108/IMDS-09-2016-0391.

# The role of technology in the connected ecosystem

## 3

**Ed Wogan, MS**

*Vice President, Brand Development-Retail Expansion, Catalina USA, Gloucester, MA, United States*

## Background

Providing food to consumers, in spite of rapidly changing technology, efficiencies in supply chain, logistics, and manufacturing, has become more complicated than ever before. As of recent, a seismic shift in the grocery landscape has resulted in approximately 44% of food sales now taking place inside of the traditional grocery store, down from approximately 90% just 30 years ago (Boyle, 2019).

Some 60% of grocers surveyed reported that fresh products are extremely important to their business, yet two-thirds say they are losing over 1.5% of annual revenue due to expired or spoiled fresh products (Progressive Grocer, 2019). In addition to the case to be made for controlling waste and keeping food out of landfills (one estimate is that 40% of food produced in the United States ends up there), the need for stringent adherence to a system of enforceable checks and balances is paramount for mitigating waste, securing the food distribution ecosystem, and ensuring the safety of the consuming public.

Other influential factors include consumers' growing penchant for food experiences with product sourced outside of the traditional grocery venue and consumed outside of the home and from a myriad of creation and processing venues. Beyond the scope of traditional grocery retailers, consumers now have more options than ever before to access and consume food, much of it perishable and less processed than ever (such as hybrid retail establishments, food-ordering apps, and modern food delivery options.) The vast variety of natural and organic products requiring less processing, farm-to-table alternatives, and dietary choices/needs (such as keto, gluten-free, and lactose-free among others) while creating expansive choices for consumers have created even more challenges for retailers, purveyors, and the people responsible for monitoring safety and standardized handling practices. The lack of presence of preservatives and additives to maintain extended shelf life, and consumer demand, has made the need for stringent food safety standards more compelling than ever. The president of a Northeast regional grocery chain shared at the Food Marketing Institute (now going by the name "FMI") Midwinter Executive Conference that her concerns around lack of controls and discipline around food safety handling and monitoring protocol for food sourced from farm to table, regional purveyors, and outside traditional supply chain methods "leave me terrified about the safety of the consumer and our exposure as a retailer" (Spire, J personal communication 2019).

## Emerging retail venues and product access methods

Convenience Stores are the only brick and mortar retail venue to show a consistent positive growth trajectory in store count and same store comparative sales (in stores open more than 1 year, a retail industry standard Key Performance Indicator), and their commitment to perishables and "foods to go" has continued to expand exponentially. Of approximately 153,000 convenience store locations operating in the United States, roughly 62% are independently owned or franchised, the balance operated by chain stores (Lenard, 2019). Convenience stores (often referred to as "C-stores") have continued to evolve their physical store formats to encompass fresh products, expansive bakery, foods and meals to go, and product prepared and assembled or delivered to the store. C-store utilization of food service products as a percentage of their total store sales has risen to greater than 23% according to the National Association of Convenience Stores State of the Industry report of 2018 (National Association of Convenience Stores, 2018). This is an industry record and is not projected to diminish. C-store operators, chronically faced with high employee turnover and thin gross margins, must learn to maximize the opportunities available to them in offering fresh-centric products while adhering to food safety product standards and operational efficiency. With that expansion comes a need for discipline and accountability in the areas of production, assembly, and ingredients, inclusive of a system of visibility, reporting, and checks and balances.

The right **technology platform** and software can help convenience store retailers (and those in any retail vertical, for that matter) keep a finger on the pulse of food safety and other production concerns. **Software** can also provide insights into individual store behavior, how they benchmark against others in a chain environment, and adherence to company standards, practices, and protocol. **Automation** and customization of software-driven reporting, inclusive of exceptions and alerts, can eliminate the need to sift through reams of paper-driven reports, and deviation from acceptable behavior, product testing, and reporting deadline exceptions can all be automated to call out issues, which can now be quickly identified and corrected. That is where technology comes into the picture, 48% of retailers state they are looking at increasing technology budgets, inclusive of tech-centric food safety practices and protocol (Kodali, 2019).

**Disruptive technology** and **innovation** are alive and well in the grocery retail and supply chain space, as demonstrated by the myriad of ways that consumers can access food, inclusive of home delivery and curbside pickup. A growing trend in home delivery of products directly from a retailer-controlled distribution resource or via a partnership with a same-day grocery delivery service company like Instacart or Shipt (owned by Target Corporation) creates a whole new level of complexity around ensuring food safety standards are maintained. Many retailers offer a "click and collect" solution where a third-party or company employee selects orders in stores-which are then delivered or picked up are paying close attention to product safety standards, especially around perishables and maintenance of acceptable temperature ranges. These purveyors are now in the competitive mix with Amazon Fresh, as retailers continue to identify and embrace new ways to compete. The challenge becomes the uncertainty that results when the product is out of the hands of the retailer and in transit to the consumer's home, thus resulting in "you can't manage what you can't measure." Cost-effective options are being developed to include low-cost **sensor technology** that is embedded in the cooler units that are used to store the product during distribution, much of it wireless, which keeps track of temperature fluctuations outside of acceptable norms and provides an alert and requires a corrective action.

## Greater options can offer greater exposure

Leading grocery retailer the Kroger Company, based in Cincinnati, OH, operates over 2700 stores in the United States, and recently entered into a pilot agreement with Walgreens as a pickup destination. The consumer can go online to Kroger's website and order groceries, drive to a designated Walgreens location, and have the order loaded into their car curbside. The pilot was so well received that Kroger and Walgreens have expanded the service offering, and, according to a 2019 statement in *Supermarket News* by Jeff Talbot, Vice President of new business development at Kroger, "Our growing relationship with Walgreens is just one more way Kroger is making life easier and better for even more customers, because everyone deserves to have affordable, easy-to-enjoy, fresh food" (Redman, 2019). A service option where the consumer picks up the order from the retail store provides more visibility and assumed security to the retailer and the customer.

### State, local, and industry association engagement

Industry associations like FMI act as watchdogs and harbingers of information, leading-edge technology, use cases, and best practices on a large scale. Equally as important on a local or regional level, support and commitment exist in critical industry organizations like The Massachusetts Food Association (MFA). This nonprofit trade association for supermarkets and grocery industry membership includes retailers, food brokers, manufacturers, wholesalers, and distributors. Senior Vice President, Government Affairs and Communications, Brian Houghton, is a strong proponent for ensuring the membership is well versed on industry and government affairs. He is a past-chair of the Food Establishment Advisory Committee (FEAC) under the MA Department of Public Health's Food Protection Program (FPP). FEAC's mission statement is to identify food safety and defense issues and assign priority status to resolution based on public health significance relative to

105 CMR 590.000; State Sanitary Code Chapter X-Minimum Sanitation Standards for Food Establishments. Priorities are to

1. Propose solutions to issues based on current science and technology,
2. Promote education, communication, and uniformity within the regulatory agencies and the food industry, and to
3. Advise the Director of FPP regarding implementation.

According to Houghton,

> *The commitment on behalf of the MFA to ensuring the membership is appraised, educated and represented is a 110+ year old legacy, (founded in 1907) and includes food safety standards, best practices and emerging technologies, among other industry priorities*

**Houghton, B., Personal Communication, 2020.**

## Retailer's commitments-why it is a critical component

The challenges around the management and efficient utilization of the expansive amounts of **data** generated within a retail operation, manufacturing or production environment, or any step of the supply chain are formidable. The impact of **decentralization** within the food supply and distribution ecosystem and the need for transparency and insights into **immutable** data that is actionable are significant.

Ricky Singh is the Director of Food Science for 400+ Sprouts Farmer Market stores. He believes that

> *Food Safety will always be of primary importance in our retail industry, and emerging technologies will transform how we view data, and communicate safety and quality to our end consumers. Our consumers demand transparency, safety, and quality in fresh, prepared or packaged foods*

**Singh, R, Personal Communication, 2020.**

The challenge also becomes management and efficient utilization of the expansive amounts of data generated within a retail operation, manufacturing or production environment, or any step of the supply chain.

### Wholesale distribution-supply chain standardization

From the perspective of wholesale food distribution and supply chain, food safety protocol requires an ongoing commitment to safety standards and utilization of technology. According to Senior Vice President Edward Rawson of Associated Grocers of New England,

> *... it is all about cold chain integrity- that is where everything starts and ends. It is critical that all products received into our distribution facility do so in its proper and safe environment. We take extensive precautions to ensure integrity is*

*maintained, inclusive of monitoring product temperature with sensors, recording data, and monitoring inbound and outbound deliveries inclusive of physical inspection. Additionally, we pay close attention to adherence upon arrival at a grocery retail outlet, and that deliveries are received in a timely fashion. Being able to track and record provides visibility and accountability through every step of the product journey*

**Rawson, E., Personal Communication, 2020.**

## Additional complexities drive innovation and set standards for food safety

As a result of legal, media, and consumer-driven pressures, technology plays an even more critical and functional role in the administration of food safety policies, procedures, and protocol. The 2011 **FDA Food Safety Modernization Act ("FSMA")** (Pub.L. 111−353, 124 STAT 3885) creates a system of processes for the FDA to better protect the health of the general public by strengthening the food safety system. It is designed to enable the FDA to focus on preventive measures rather than relying on reacting to problems after the fact. FSMA, an implementation which has been postponed several times over the past several years, is critical in its application and the value that it can immediately bring. In 2019, over 50% of product recalls were preventable (FDA, 2019), a statistic that begs for creation and implementation of standards and adherence. As compliance to safety standards becomes more complex, and media and public scrutiny continue to expand exponentially, a single recall can be potentially devastating to a brand, retailer, or purveyor.

## What does it ultimately mean for the industry?

A solid technology partner can ultimately help an operator improve efficiency and profitability, mitigate waste, and improve safety standards. Obtaining visibility into operational activity, adherence to company, and industry acceptable policies and procedures and creating an acceptable reporting protocol helps mitigate risk, improve safety standards, and positively support the great lengths that retailers, purveyors, and manufacturers go to in the areas quality and safety.

## What does it ultimately mean for the consumer?

Data-driven, visible, and accountable food safety processes and standards do more than ensure acceptable standards are adhered to and that no one becomes ill or worse. Retailers in all verticals that deliver consumable products to the consumer, manufacturers, and distributors continue to work harder and harder to ensure avoidance of food safety issues and illness outbreaks, and that the consumer perception of their brand remains intact and is not tarnished.

## Why is it important?

As technology, communications, and media (both conventional and social) continue to evolve, the impact of data and information in a useable context becomes even more critical. Further migration into the Customer Experience (CX) Economy minimizes any margin of error, and this, combined with the safety of the public, makes accountability, visibility, and creation of a culture of operational excellence paramount. Chipotlé Mexican Grille, as a result of a string of high-profile outbreaks caused by their lack of adherence to consistent and accountable standards, serves as an example of how even "bell-weather brands" are not immune to the devastating impact of food safety failures. Beyond just bad public relations and press, the blemish to their brand in the area of freshness, safety and security is forever present, and also delivered a negative impact to their brand image, public perception, sales volume, and Wall Street evaluation as a result of reported lack of protocol. A case cannot be made and justified in the court of public opinion that this was an acceptable deviation from standards, sadly judgment is passed not on what is done well, but what is not. Creation of an infrastructure inclusive of clearly define standards, technology to support those standards and provide real time visibility, and the ability to implement corrective actions is the best preventive measures any retailer or purveyor can invest in to ensure the safety and well-being of their customers, employees, and ultimately the viability of their business practice and brand.

## Conclusion

By the year 2050, the global population is expected to reach or exceed 9 billion people (U.N., 2017), which creates a myriad of challenges and will require a commitment to sustainability and environmental efficiency by every inhabitant. The global challenge to feed everyone and maintain high levels of food safety and nutrition will be one that everyone is personally invested in. Food safety and sustainability will need to be addressed at every stage of the supply chain, and application of efficient **Blockchain** principles will be mandatory. Some retailers are taking a forward leaning approach to the Global Food Safety Initiative. Ahold Delhaize, operator of over 67,000 stores in more than 10 countries (2000 or so in the United States operating under multiple banners like Stop & Shop, Food Lion, Giant, Hannaford, and Peapod, to name a few) is utilizing some unique Blockchain principles to ensure product quality, safety, sustainability, and fair labor practices are adhered to in the production of their orange juice product. By combining visibility and discipline from state of origin to consumption, Ahold is ensuring that manufacturing processes are understood from "grove to store shelf."

The **bar code** is a machine-readable optical label that contains information about the item to which it is attached. In 1966, the Kroger Company published a "Wish for a better future" booklet, stating "Just dreaming a little … could an optical scanner read the price and total the sale …. Faster service, more productive service is needed desperately" (Weightman, 2015). A few years later, on June 26, 1974, a worker at a Marsh supermarket in Troy, Ohio, swiped a 10-pack of Wrigley Juicy Fruit gum— the first item scanned for its **Universal Product Code** (Hirst, 2014). Today, via a **Quick Response (QR) code,** the product can be tracked along every step of the processing and supply chain journey, inclusive of the consumer. QR codes have come a long way from their inception in 1994 for use in the automotive industry in Japan. This is just one example of the innovation that the industry and subsequent need are driving; the creation of an infrastructure inclusive of clearly define standards, technology to support those standards and provide real time visibility, and the ability to implement corrective actions is the best preventive measures any retailer or purveyor can invest in to ensure the safety and well-being of their customers, employees, and ultimately the long-term viability of their business practice and brand.

The role of technology in the practice of food safety standards is to access real-time data to validate and reinforce acceptable behavior and to mitigate foodborne illness risk. Application of Blockchain principles to record data chronologically and make it available for public inspection or access will continue to evolve, driven by the need for industry standardization. Having access to extensive quantities of data becomes moot in the event that you cannot harness it or leverage it in a way to support risk mitigation. It is one thing to have access to all kinds of data and reporting capabilities that provide visibility, but the big question is what is your organization prepared to handle if a food safety incident happens real time?

## Data reinforcing growth of internet sales and impact on retail in general

According to a recent economic report in *The New York Times,* physical retailers closed more than 9000 stores in 2019-despite a strong consumer economy (Goolsbee, 2020). Some people call what has happened the "retail apocalypse," as Amazon.com and other online retailers have changed consumer behavior radically, and other big retailers like Walmart and Target have tried to beef up their online presence. While e-commerce is growing sharply, it may not be as large as some think. Online sales have risen from $5 billion per quarter to almost $155 billion per quarter today, yet Internet shopping still represents only 11% of the entire retail sales total. Furthermore, more than 70% of retail spending have had slow encroachment for the Internet either because of laws or regulations that govern distribution. This includes spending on automobiles, gasoline, home improvement and supplies, drugs, pharmacy, food, and beverages (Goolsbee, 2020).

New technologies, along with new policies, are needed to strengthen efforts to mitigate the increase in opportunity for failures and for crime (such as food fraud, counterfeiting, economically motivated adulteration, etc.)-along with their impact on food safety and reputation as a whole-that comes with this growth in online shopping.

# References

Boyle, M. (2019, December 3). *Robots in aisle two: Supermarket survival means matching Amazon*. Bloomberg News. Retrieved from https://www.bloomberg.com/features/2019-automated-grocery-stores/.

FDA. (2019, September 30). *Food Safety Modernization Act (FSMA)*. Retrieved from https://www.fda.gov/food/guidance-regulation-food-and-dietary-supplements/food-safety-modernization-act-fsma.

Goolsbee, A. (2020, February 13). Never mind the Internet. Here's what's killing malls. *The New York Times*. Retrieved from https://www.nytimes.com/2020/02/13/business/not-internet-really-killing-malls.html?searchResultPosition=1.

Hirst, E. (2014, June 26). 40 years ago today: Wrigley gum the first product to have its bar code scanned. *Chicago Tribune*. Retrieved from https://www.chicagotribune.com/business/chi-bar-code40-years-old-wrigley-gum-20140626-story.html.

Kodali, S. (2019, March 11). *The state of retailing online 2019: Omnichannel, marketing, and personalization*. National Retail Federation. Retrieved from https://cdn.nrf.com/sites/default/files/2019-03/StateOfRetailingOnline%202019_Omnichannel_Marketing_And%20Personalization_030719.pdf.

Lenard, J. (2019, December 31). *Fact sheet: Scope of the industry — U.S. Convenience store count*. National Association of Convenience Stores. Retrieved from https://www.convenience.org/Research/FactSheets/ScopeofIndustry/IndustryStoreCount.

National Association of Convenience Stores. (2018). *NACS state of the industry report® of 2018*. Retrieved from https://www.convenience.org/Solutions/Store/Products/NACS-SOI-Report-of-2018-Data-Hard-Copy.

Progressive Grocer. (2019, November). *US grocery supply chain*. Research by RELEX Solutions. Retrieved from https://progressivegrocer.com/file/PG15df7bde158c0e236661515/us-grocery-supply-chain-2019.

Redman, R. (2019, August 19). *Kroger, Walgreens expand retail pilot: Walgreens health and beauty products to debut in Kroger stores*. Supermarket News. Retrieved from https://www.supermarketnews.com/retail-financial/kroger-walgreens-expand-retail-pilot.

U.N. (2017, June 21). *World population projected to reach 9.8 billion in 2050, and 11.12 billion in 2100*. Department of Economic and Social Affairs. Retrieved from https://www.un.org/development/desa/en/news/population/world-population-prospects-2017.html.

Weightman, G. (2015, September 23). The history of the bar code. *Smithsonian Magazine*. Retrieved from https://www.smithsonianmag.com/innovation/history-bar-code-180956704/.

# Food quality and technology

# Introduction

**Darin Detwiler, LP.D**

*Assistant Dean and Associate Teaching Professor, Northeastern University, Founder and CEO of Detwiler Consulting Group, LLC., Boston, MA, United States*

Though scientists, technologists, and legislators have made significant progress in making our food safer over the last 100 years, no consumer, regardless of where they live, should become sickened or die from food. Further, safe food should be available to everyone. The frequency and quantity of food recalls, along with the number of outbreaks, illnesses, and deaths, indicate that problems still exist somewhere along the farm-to-fork process. At the same time, a large portion of foodborne illnesses could be prevented. When it comes to protecting our food, and making sure that everyone is fed, one fear is that progress has plateaued.

We are at a turning point in our approach to food growth, production, protection, and distribution. There will be approximately 2 billion more people in 2050 than today, for a total of 9.7 billion people (UN, 2019). Harmonization and standardization are critical to protecting the world's food supply both today and in the future. Food quality is an important element of food safety, in that many of the same forces involved in food quality failures are at play when it comes to food safety failures. Much food is wasted or destroyed due to food safety and quality failures, with the collateral negative impact on food availability.

Food quality has multiple definitions, depending on the source, with next- or end-use consumers typically having the final definition. Common to most definitions is that food quality involves processes to support consistent specifications to meet the consumers' desires for premium end product (density, color, smell, texture, viscosity, etc.)

Food authentication dates back to the earliest days of bartering and markets. Organoleptic testing, which uses sensory organs for evaluation of odor, flavor, and texture of food, served for nearly a century as the foundation of the USDA's detecting foodborne pathogens before the creation of modern methods (such as whole genome sequencing). Authenticity concerns are nothing new: only the detection methods for safety and quality have changed.

One new element of food quality that needs to be considered is quality associated with certifications-including, but limited to, halal, kosher, vegan, and vegetarian. For these certifications, many of the same concerns exist as in other food reputations, food safety included.

**Building the Future of Food Safety Technology.** https://doi.org/10.1016/B978-0-12-818956-6.00004-X

Kosher-certified products provide a great example of where demand has increased significantly over the past few decades. Kosher is a major food trend, but not solely for the consumers as one might predict.

*While Jewish consumers have long been devoted to Kosher-designated foods, many non-Jewish consumers have come to appreciate Kosher as well. It relies on unprocessed ingredients, requires high standards of cleanliness, and traceability is a key part of production processes. Many consumers choose these products as an alternative to buying other 'untrusted' brands.*

**Global Food Safety Resource, 2020.**

Halal-certified products are another example of certified products-in this case, ones that are allowed under Islamic dietary guidelines, according to Muslim customs and as prescribed in the Quran. Muslims cannot eat *haram* foods, which means unlawful or prohibited, that include ingredients such as alcohol, animal fats, vanilla extract, gelatin, animal rennet, pepsin, lipase, pork and pork products (ham, sausage, bacon), and any noncertified meat and poultry (Gagne, 2020).

In Dubai, UAE, an international city with a population of 3.38 million people as of March 2020 (Dubai Statistics Center, 2020), has seen the number of restaurants in the city quadruple from about 3000 in 2013 (Alwadi, 2013) to 11,813 five years later (Emirates 24/7, 2019). The Dubai Municipality Food Code requires halal certificates for the sale, import, and export of food. Food service establishments are also required to identify foods with allergens or nonhalal ingredients in their menus. Storage, preparation, and serving of nonhalal foods also come with regulatory guidance (Food Code, 2014).

Dubai imports about $200 billion of food annually from nearly 200 countries (Saseendran, 2017). In 2017, during the opening ceremonies for the 11th Dubai International Food Safety Conference, Hussain Nasser Lootah, Director General of Dubai Municipality, launched "Food Watch," a digital platform that aims to completely digitize the food safety and nutritional information of all edible items served through the 20,000 or more food establishments in the Emirates (Detwiler, 2018).

In this example, the future of food safety technology related to traceability and transparency is being applied not only to food safety but also to food quality and beyond. Another example of this can be found in Blockchain-often described as being able to improve food safety. These messages typically include how it would improve traceability and decrease recall timelines. While this increased reactive focus on data collection has a definite place in response to failures in food safety, they still take place after incidents or crises have occurred; people have been harmed; and consumers have become victims, hospital patients, and worse.

Much like a car's airbag, Blockchain definitely may be part of the solution, but deployment after an incident has already happened, regardless of its efficiency, forces us to accept that harm already has occurred.

Over time, after-the-fact responses reduce a company's options to identify, stop, and correct a failure while the liabilities of that company continue to increase. Thus,

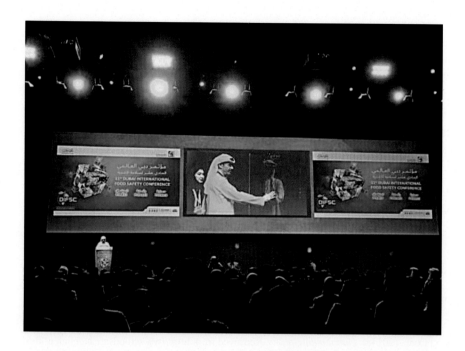

Photo of Dubai officials launching Foodwatch app to completely digitalize food safety and nutritional information of all food items served throughout Dubai.

*Photo taken by Darin Detwiler during the Dubai International Food Safety Conference November 19, 2017, at the Dubai International Convention and Exhibition Center.*

this is where hindsight and insight usually include lawsuits, court trials, and sometimes even changes in legislation. According to a 2012 study, many companies will experience a sharp drop in their NYSE stock value over a quarter of trading, which then requires at least three-quarters to return to preincident values (Seo et al., 2013).

Consumers may not be aware that new technologies and food safety practices come with a price that increases the grocery bill. But what are the costs if these steps fall short of protecting us? Consider also, that while companies frequently recover (or at least survive) after these incidents, those consumers and their families most impacted by a foodborne illness or food allergen crisis never fully recover.

Industry's use of Blockchain must include a parallel focus on its use to predict and prevent failures before public harm arises. Here, the detection and analysis of evidence and issues before there is a public health crisis is key. This approach brings additional options for mitigation while minimizing (if not eliminating) liabilities. The impact on consumer safety adds great value to technology used proactively. Further, this is where Blockchain has the capacity to make a positive impact on food quality, authenticity, defense, and security.

Not all failures can be identified and stopped before it is too late. However, if industry leaders fail to develop practices, and a culture that embraces predictive analytics driven by a balance of data/technology literacy and human literacy (understanding the true burden of disease, asking the right questions, prioritizing consumers' safety), then families will ultimately pay for the newest technology that protects industry more than it protects consumers (Detwiler, 2018).

## References

Alwadi, A., & quoted in Malek, C. (2013, March 26). Dubai food code tightens the rules on non-halal food sales and allergens. *The National, UAE*. Retrieved from https://www.thenational.ae/uae/dubai-food-code-tightens-the-rules-on-non-halal-food-sales-and-allergens-1.333781.

Detwiler, D. (2018, February 27). Blockchain in food safety: One nation's move to increase food safety with Blockchain. *IBM Blockchain Blog*. Retrieved from https://www.ibm.com/blogs/Blockchain/2018/02/one-nations-move-to-increase-food-safety-with-Blockchain/.

Dubai Statistics Center, & quoted in Dubai Online. (2020, March 2). *Current population statistics*. Retrieved from https://www.dubai-online.com/essential/population/.

Emirates 24/7. (2019a). *Number of restaurants and cafes in Dubai increase by 9.7% in 2018*. Retrieved from https://www.emirates247.com/business/number-of-restaurants-and-cafes-in-dubai-increase-by-9-7-in-2018-2019-02-07-1.679279.

Food Code. (2014a). *Dubai municipality*. Retrieved from http://www.foodsafe.ae/contentfiles/uploads/Food_Code_English_interactive.pdf.

Gagne, A. (2020a). Eating according to religious practices: Kosher and halal. *Gordon Food Service*. Retrieved from https://www.gfs.com/en-us/ideas/eating-according-religious-practices-kosher-and-halal.

Global Food Safety Resource. (2020). *Safety and quality drive increased demand for kosher certification*. Retrieved from https://globalfoodsafetyresource.com/kosher-certification/#.

Saseendran, S. (2017a). Dubai launches high-tech Food Watch programme. *Gulf News*. Retrieved from https://gulfnews.com/uae/health/dubai-launches-high-tech-food-watch-programme-1.2126769.

Seo, S., et al. (2013a). The impact of food safety events on the value of food-related firms: An event study approach. *International Journal of Hospitality Management, 33*, 153–165.

UN. (2019, June 17). *Growing at a slower pace, world population is expected to reach 9.7 billion in 2050 and could peak at nearly 11 billion around 2100*. Department of Social and Economic Affairs. Retrieved from https://www.un.org/development/desa/en/news/population/world-population-prospects-2019.html.

# International food quality and safety technology in action: Dubai's Foodwatch

**Bobby Krishna, MSc**

*Senior Specialist for Food Permits and Applied Nutrition Section, Dubai Municipality, Dubai, United Arab Emirates*

## FoodWatch

Dubai is globally recognized as a city that nurtures innovation, and, in the heart of Dubai's vision is a desire and willingness to embrace and harness advanced technologies. One such area of innovation is in the use of digital technology for public health management, particularly in enhancing food safety. With organizations rapidly adopting technologies such as the Internet of things (IoT), artificial intelligence (AI), robotics, data analytics, and visualization tools, the Food Safety Department of Dubai Municipality recognized the immense opportunities to use such technologies to improve the quality of public health systems in the city. The Department realized that digital technology has the potential to affect every aspect of food safety, enabling both the government and the food industry to identify and manage risks more precisely. While such technologies have impacted the way we interact, learn, work, and perceive things around us, there are very few used case references for technology use in public health management, which makes Foodwatch platform the first of its kind.

The Foodwatch platform, launched in 2018, facilitates data exchange between authorities, food businesses, service providers, and consumers to verify products and services with certainty across the food system. Foodwatch maintains verified profiles of every organization and associated individual within the food safety ecosystem of Dubai, each of which has a set of "permissions" associated with it. These permissions serve as "legal permits" that allow organizations to carry out particular processes (e.g., serve raw animal products) or persons to provide particular services (e.g., a trainer to deliver training). Every outcome is converted into a digital "token" that the organization can use as evidence of an action (e.g., training certificate). Every transaction within the system leaves an immutable digital footprint that can be traced back any time. Persons in charge (PICs) of food safety in a business, contractors, consultants, trainers, and auditors have their detailed profiles on Foodwatch, and they are linked to a unique, safe, and secure digital identity that serves as a "key" to exchange trusted information. The system also maintains a record of the activities of these individuals and their organization that drives the

**Building the Future of Food Safety Technology.** https://doi.org/10.1016/B978-0-12-818956-6.00005-1

system that in turn identifies their training and development needs. For instance, a PIC in a large catering facility may have additional training requirements compared to a PIC in a coffee shop.

While the government uses Foodwatch for regulatory purposes, food businesses have a very different value proposition in the form of better and effective food safety management. Food safety management systems have been largely paper-based, and it costs both the food industry and the government enormous time and resources to maintain and verify records and documents related to these systems. Foodwatch transformed this by building trust around digital, immutable, permanent, and auditable record-keeping. Documents related to supplier verification, certification, product and process information, training, temperature monitoring records, pest monitoring, cleaning and disinfection, etc., are some examples of documents that have been fully digitalized. The Foodwatch connect app that could be set up on any mobile device helps PICs of food businesses manage their food safety program very easily. Compatibility with various IoT devices used for temperature monitoring is being tested now, which will allow monitoring and tracking devices to directly connect with the Foodwatch platform and any exception (e.g., a temperature deviation) can be made actionable. Through digitalization, Foodwatch has significantly reduced document transaction costs by reducing duplication, reconciliation, and record-keeping tasks. The valuable time saved can now be used for more effective on-site verification of food safety systems, or for training and development. A business usually spends over USD 3000 per year to maintain a traditional food safety management system, purely for record-keeping, management, and verification of data. With the shared value model, the platform is available to food businesses in Dubai at slightly more than 1 USD per day.

An important aspect of the Foodwatch platform is its ability to verify and evidence compliance to food safety requirements using the transparency model. Public health measures in many countries are verified through routine food inspections with the support from service providers such as training centers, laboratories, hygiene suppliers, pest management companies, and so on. Effectiveness of the public health management is evidenced through documentation, paper-based record-keeping, certifications, and on-site audits and verifications that are time, cost, and resource intensive. Most importantly, the traditional regulatory approaches are more reactive and less predictive and preventive. Food and environmental health inspection reporting was digitalized in many countries over the last 2 decades. However, there are very few public health agencies that have capitalized on the power of data science for public health decision-making. With the exception of the Chicago Health Department, no use cases of data-driven food safety management systems existed until now. By moving to digital records, Foodwatch has already opened up information silos and enabled data sharing and connectivity with other digital ecosystems. Over 20,000 food businesses use Foodwatch and around 60,000 users contribute to the data. The system connects with other regulatory systems used for food inspection, food import, and other public health inspections to monitor waste and environmental management, pest activities, etc. Foodwatch is connected with the business licensing authority that authorizes organizations to carry out specific activities in Dubai. Built-in rules and algorithms help in real-time verification and authorization and when necessary initiate an action to prevent a food business or a service provider from providing unsafe products or poor service. This has significantly improved the services offered by the Food Safety Department and has provided enhanced visibility and accountability throughout the food supply chain. Interoperability is another important feature of Foodwatch platform. For instance, the platform is connected to the Road and Transportation Authority, and this helps in tracking food transportation vehicles and their performance. With the two-way communication with the vehicle licensing authority, food establishments can now use the vehicle tracking facility to verify their food deliveries and report vehicles that do not comply with the food safety requirements.

At the backend, Foodwatch uses powerful big data analytical tools that are connected to many datasets within the regulatory environment including food and public health inspections, consumer complaint system, food import data, laboratory testing data, and customer services data. With organizations rapidly adopting technologies beyond IoT and AI, Foodwatch will serve as an ideal digital framework for the government and the industry to transition to more advanced systems as they become available. Foodwatch will continue to integrate disparate systems and move to a more advanced stage of digital capability in the coming years creating value for the government, industry, and above all for the consumers.

# Application of technology to food quality and food safety

**Darin Detwiler, LP.D** [1], **Wendy Maduff, PhD** [2]

[1]*Assistant Dean and Associate Teaching Professor, Northeastern University, Founder and CEO of Detwiler Consulting Group, LLC., Boston, MA, United States;* [2]*Vice President of Corporate Food Safety and Quality, The Wonderful Company, Los Angeles, CA, United States*

## With early technological revolutions came new concerns

Food safety as it pertains to the final consumer was not recognized by the United States government until Peter Collier (first head of the Chemical Division if the new US Department of Agriculture, appointed in 1862) voiced his concerns about food adulteration in 1880. This took place during the "Second Industrial Revolution" (between 1870 and 1914), when development of the internal combustion engine, along with production of steel, oil, and electricity, resulted in urbanization which resulted in increased food distribution distances as well as the increase in imported foods (Detwiler, 2020).

In 1883, the USDA appointed Harvey W. Wiley, MD, as its Chief Chemist (USDA, 2018). Wiley focused his attention and government funding toward the investigation of food adulteration (Harvey Washington Wiley, 2018), which generated a published series of technical bulletins on foods and food adulterants (USDA, 1887), proposals of various versions of pure food legislations to Congress, unsuccessfully, between 1897 and 1901 (Harvey Washington Wiley, 2018), and even experimented with live volunteers, referred to as his "Poison Squad," to determine the effects of preservatives on humans (Blum, 2018).

During this period, food safety concerns and the USDA grew, leading to the eventual formation of the FDA via the 1906 Pure Food and Drug Act, made largely possible due to consumers' reactions to Upton Sinclair's 1906 novel *"The Jungle,"* which focused on exploitation of immigrants and harsh working conditions (FDA, 2018; Saxowsky, 2008). Even though Sinclair's intended message was to support socialism, readers took note of the two chapters in which he described the detailed conditions under which meat was prepared. The book changed consumers' perspectives of food safety and quality, unifying them to demand new regulations for purity and inspections. As a result, Congress passed the Pure Food and Drug Act of 1906 (Pub. L. 59−384, 34 Stat. 768, Chapter 3915) as well as the Federal Meat Inspection Act of 1906 (Pub.L. 59−242, 34 Stat. 1256). Sinclair and other writers and investigative reporters (referred to as "Muckrakers" and "Progressives") pushed social activism and political reform to eliminate problems caused by industrialization, urbanization, immigration, and political corruption (Detwiler, 2020).

The FDA's early concerns aligned with these progressives' concerns over adulteration (intentional use of unsafe preservatives and additives), food processing facility conditions, and intentional imitation food (e.g., margarine being sold as butter, unless labeling clearly addressing the differences). Though these issues remain today, new challenges such as microbial adulteration, safety expectations on the farm, and more deliberate crimes of counterfeit food are also incorporated into modern food safety expectations (FDA, 2020).

## A more modern view

Most people in the food safety industry are familiar with the food safety basics established over 45 years ago. However, food safety continues to evolve. An example is Hazard Analysis Critical Control Points (HACCP) that was developed in the 1950s. In 1974, the FDA integrated the three HACCP principles into its low-acid and acidified foods regulations. HACCP became the leading food safety system in the late 1980s, and by 1997, HACCP had added four principles beyond the original three. Advancement of HACCP can also be found in the FDA Food Safety Modernization Act (FSMA), which President Barack Obama signed into law in 2011 (FDA, 2019; Surak, 2009).

FSMA maintains the existing food safety foundation and adds focus to preventative food safety challenges and extends food safety expectations globally as many ingredients and food products are sourced internationally.

## Examples of new technologies with implications for food quality and safety

Over the years, guidance has been optimized for different food production and handling "sectors":

| Farming | Processing | Manufacturing | Retail | Consumer |
| --- | --- | --- | --- | --- |

Each of these sectors offer a glimpse at several areas of concern (all areas of concern listed below may not apply to each sector, for example, microbial limits in agricultural, rinse, ingredient, and drinking water may be different).

(1) **Data Systems (Hardware, Software) for Traceability:** Traceability has been a focus for years. The old adage for traceability used to be *"One step back and one step forward."* Now the expectation is to know the entire history of all the food components, from seed to the end user/consumer. Currently, this issue has two main contributing factors: hardware/data management and willingness of

companies to share their data. The recent improvements to software and technology combined with the ubiquity of mobile devices, especially phones, allow for food safety and quality data (along with information related to authenticity and defense) to be easily collected along the entire supply chain and stored in readily accessible servers at a minimal cost (Mearian, 2017). Additionally software programs now run on advanced mobile devices which permits easy, real-time data entry.

Despite many food safety software systems having the ability to be integrated, some suppliers and customers do not want total transparency for financial reasons.

For example, if a supplier had a foreign matter issue in an ingredient for customer A, the supplier may not want customer B to know about it despite their ingredient running on the same or different lines because they do not want to lose sales. Also if the two customers are competitors, maybe the supplier does not care about sharing the data, but customer A cares because if an alternate supplier learns they need the ingredient, the alternate supplier may raise the price of the ingredient and/or customer B might buy all available ingredient from the alternate supplier so customer A cannot produce their product. Therefore the supplier will not, or cannot, grant full access to their traceability data of all items to all customers.

An ideal traceback of a piece of annually planted produce, such as lettuce, would include all safety information from the seed supplier, irrigation water source, soil amendment components, pesticides if used, harvesting equipment (locations used between washes), wash water/solutions, workers, pack houses (the lines the item ran on), packaging supplier, transportation, distribution centers (cross docs), the retail facility, temperatures along the chain, and the final consumer in only a few minutes. Years ago, manually collecting this data usually required 3–10 business days, depending on the number of components and often the information was incomplete due to poor record-keeping.

(2) **Food Treatments:** Though new lethality treatments for food are slow coming, existing treatments are being and will likely be improved (more even heating, faster cooling, flash cooking, etc.) for higher microbial reduction and growth prevention. Some of these advances will also benefit food quality.

(3) **Food Safety Systems:** In the past, food safety was compartmentalized, and certain areas received more consideration; however, today all areas are reviewed equally. HACCP plans have evolved into food safety plans which, in theory, encompass all potential food safety risk areas. In the past 20 years, numerous best practices have become requirements, such as environmental monitoring programs (EMPs), allergen programs, and raw material receiving. Additionally, each program has become more elaborate. For example, environmental testing has been used for decades in production facilities. Over time, additional expectations have been added; today, EMPs included standard considerations, zoning, using standard swabbing (surface area sample sizes), determining the proper swab type, and incorporating air samples and often

have different action limits in the different zones. Today's pathogen environmental monitoring program (PEMP) includes different criteria than the EMP. Another newer development is if a bacterium of interest or a pathogen is found, a formal investigation procedure (vector swabbing) is performed.

**(4) Food Packaging**: Packaging is continually evolving. In the recent past, packaging materials have had different goals, such as extending quality and shelf life, being recyclable, and being sustainable. Currently, much effort is being placed on developing and improving sensors in packaging so people may skip lines and simply walk out of the establishment-currently being tested in Amazon Go stores-in hopes of eliminating checkout waiting and shoplifting (Plastics, 2018; Show & Show, 2020). Though not the motivator for developing this technology, having the information of who bought what food products is extremely valuable information in the event of a recall. Currently, there does not appear to be much research focused on antimicrobial packaging.

**(5) Wearable Technology:** Wearable technology is in its infancy. Currently, headsets and head-mounted cameras are being tested in the retail sector (Clark, Crandall, and Shabatura, 2018). The potential exists for real-time correction systems to be in place. For example, to alert a restaurant worker if he/she follows an incorrect cooking procedure, if it is time to wash his/her hands, if food is being placed in the wrong holding temperature, or if a temperature in a cooler is incorrect, the system could warn the employee it is not safe to use.

**(6) Food Testing:** Food testing has steadily improved over time, from improving the limit of detection to test sophistication (whole genome sequencing, WGS). For many years, the time to results usually required a minimum of 24—36 h. A new analytical test method exists with a four-cell limit of detection for *Listeria*-one that can produce results in under an hour (NEOGEN, 2018). The manufacturing company is improving it (one cell limit of detection, reducing organic matter interference, etc.) and working on making this test for other pathogens. Currently, WGS requires 2—5 days for results; however, sequencing times are decreasing for multiple reasons, so it is reasonable to expect sequencing times could decrease from two to 5 days to a few hours in the future.

Many people are hoping for the development of real-time results, but the most anticipated advancement is when metadata (relatedness) can unequivocally determine relatedness of microorganisms for tracking and outbreak attribution purposes.

**(7) Consumer Education:** Consumer education is potentially the most impactful area of future food safety as many companies focus on providing what their customers want, no matter the repercussions. Many US consumers do not understand the consequences of their requests, especially as it may impact other countries. Some decisions made from consumer beliefs include

- GMO-free
- Antibiotic-free
- Grass-fed
- Cage-free

- Organic
- "Natural"
- Safe handling of their own food
- Definitions on labels ("best by dates," "use by dates," etc.)

For example, industry is reluctant to share pathogen occurrence information primarily because of public judgment. Ideally, consumers would appreciate sharing this information, with the assumption that this could prevent further product contamination. Unfortunately, consumers would be surprised to learn that-outside of large recalls and deadly outbreaks such as Peanut Corporation of America (CDC, 2009), Jensen Farms (CDC, 2012), Chipotle Mexican Grill restaurants (CDC, 2016), and Blue Bell Creamery (CDC, 2015)-this information is rarely a reflection of negligence.

Areas of opportunity to educate consumers:

- **Refrigerate foods** that will be consumed later, including
  - Foodborne outbreaks at church functions (Beach, 2018)
  - Kids sports activities
  - Buying a sandwich in the morning for lunch or dinner
- **Food on the table-**if food is cooked and put out for consumption, it may be safe at first, but as it cools and bacteria can start to grow it may not be safe-messaged repeatedly (Pereira, 2020)
- **Leftovers** and food safety (USDA, 2016).
- **Food quality-**when does this become a food safety issue
- **Food with multiple components** (seasoned chips, frosted cakes, adding garnish to cooked meat)
- **Guidance-**stratification of communicating to different generations

Specific examples:

- **Cage-free eggs-**cage-free chickens often endure more stress from cramped living conditions and endure pecking. People think it means range-free.
- **GMO-free-**more than a third of children in need have a vitamin A deficiency severe enough to cause blindness and/or contribute to death (UNICEF, 2019).
- **Golden rice-**genetically modified to carry the β-carotene gene, a precursor to vitamin A (Tang, Qin, Dolnikowski, Russell, and Grusak, 2009).

## The potential impact of technology on food safety and food quality in the future

Discussing what might happen in the future is always a challenge. Much like science fiction writing, sometimes new technologies come to fruition; 3D printers (Star Trek), hoverbikes (Star Wars), and video chat (2001: A Space Odyssey); and others have not (yet) become a reality-such as teleportation and lightspeed travel. Undoubtedly, some new forms of data collection and analysis technologies, as well as those related to traceability and transparency within the food supply system, will happen in the next 30 years. These will not replace existing operations or workforces but will enable them to be stronger and more capable of mitigating failures while protecting brand reputation. Any future advancement of new technologies depends on the digitization of documents across food's entire journey from farming to consumer. Nonetheless, regardless of new technologies, the power of consumers cannot be overlooked.

Consumer education could have a huge impact on the future of food safety because people heavily influence industry and the government. Similar to the formation of the FDA from public pressure (as a result of Sinclair's novel *The Jungle* in the early 1900s), modern consumers have the same gang effect often instigated by crowd-sourced data and postings on social media.

Unfortunately, the focus of people's efforts are often driven by misrepresented, poorly researched, and/or non-science-based claims. Advocates can become activists whose beliefs are often so strong that they resort to blackmail by threatening negative social media to get their desired result(s). The multiple outbreaks tied to Chipotlé Mexican Grille (CDC, 2016; Marler, 2015) and *Listeria* outbreak and recall of Blue Bell Creamery's Ice Cream products (CDC, 2015) saw a clash between consumers who lost trust in the brands and those who stood strong with their loyalty to the brands. A simple look at memes related to these two events reveals a polarized set of consumer opinions. When almost anything can be posted online without repercussion or fact-checking, information gained by followers, subscribers, or simply casual readers becomes impossible to label as fact or fiction. These examples are not alone. While social media can be an effective platform for change, many examples exist of people who are only seeking fame with brazen disregard to the validity of their cause/claim. If the public learns the true situation, potential side effects of situations, and input from reputable science, the opportunity to support well-founded causes should prevail, though the initial harm to an industry or company has been done.

## References

Beach, C. (2018, November 19). Church BBQ outbreak serves as food safety reminder for charitable events. *Food Safety News*. Retrieved from https://www.foodsafetynews.com/2018/11/church-bbq-outbreak-serves-as-food-safety-reminder-for-charitable-events/.

Blum, D. (2018). *The poison Squad*. New York: Penguin Press.

CDC. (2009, May 11). *Multistate outbreak of* Salmonella typhimurium *infections linked to Peanut butter, 2008–2009 (final update)*. Retrieved from https://www.cdc.gov/salmonella/2009/peanut-butter-2008-2009.html.

CDC. (2012, August 27). *Multistate outbreak of listeriosis linked to whole cantaloupes from Jensen farms, Colorado (final update)*. Retrieved from https://www.cdc.gov/listeria/outbreaks/cantaloupes-jensen-farms/index.html.

CDC. (2015, June 10). *Multistate outbreak of listeriosis linked to Blue Bell Creameries products (final update)*. Retrieved from https://www.cdc.gov/listeria/outbreaks/ice-cream-03-15/index.html.

CDC. (2016, February 1). *Multistate outbreaks of shiga toxin-producing* Escherichia coli *O26 infections linked to Chipotle Mexican grill restaurants (final update)*. Retrieved from https://www.cdc.gov/ecoli/2015/o26-11-15/index.html.

Clark, J., Crandall, P., & Shabatura, J. (2018). Wearable technology effects on training outcomes of restaurant food handlers. *Journal of Food Protection, 81*(8), 1220–1226. Retrieved from https://meridian.allenpress.com/jfp/article-abstract/81/8/1220/174981/Wearable-Technology-Effects-on-Training-Outcomes?redirectedFrom=fulltext.

Detwiler, D. (2018, February 27). Blockchain in food safety: One nation's move to increase food safety with Blockchain. *IBM Blockchain Blog*. Retrieved from https://www.ibm.com/blogs/blockchain/2018/02/one-nations-move-to-increase-food-safety-with-blockchain/.

Detwiler, D. (2018, December 12). Who would Blockchain really benefit? *Quality Assurance and Food Safety Magazine*. Retrieved from: https://www.qualityassurancemag.com/article/who-would-blockchain-really-benefit/.

Detwiler, D. (2020). *Food safety: Past, present, and predictions*. Cambridge: Elsevier Academic Press.

FDA. (2018, January 31). *Background: Research tools on FDA history*. Retrieved from https://www.fda.gov/about-fda/research-tools-fda-history/background-research-tools-fda-history.

FDA. (2019, September 30). *Food Safety Modernization Act (FSMA)*. Retrieved from https://www.fda.gov/food/guidance-regulation-food-and-dietary-supplements/food-safety-modernization-act-fsma.

FDA. (2020, February 13). FSMA rules & guidance for industry. Retrieved from https://www.fda.gov/food/food-safety-modernization-act-fsma/fsma-rules-guidance-industry.

Food Code. (2014). Dubai municipality. Retrieved from http://www.foodsafe.ae/contentfiles/uploads/Food_Code_English_interactive.pdf.

Global Food Safety Resource. (2020). Safety and quality drive increased demand for kosher certification. Retrieved from https://globalfoodsafetyresource.com/kosher-certification/#.

Harvey Washington Wiley. (2018). *Science history institute*. Retrieved from https://www.sciencehistory.org/historical-profile/harvey-washington-wiley.

Marler, B. (2015, November 1). A bit(e) of history of chipotle food poisoning outbreaks. *Marler Blog*. Retrieved from https://www.marlerblog.com/case-news/a-bite-of-history-of-chipotle-food-poisoning-outbreaks/.

Mearian, L. (2017, March 23). CW@50: Data storage goes from $1M to 2 cents per gigabyte. *Computer World*. Retrieved from https://www.computerworld.com/article/3182207/cw50-data-storage-goes-from-1m-to-2-cents-per-gigabyte.html.

NEOGEN. (2018). Listeria *right now*. Retrieved from https://foodsafety.neogen.com/pdf/catalogs/listeriarightnow_brochure.pdf.

Pereira, L. (2020, January 28). *Your winning game plan for super bowl party food and leftovers*. Foodsafety.gov. Retrieved from https://www.foodsafety.gov/blog/your-winning-game-plan-super-bowl-party-food-and-leftovers.

Plastics Make It Possible. (2018, January 5). *Plastic packaging history: Innovations through the decades*. Retrieved from https://www.plasticsmakeitpossible.com/about-plastics/history-of-plastics/plastic-innovations-in-packaging-through-the-decades/.

Saxowsky, D. (2008, January 5). *History of US government response*. NDSU Department of Agribusiness and Applied Economics. AG Law Text. Retrieved from https://www.ndsu.edu/pubweb/%saxowsky/aglawtextbk/chapters/foodlaw/HistoryFS_000.html.

Seo, S., et al. (2013). The impact of food safety events on the value of food-related firms: An event study approach. *International Journal of Hospitality Management, 33*, 153–165.

Show, G., & Show, U. (2020, February 29). Amazon Go Grocery launches in Seattle's Capitol hill with no cashiers. *MyNorthwest*. Retrieved from https://mynorthwest.com/1739880/amazon-go-grocery-launches-seattle-capitol-hill/.

Surak, J. (2009 February 1). The evolution of HACCP. *Food Quality & Safety Magazine*. Retrieved from https://www.foodqualityandsafety.com/article/the-evolution-of-haccp.

Tang, G., Qin, J., Dolnikowski, G., Russell, R., & Grusak, M. (2009, April 15). Golden rice is an effective source of vitamin A. *American Journal of Clinical Nutrition, 89*(6), 1776−1783. Retrieved from https://www.ncbi.nlm.nih.gov/pmc/articles/PMC2682994/.

UNICEF. (2019, February). *Vitamin A*. Retrieved from https://data.unicef.org/topic/nutrition/vitamin-a-deficiency/#:%:text=The%20World%20Health%20Organization%20has,Asia%20(44%20per%20cent.

US Department of Agriculture. (1887). Technical bulletin 19330 − number 13: Foods and food adulterants. Retrieved from https://archive.org/details/foodsfoodadulter13unit/page/n10.

US Department of Agriculture. (2016, December 20). *Keep food safe! Food safety basics*. Retrieved from https://www.fsis.usda.gov/wps/portal/fsis/topics/food-safety-education/get-answers/food-safety-fact-sheets/safe-food-handling/keep-food-safe-food-safety-basics/ct_index#:%:text=Discardanyfoodleftout,within3to4days.text=Reheatleftove.

US Department of Agriculture. (2018). *FSIS history*. Retrieved from https://www.fsis.usda.gov/wps/portal/informational/aboutfsis/history.

# Food safety and technology

# Challenges in the prevention of foodborne illness

7

**Gary M. Weber, PhD**

*Senior Director Food Safety and Contamination Prevention, Worldaware, Washington, D.C., United States*

## Prologue

When Dr. Detwiler, author of *Food Safety: Past, Present, and Predictions* (Elsevier Academic Press, 2020), asked me to write a section focusing on prevention for his next book, I was both honored and concerned. I was concerned because while I am a vocal proponent and "practitioner" of prevention, I know it is easier said than done in practice, as well as in writing how to accomplish it.

Prevention is a strange challenge because when prevention is achieved, nothing happens. People then ask "Why are we concerned about nothing, why are we spending money to accomplish nothing?" Think about measles, reported to be eradicated from the United States in 2000. Then, because nothing was happening, the antivaccination movement emerged, and something happened again. The CDC confirmed at least 1282 cases of measles in 2019 (CDC, 2020). I grew up in an era of fear of polio, measles, mumps, and chicken pox. Today, because of prevention, accomplished through vaccination, my children and grandchildren need not be afraid. But wait, now they do because since nothing is happening, with respect to these diseases, people are questioning why we invest in prevention of "nothing."

The same risks exist in companies. It is easy to invest in prevention after foodborne illnesses or deaths occur, or a product is recalled, especially when there is loss of brand equity and profits. After a few years without a problem, the budget line items for prevention are questioned. Thankfully, the regulatory agencies and customers keep the heat on.

I struggle with the best way to discuss prevention as a concept, a belief, a culture, if not a "religion." Why a religion, because the very nature of religions is to believe in something you cannot see or prove, but you keep the faith and practice, nonetheless. I also know that real world examples and case studies are the time-tested way to tell a story and to share knowledge. Even more important, these stories integrate the lessons learned into the cognitive processes of those who will listen and believe.

Please join me as we take a walk back in time, turn around, and head back to the present to imagine the future for prevention.

**Building the Future of Food Safety Technology. https://doi.org/10.1016/B978-0-12-818956-6.00007-5**

## A history of prevention

Looking back at the history of an issue is worth the trip. History includes many milestones in the evolution of the prevention mindset. One of the first to focus on prevention, and to write about the pursuit, was Sir John Simon (A.N., 1905). In 1848, the Corporation of the City of London applied to Parliament for funds to appoint a medical officer of health. Sir John Simon was selected for this position at the age of 32. He wrote reports of his observations and opinions, and, by 1854, reprints of his reports gained high demand.

Sir Simon wrote "I have no hesitation in saying that sanitary mismanagement spreads very appreciable evils in the middle ranks of society; and from some of the consequences, so far as I am aware, no station can call itself exempt." He went on to say "The fact is, except against willful violence, life is very little cared for by the law" (A.N., 1905). For 20 years, Sir John Simon worked to address the "sanitary mismanagement" that led to much sickness and the loss of life. He ushered in a more focused approach to prevention.

The organized focus on prevention continued with Dr. Charles-Edward Amory Winslow, MD, who took on the challenge himself. His lectures and papers are arguably some of the most significant illustrations of the foundation of public health prevention philosophy and practice today. Just as his thought process and passion guided the establishment of Yale Department of Public Health within the Yale Medical School in 1915, his writings still guide us today.

Much like the times we live in today with rapid technological breakthroughs in genomics and whole genome sequencing (WGS), he lived in an era of great advances in bacteriology and other fields of science. During his time, he emphasized a broader perspective on causation and adopted a more holistic perspective to public health. Today, we can embrace Dr. Winslow's leadership, ideals, and ideas as a guide to addressing the current challenges of prevention today, specifically the prevention of foodborne illness.

One hundred years ago, on January 2, 1920, Dr. Winslow expressed his views on "The Untilled Fields of Public Health" at a lecture in St. Louis, Missouri. He stated

*Public health is the science and art of preventing disease, prolonging life, and promoting health through the organized efforts for the sanitation of the environment, the control of community infections, the education of the individual in principles of personal hygiene, the organization of medical and nursing service for the early diagnosis and preventative treatment of disease, and the development of the social machinery which will ensure to every individual in the community a standard of living adequate for the maintenance of health*

**Winslow, 1920**

Today, this is still the way forward, the guideposts needed to reduce the ever-present threat of foodborne diseases. We can translate how Dr. Winslow addressed the public health challenges of his day to create a contemporary focus on prevention of foodborne illness through accomplishing the following:

1. **Embrace** the principles of preventing foodborne illness, including the science and art of risk reduction, development and enforcement of regulations, establishment of food safety cultures, and a holistic approach.
2. **Address** hazards and prevention approaches to control pathogens in the agricultural and food production environment to reduce food contamination risk.
3. **Educate** the individual in support of personal, food manufacturing, food processing, transportation, cooking, and handling practices.
4. **Utilize** technology to rapidly detect foodborne illness cases and identify suspect food vehicles to reduce the number of individuals who become ill.
5. **Utilize** technologies and communication to support the rapid and efficient recall of contaminated food.

The world Simon and Winslow tried to change by guiding the principles of prevention has indeed changed in most developed countries. However, in every country, developed or not, threats remain too great to not embrace the prevention culture or "religion." Today, we know food safety threats beyond bacteria, parasites, fungus, and viral risks. The following risks must also be the subject of prevention:

1. Chemical residues such as pesticides, herbicides, fungicides, antibiotics, mycotoxins, and heavy metals
2. Allergens
3. Physical contaminants, such as stones, glass, metal, or hard plastic
4. Zoonotic diseases such as BSE, TB, brucellosis, and avian influenza strains, etc.
5. The emergence of antimicrobial resistance in human and animal pathogens
6. Human behaviors that result in consuming raw foods labeled as intended to be cooked or, in the case of milk, pasteurized
7. Human behaviors that result in feeding raw meat contaminated with pathogenic bacteria to pets.

## Evolution of prevention in the USDA's food safety and inspection service

As we look back, we can see the evolution of the prevention mindset when we think of Upton Sinclair's 1906 novel *The Jungle*. Consistent with the "Law of Unintended Consequences," Sinclair is reported to have written the novel to portray the harsh conditions and exploited lives of immigrants in Chicago and other cities. His primary purpose in describing the meat industry was not to address prevention of foodborne illness but to prevent the harsh working conditions and advance his agenda, socialism (Slotnik, 2016). However, his novel led to the passage of the Meat Inspection Act in 1906 (USDA, 2014).

In 1993, the Jack-In-The-Box *Escherichia coli* O157:H7 tragedy resulted in 732 people being infected. Most of the victims were under 10 years old. Four children died and 178 other victims were left with permanent injuries including kidney and brain damage (Griffin, Tauxe, Swaminathan, and Bell, 2017). Riley Detwiler, only 16-month-old at the time, was among those who died (Detwiler, 2020; New York Times, 1993).

In 1994, resulting directly from the landmark 1993 outbreak, the USDA declared *E. coli* O157:H7 an adulterant in ground beef (Taylor, 1994). In 1996, these events resulted in the passage of comprehensive reform of the 1906 Federal Meat Inspection Act (USDA, 1997). I was actively involved in this effort. In my capacity representing cattle producers, I submitted testimony before Congress and USDA on these matters and submitted written remarks (How Should our Food Safety, 2000; USDA, 2000, p. 145). The reforms included the Hazard Analysis and Critical Control Points (HACCP) approach and required the establishment of microbiological performance criteria. There are seven principles of HACCP:

1. Conduct a Hazard Analysis
2. Identify the Critical Control Points (CCPs)
3. Establish Critical Limits
4. Monitor CCPs
5. Establish Corrective Action
6. Verification
7. Record-keeping

The reform of the Federal Meat Inspection Act, especially the focus on HACCP and application of microbial performance standards, has significantly reduced meat-related foodborne illness, especially related to shiga toxin producing *E. coli* (STEC) strains.

## Evolution in prevention at the Food and Drug Administration

At least 80% of the foods we eat are regulated by the Food and Drug Administration (FDA). As mentioned before, 1906 was a year of dramatic change in the prevention landscape. The first comprehensive federal consumer protection law was the 1906 Pure Food and Drugs Act (Pub.L. 59–384, 34 STAT 768), which prohibited misbranded and adulterated food and drugs in interstate commerce.

Even after passage of the Pure Food and Drug Act, gaps in the prevention safety net were well understood, and as is often the case, there was growing national outrage over some consumer products that poisoned, maimed, and killed many people. This all came to a head in 1937, when an untested pharmaceutical killed many patients, including many children. The enactment of the 1938 Food, Drug, and Cosmetic Act (Pub.L. 75–717, 52 STAT 1040) tightened controls over drugs and food, cosmetics, and medical devices. This law, now amended, is still in force today. In 2011, the comprehensive amendments to the Food Drug and Cosmetic Act was passed by Congress and signed into law by the President. These amendments are known as the FDA Food Safety and Modernization Act (Pub.L. 111–353, 124 STAT 3885).

The regulations promulgated under the Act, guidance to industry, enforcement, and compliance by industry continue to be a work in progress. The rules cover a wide range of food production sectors and actions, including

1. The Hazard Analysis and Risk-Based Preventive Controls Rule for Human and Animal Food
2. Foreign Supplier Verification Rule
3. Standards for Growing, Harvesting, Packing, and Holding Produce for Human Consumption and subpart Sprouts Safety Rule
4. The Sanitary Transport Rule.

Similar to HACCP, the rules include a focus on hazard analysis. However, they diverge into a degree of greater prevention-oriented requirements including

1. Establishment of preventive controls, corrective actions, and preventive actions
2. Development and application of registered scheduled processes and validation of risk reduction steps
3. Environmental monitoring requirements for ready-to-eat food exposed to the environment before packaging potential postprocessing contamination of food
4. Sanitation preventive controls to reduce the potential contamination of food by environmental contaminants and allergen cross-contact
5. Allergen controls and labeling
6. Required worker training and records
7. Required record-keeping for preventive controls
8. Supply chain and foreign supplier verification programs
9. Food defense and intentional adulteration plans
10. Recall plans
11. Sanitary transportation of human and animal food.

The FDA reports that there are more foreign food production firms that export food to the United States than domestic production firms. FSMA has also created a significant number of prevention-oriented requirements on a global scale.

## Challenges in identification of food vehicles early in illness clusters

A critically important and often overlooked prevention tool is the technology and process used to identify human illness quickly and identifying suspect food vehicles before individual illnesses and clusters become an outbreak. The process of interviewing patients with confirmed foodborne illness is a time-consuming process. The time-consuming process of collecting food histories, addressing the challenges of patients' memories regarding what they may have consumed days or weeks earlier, and evaluating probability estimates for potential food vehicles makes identification of suspect food vehicles a challenge. With the advent of genomic technologies and WGS, the process of matching human illness isolates to current or historic product isolates or facility or environmental isolates allows us to shorten the time it takes to identify illness causing foods. The use of WGS and uploading of patient isolates in PulseNet hopefully will increase the speed of identifying suspect food vehicles (Carleton, 2019). The FDA can take no action to recall a product until the evidence is in. Recalling the wrong product has happened in the past, so being wrong has implications to public health (Zhang and Adamy, 2008).

The importance of rapid identification of the contaminated food vehicle is the responsibility of the States and the Centers for Disease Control and Prevention (CDC). The CDC established FoodCORE (Foodborne Diseases Centers for Outbreak Response Enhancement), improving foodborne disease outbreak response capacity in state and local health departments in 2010 (Biggerstaff et al., 2013).

Here are four examples of the time required for the CDC to provide the FDA the necessary information so the FDA can investigate the firms causing the food contamination and potentially require a recall.

### Multistate outbreak of listeriosis linked to Blue Bell Creameries products

This resulted in 10 cases across four states: 10 hospitalizations with three deaths (CDC, 2015). First case was in 2010, two cases in 2011, one case in 2012, five cases in 2014, and one case in 2015. On April 20, 2015, after an ice cream sample tested by South Carolina was found to be contaminated with the strain of *Listeria monocytogenes*, with a matching WGS to patient isolates, the FDA was able to request a recall of all ice cream products. This was a 5-year illness event.

### Multistate outbreak of Salmonella Poona infections linked to imported cucumbers

This resulted in 907 cases across 40 states: 204 hospitalizations with six deaths (CDC, 2016a). The first case was uploaded into PulseNet on July 1, 2015, and the food vehicle was confirmed and FDA initiated a recall 35 days later.

### Multistate outbreak of listeriosis linked to frozen vegetables

This resulted in nine cases across four states: nine hospitalizations with three deaths (CDC, 2016b). The first illness isolate was uploaded into PulseNet in September of 2013. There were five patient WGS isolates uploaded in 2015 and three more in 2016. The last was in May 2016 and the FDA requested the frozen vegetables be recalled on June 2, 2016. These illnesses continued for 22 months before FDA was notified of the confirmed food vehicle.

### Multistate outbreak of shiga toxin-producing *Escherichia coli* O157: H7 infections linked to I.M. Healthy brand SoyNut butter

This resulted in 32 cases across 12 states: 12 hospitalizations with no deaths (CDC, 2017). The first illness isolate linked to this eventual outbreak was uploaded into PulseNet on January 5, 2017. The FDA was informed of the confirmed food vehicle and asked the company to recall all their production on March 3, 2017, 43 days after the first illness.

Clearly, there is a need for the CDC FoodCORE project to reduce the number of days it takes to inform the FDA of an implicated food vehicle. This is currently the most rate-limiting step in the prevention continuum.

## Implications for improved traceability and blockchain as a prevention tool

Those inside and outside of the food industry hear and read a lot about traceability, Blockchain specifically (Detwiler, 2018). If you listen to most of what is said about the technology, you hear things like "more secure," "smarter," or "faster." Think back to what we have discussed here about prevention. The first task in preventing foodborne illness is preventing the food from being contaminated, recontaminated, cooked, or handled improperly. If a food is causing an illness, the next most important task is to quickly identify the food vehicle. Then and only then can FDA engage companies, review records, and request firms to initiate a recall. Recall plans are required under the Preventive Controls Rule for Human and Animal Food (FDA, 2018), and they are examined by the FDA during inspections. Many third-party audit schemes require all products in a mock recall to be found at distribution centers within 2 hours. Large food companies have elaborate records that document where their food originated. Even with all the records and perfect traceability, the implicated product may no longer be on the shelf. This is especially the case with a short shelf life, perishable product. That said, the FDA and the states will always conduct a for-cause inspection at the firms implicated by the outbreak analysis. While enhancing traceability can be helpful, it is not the weak link in the prevention continuum.

## What can case studies tell us about prevention?

Let us look a little deeper into the four illness outbreaks discussed earlier for prevention clues.

### Multistate outbreak of listeriosis linked to Blue Bell Creameries products

The root cause of this outbreak resides in four compartments, including

- Without WGS of patient and product isolates, we probably would never have known this was occurring.

- FDA policy on *L. monocytogenes* (LM) at the time did not view LM in a frozen food like ice cream as a hazard.
- LM environmental contamination at the manufacturing facilities was most likely spread to containers during cleaning and sanitizing operations that spread the pathogens through aerosols.
- The standard of care for immunocompromised patients in hospital was not conservative enough in terms of the foods being consumed in the hospital.

The key to preventing this is elimination of LM in the ice cream production environment.

### Multistate outbreak of Salmonella Poona infections linked to imported cucumbers

- Prior to harvest of the cucumbers in Baja Mexico, they were hit by record rainfall due to a tropical storm. It is likely the cucumbers were contaminated by surface water/soil/splash in the fields or the cucumbers were washed with unsafe water.
- The outbreak continued long after the recall likely due to contaminated reusable plastic containers or retail displays.
- The prevention lesson is about recognizing how weather events represent a risk, as does the quality of surface water, soil conditions, and the potential for contaminated water to contact produce.

### Multistate outbreak of listeriosis linked to frozen vegetables

- This outbreak was the result of LM contaminated postblanching chilling water or environmental LM spread during cleaning to products before they entered a spiral freezer.
- Complicating the issue was the fact consumers were increasingly consuming frozen vegetables, intended to be fully cooked, by adding them to salads and smoothies.

The prevention lesson is elimination of LM from the production environment and for consumers to read and follow cooking instructions.

### Multistate outbreak of shiga toxin-producing *Escherichia coli* O157: H7 infections linked to I.M. Healthy brand SoyNut butter

- This outbreak is one of the most puzzling. We know salmonella is a potential contaminant of peanut butter, but STEC is a new one.
- We know the facility was not cleaning equipment because cleaning is difficult with this type of product.
- The STEC most likely was a postroasting contaminant.

- The prevention lesson is difficult to grasp, other than that processors should consider many different pathogens as a risk. The fact this product was marketed for children amplified the risk.

## Summary

Prevention clearly has always been the most important public health goal. It takes thought, organization, and investment to reduce the risk to the public from human and zoonotic disease or diseases spread through food.

Public health officials, government agencies, and companies end up at risk when the success of their work is countered with questions, at many levels, such as: "Why do we spend so much to achieve nothing?" "Nothing" as in we eradicated measles or polio so why do we need to continue vaccinations? In regulatory agencies and the CDC, it is likely they too can become a victim of their success when funding requests are challenged because Congress or the President does not see an urgent need. Companies face similar pressures when there is no recent evidence of a threat, when there are no recalls, or other issues. The questions begin "Why are we spending so much on prevention or why do we need to carry so much insurance?"

Prevention is not all that difficult, but it can become nearly impossible to convince others to maintain the focus once you have achieved success. That is why food safety culture is a thing and why to some it is a religion. We must never give up investing in prevention, but we must be careful to focus on and invest in the most important things that truly drive prevention.

## References

A.N. (1905). The life work of Sir John Simon. *The Journal of Hygiene, 5*(1), 1—6. Retrieved from www.jstor.org/stable/3858726.

Biggerstaff, et al. (2013, August 8). *FoodCORE (Foodborne Diseases Centers for Outbreak Response Enhancement): Improving foodborne disease outbreak response capacity in state and local health departments, year one summary report*. CDC. Retrieved from https://stacks.cdc.gov/view/cdc/20794.

Carleton, H. (2019, May 23). *Advanced Molecular Detection (AMD)*. "2019: PulseNet laboratories transition to whole genome sequencing.". CDC. Retrieved from https://www.cdc.gov/amd/whats-new/pulsenet-transition.html.

CDC. (2015, June 10). *Multistate outbreak of listeriosis linked to blue Bell creameries products (final update)*. Retrieved from https://www.cdc.gov/listeria/outbreaks/ice-cream-03-15/index.html.

CDC. (2016a). *Multistate outbreak of Salmonella Poona infections linked to imported cucumbers (final update)*. Retrieved from https://www.cdc.gov/salmonella/poona-09-15/index.html.

CDC. (2016b). *Multistate outbreak of listeriosis linked to frozen vegetables (final update)*. Retrieved from https://www.cdc.gov/listeria/outbreaks/frozen-vegetables-05-16/index.html.

CDC. (2017, March 4). *Multistate outbreak of shiga toxin-producing* Escherichia coli *O157: H7 infections linked to I.M. Healthy brand SoyNut butter (final update)*. Retrieved from https://www.cdc.gov/ecoli/2017/o157h7-03-17/index.html.

CDC. (2020, February 3). *Measles cases and outbreaks*. Retrieved from https://www.cdc.gov/measles/cases-outbreaks.html.

Centers for Disease Control and Prevention. (2018, November 5). *Estimates of foodborne illness in the United States*. Retrieved from https://www.cdc.gov/foodborneburden/index.html.

Detwiler, D. (2018, February 27). Blockchain in food safety: One nation's move to increase food safety with Blockchain. *IBM Blockchain Blog*. Retrieved from https://www.ibm.com/blogs/blockchain/2018/02/one-nations-move-to-increase-food-safety-with-blockchain/.

Detwiler, D. (2020). *Food safety: Past, present, and predictions* (1st ed.). Cambridge, MA: Elsevier Academic Press.

FDA. (2018, September 12). *FSMA final rule for preventive controls for animal food*. Retrieved from https://www.fda.gov/food/food-safety-modernization-act-fsma/fsma-final-rule-preventive-controls-animal-food.

Griffin, P., Tauxe, R., Swaminathan, B., & Bell, B. (2017, october 11). *We were there* — E. coli *O157: How deadly burgers made food safer* — *the impact of the 1993* E. coli *O157 outbreak*. CDC. Retrieved from https://www.cdc.gov/od/science/wewerethere/ecoli/index.html.

*"How should our food safety systems address microbial contamination?": Hearing before the Committee on U.S. Senate, Committee on Agriculture, Nutrition, and Forestry, 106th cong. 139.*(2000) (testimony of Gary Weber). Retrieved from https://www.govinfo.gov/content/pkg/CHRG-106shrg71374/html/CHRG-106shrg71374.htm.

IBM. (n.d.). What is blockchain technology?. Retrieved from https://www.ibm.com/blockchain/what-is-blockchain.

Sinclair, U. (1906, February 26). *The jungle*. New York: Doubleday.

Slotnik, D. (2016, June 30). Not forgotten: Upton Sinclair, whose muckraking changed the meat industry. *Obituaries. The New York Times*. Retrieved from https://www.nytimes.com/interactive/projects/cp/obituaries/archives/upton-sinclair-meat-industry.

Taylor, M. (1994, September 24). *Change and opportunity: Harvesting innovation to improve the safety of food*. San Francisco, CA: Speech before the American Meat Institute Annual Convention. Retrieved from https://www.foodsafetynews.com/AMI%20Speech%20September%201994.pdf.

The New York Times. (1993, February 22). *17-Month-old is 3rd child to die of illness linked to tainted meat*. Retrieved from http://www.nytimes.com/1993/02/22/us/17-month-old-is-3d-child-to-die-of-illness-linked-to-tainted-meat.html.

USDA. (1997, September). *Annual report is submitted to the Committee on Agriculture of the U.S. House of Representatives and to the Committee on Agriculture, Nutrition, and Forestry of the U.S. Senate*. Food Safety and Inspection Service. Retrieved from https://www.fsis.usda.gov/wps/wcm/connect/f05cfba9-9906-4443-95eb-841bf8003bb0/rtc96.pdf?MOD=AJPERES.

USDA. (2000, February 29). *Recent developments regarding beef products contaminated with* Escherichia coli *O157:H7*. Food Safety and Inspection Service. Retrieved from https://www.fsis.usda.gov/wps/wcm/connect/30138f4d-710f-4e04-8038-c76fad875dbe/ecolimtg.pdf?MOD=AJPERES.

USDA. (2014, February 21). *Celebrating 100 Years of FMIA*. Retrieved from https://www.fsis.usda.gov/wps/wcm/connect/fsis-content/fsis-questionable-content/celebrating-100-years-of-fmia/overview/ct_index.

*VA Medicinal Cannabis Research Act of 2019, H.R. 712, 116th cong.*(2019).

*Veterans Medical Marijuana Safe Harbor Act, H.R. 1151, 116th cong.*(2019).

Winslow, C. (1920, January 9). The untilled fields of public health. *Science, 51*(1306), 23–33. https://doi.org/10.1126/science.51.1306.23. Retrieved from https://science.sciencemag.org/content/51/1306/23/tab-pdf.

Zhang, J., & Adamy, J. (2008, July 23). Salmonella outbreak exposes food-safety flaws: Lack of preparation and poor records cause delays, errors. *The Wall Street Journal*. Retrieved from https://www.wsj.com/articles/SB121677198766575559.

# Retail Food safety

**Jeremy Zenlea, MBA**

*Head of Food Safety for EG America, Westborough, MA, United States*

Historically, the guiding principle behind a successful retail food establishment ("Retail Food") was the ability to sell goods at a price that was attractive to both the purveyor's profit margin and the consumer's wallet. For the purposes of this section, **Retail Food** refers to any entity that is permitted as a food establishment and engages in the sale of fresh and/or prepared food directly to the end consumer (i.e., grocery, convenience, food service, quick service restaurants). Because of this, many of the food-related technologies created for the retail market focused primarily on profitability and efficiency and *not* on quality and food safety. This principle reigned for many years, until the value proposition of food items was altered with the advent of the Internet and popularization of e-commerce and social media.

Now, unlike any other time in history, the consumer has the ability to access a wide variety of purchasing avenues for a particular food item, instead just being limited to purchasing it at their local brick and mortar retailer. With greater choice comes greater competition, leading many of the largest Retail Food companies to differentiate themselves by redefining the word *value* to include quality and food safety in addition to price. The modern consumer's decision to purchase an item from a specific retailer is not only influenced by price but it is also influenced by brand integrity. **Brand integrity** refers to the ability of a brand or company's products, reputation, and image to influence their consumer's perception and ultimately their purchasing decision.

In the Retail Food market, brand integrity has a direct, positive correlation with food quality and safety as both can now be easily evaluated via consumer reviews, blogs, apps, and social media. Therefore, a need has arisen in the Retail Food market for corporate and store-level technologies that focus on prediction, prevention, and reaction. Retail Food now needs to predict when, where, and why, and how a significant food safety event will occur, what preventative measures, once predicted, to take, and how to best react in a way that minimizes the impact to the consumer and brand integrity.

**Building the Future of Food Safety Technology. https://doi.org/10.1016/B978-0-12-818956-6.00008-7**

## Gold standard of Retail Food safety technology

The ability to turnover inventory quickly in the Retail Food industry means that food offerings and their components have to move through the supply chain and into the consumer's hands at breakneck speeds. The consumer's ever growing want for fresh, short coded foods has further sped up the consumption process. A fresh sandwich can have as little as a 4-day shelf life, thus, to maximize delivered shelf life, the sandwich flows from a commissary to a distribution center to a store within 24 h. The fresh sandwich then is purchased and typically eaten by a consumer within 72 h. Because of this, **recalls** in Retail Food are only as good as the speed to which they can be issued and are often not very effective in preventing consumers from purchasing and eating the recalled product. Consequently, recalls in Retail Food are solely a reactive measure as they do little good in protecting the consumer, thus food safety technology must focus on prevention and more importantly prediction.

This brings us to the gold standard of Retail Food safety technology, a program that has the ability to take large amounts of data from existing data streams, compile it all together, and make a risk profile. Using a risk profile, the firm can assign a grade or score to each of its locations that denotes the likelihood of a significant food safety event. To illustrate how this can be achieved, we are going to create a risk profile for a fake Retail Food firm named Zenlea's Food Market (ZFM). ZFM is a chain of food establishments that offer made-to-order, heat-to-order, and grab-and-go fresh prepackaged foods made in the firm's commissary.

1. **Existing Data Streams**: The integrity of a risk profile and its ability to be used to predict significant food safety events depends on the information being fed into it. The data points incorporated into the risk profile are foundational and consequently need to be carefully chosen. The level of difficulty to achieve this task relies on which data streams already exist within an organization and which do not. In the modern Retail Food company, most operations, i.e., communications, marketing, sales, and inventory data, are already transmitted in real time from a remote location, received, and stored on the firm's servers or in the cloud. Because of this, all of these data are accessible to anyone, provided they have been given sufficient access rights, within the company. The challenge is to decide which of the existing data streams can be pieced together like pages in a book to tell a story of a given location.

   Upon analyzing all of the different existing data streams available, ZFM decided to focus on those that relate to public health both directly and indirectly. ZFM decided to utilize the following data streams: consumer complaints, health inspection scores, sanitation chemical usage rates, potable water temperatures, display case temperatures, cooking temperatures, storage room temperatures, and number of employee reportable illnesses per location. Furthermore, ZFM verified that each of these data streams are continuously and accurately collected from each location.

2. **Nonexisting Data Streams**: The firm may decide that the existing data streams available to them are not enough to create an accurate risk profile. For instance, if ZFM wants to better assess handwashing practices at store level, they may install Wi-Fi-connected handwashing equipment that can transmit data from each handwashing station. This may be done by tracking the number of uses of a hand soap dispenser or how many times an employee uses a handwashing sink by installing a badge reader or keypad at each handwashing station. Of course, anytime a new data stream is introduced at the store level, it will take time to collect enough data and verify the accuracy of the data in order for it to become valuable. This amount of time is heavily dependent upon gaining buy-in from store personnel and can be shortened by utilizing sufficient training, clearly outlining accountability and even setting up incentive programs to drive adoption. It can be understood that setting up nonexisting data streams will take time, money, and effort some more than others depending on if the data stream is supported by new or existing technology and other factors. Thus, it is important that a Retail Food firm must first utilize their existing data streams to build the initial risk profile and then decide which nonexisting data streams need to be executed to strengthen each store's risk profile. Considering nonexistent data streams during the discovery process of the overall project of creating a risk profile can be helpful; however, trying to actually implement them right away will add unnecessary complexity and significantly impede the launch of the final product.

3. **Data Stream Enhancements**: While there are many existing data streams that may be useful for determining a Retail Food location's risk profile, some may need to be enhanced in order to pull out specific food safety-related information. ZFM decides that its risk profiles are missing crucial data—consumer feedback. Consumer feedback comes in many forms, with the two most prominent being consumer complaints and social media posts. Unfortunately, consumer complaints and social media posts can be about a wide array of topics, from a consumer treated unfairly by an employee to a consumer suggesting a new product idea. Thus, the challenge is how to sift through large amounts of information and pick out that which is only pertinent to food safety. Existing Retail Food firms have met this challenge by developing software that uses new-age technologies like artificial intelligence to search and identify certain keywords within consumer feedback. This approach is exciting and will eventually result in a meaningful data stream, but it may be unattainable for the average Retail Food firm, as its development and maintenance requires resources that may not be available. ZFM decides to take a different, less costly approach and decides to focus on capturing data from consumer complaints, which are already documented in the firm's customer relationship management system. The firm's customer relationship management system already has the ability to capture detailed descriptions of a complaint and categorize it by store location, weather, and even time of day. ZFM decides to add a food safety category that is broken up into associated subcategories, such as foreign objects, pests, missing label information (many Retail Food stores print their own labels on site),

allergic reactions, and health/wellness. ZFM can then create a data stream from the CRM using the food safety category and recorded store location.

4. **Weighted Significance**: Not all of the data streams that are being integrated into a Retail Food store's risk profile are equal in terms of their effect on overall risk. Therefore, each stream must be assigned a weight; the data streams that have a more significant impact on overall risk will carry more weight than those that may have more of a marginal impact. ZFM determined that a data stream from the results of a third-party food safety audit may be more demonstrative of risk than that from a sanitation chemical dispenser as the audit score gives a more holistic overview of food safety at a Retail Food store.

Creating and utilizing risk profiles of Retail Food store locations is one example of the many ways that the future of food safety technology can have a real, meaningful impact on Retail Food. The ability for a Retail Food firm to use predictive analytics to forecast a significant food safety event, such as an outbreak or recall, before it occurs will enable the firm to put additional preventive measures and assets in place at locations where they are most needed, which will ultimately protect public health.

Unfortunately, developing technology that has the ability to make predictions is not scalable industry wide. The amount of data streams and the effort involved in creating and maintaining those data streams that are necessary to generate accurate future insights makes the implementation of such a program capital and resource intensive. For the larger Retail Food firms, this may be attainable, but this is unattainable for medium-sized and smaller firms who may be capital and resource deficient. Due to the immense promise of predictive technology to protect public health, not making such technology accessible to medium-sized and smaller Retail Food firms puts their consumers at a disadvantage.

## Store-level food safety technology

Given the complexity of a Retail Food operation, in order to fully understand the technological needs of Retail Food, it is important to break down the operation into three main categories: internal supply chain, external supply chain, and store-level supply chain. The internal supply chain includes company-owned warehousing, transportation, and commissary operations. The external supply chain consists of comanufactures, third-party logistics, private label suppliers, contract warehouses, and any other entity that is not company owned. Finally, store-level supply chain is just as the name of the category implies, it encompasses anything that affects food safety at store level, such as cleaning/sanitation, good retail practices, food preparation, storage, etc. For the purpose of this discussion, we will only focus on store-level food safety.

Many food safety technologies available on the marketplace are not really technologies at all in that they do not offer any real benefits that actually decrease the likelihood of a significant food safety event. Instead, they are mostly expensive and glorified document depositories that largely depend on the end user and their supply chain partners to determine how truly effective they are. Furthermore, food safety technologies, like tech-enabled traceability programs such as Blockchain, work well to augment areas of a business that previously rely on technology and automation. Software programs that assist companies with collecting and maintaining supplier food safety compliance documentation works well because they merely automate preexisting Internet-based communication. Technology-based traceability and recall systems work mostly by enhancing cloud based, preexisting warehouse management systems. While these types of food safety technology work well within the internal and external supply chain, they fail to add value to store-level food safety.

The challenge with store-level food safety is that most of the preventative processes that if not done correctly will have a negative effect on food safety executed by a human being and not by a computer or piece of sophisticated machinery. For instance, one of the programs in Food Retail that focuses on prevention is cleaning and sanitation. Most of the cleaning and sanitation technologies existing in the marketplace are usually expensive and focus on making a cleaning and sanitation task quicker and easier to perform and not necessarily on improving food safety. Correctly mopping a floor seems to be a benign and menial task, however, doing it correctly will considerably protect the spread of filth and foodborne illness. The average mopping program requires a mop, a mop bucket, and some variety of chemical-water mix depending on where the mop is being used, i.e., bathroom versus the sales floor. The task is time consuming and sometimes physically uncomfortable for the person who is performing it. As a result, many Retail Food companies have implemented automatic floor scrubber machines as they promise to make the task more effective and efficient. However, while this technology marketed as a piece of food safety technology it certainly is not. In fact, because of the size of the machines, they cannot clean hard to reach areas, and without proper care and maintenance, the automatic floor scrubbing machines can rapidly spread filth and bacteria throughout a Retail Food store in a matter of minutes.

To improve food safety at store level, the industry needs technology that focuses on simple improvements or automation of the factors that/ contribute to one's inability to effectively perform a manual task. The primary factors that contribute to someone not mopping a floor correctly are lacking training, insufficient equipment, a confusing Sanitation Standard Operating Procedure (SSOP), and inadequate chemical dilutions. It is important to note that all different types of people of all ages with differing levels of education will at one point be mopping the floor, so the technology desired must enable a high school senior with a couple of weeks experience to carry out the task just as effectively as the store manager with many years of experience. A fascinating method of controlling the primary factors via the use of technology that contribute to someone not mopping a floor correctly is by incorporating augmented reality (AR) into the task.

AR's ability to enhance a real-world environment by computer-generated perception information makes it a perfect technology to improve mopping a floor and any other manually driven store-level food safety-related task. A store employee can put on a pair of safety glasses with integrated AR that will guide them through all parts of the task. The employee will be shown how to properly dilute the floor cleaner and which equipment to use (and how to tell if that equipment is in good shape) and will be taken through the SSOP all while they are actually mopping the floor. AR technology may also be used to promote good retail practices, like superimposing a timer onto a hand wash sink to help an employee wash their hands for the proper amount of time or providing graphics of proper thermometer probe placement when taking the temperatures of foods that need time and temperature control for safety.

Most importantly, the use of AR will undoubtedly make a boring task such as mopping the floor more interesting and enjoyable to do for any type of employee, and the more enjoyable a task is to carry out, the more eager an employee will be to do it well. Along with the discussed possibilities of AR in the Retail Food environment, the technology may be an easily justifiable investment due to its ability to support any operational task, such as taking physical inventory, merchandising, or employing new planograms, and not just those that are food safety and/or quality related.

Store-level food safety technology that is currently available on the market has a long way to go before it can be realistically adopted into the Retail Food industry. Most are hard to justify the investment as they are either too focused on refining one particular task or have proven only to be marginal at best at improving a task when compared to the existing equipment, tools, or procedures available. The challenge remains that no two Retail Food locations are exactly the same. They may have different layouts, capabilities, and storage criteria. Therefore, all technological solutions must be customized to each location, making implementation costly in terms of both capital expenditure and the expenditure of internal resources.

The future of food safety technology has a lot of promise for the Retail Food industry, and the Retail Food industry is in need for better food safety technology. However, it is up to the industry itself to collaborate and voice their technological gaps and needs. Food safety is not a competitive advantage, as modern consumers tend to attribute risk factors to a whole industry rather than just a particular location or brand.

Many of us have heard a friend or family member proclaim something like *"I saw a tweet that someone got sick after eating a salad from fast food restaurant A, so I'm never eating fast food again!"* Retail Food also needs to work with their industry partners, such as developers, trade organizations, and/or the government, to make food safety technology less cost prohibitive and more accessible to all Retail Food organizations, regardless of their size. For instance, food safety-related data streams needed to create risk profiles that may be incorporated into predictive analytical software can be made more widely available by the industry if companies are willing to share their data. Data can be easily masked so that the data are kept highly confidential and formatted in a way that makes it impossible to determine the origin of that data. With data streams being more widely available, Retail Food companies will no longer have to invest in developing data streams themselves. This will remove a major barrier to the adoption of predictive analytical software for medium-sized and smaller Retail Food companies-as technology companies will now have the ability to offer lower cost, out-of-the box solutions for a complicated, but invaluable, piece of food safety technology.

In Retail Food, the consumer is what enables our existence and allows us to be successful, thus it is the job of the industry as a whole to keep creating ways to further protect the consumer. In that sense, the incorporation of robust food safety technologies into Retail Food is essential for the long-term survival of the industry.

# Cannabis-derived food products in the New Era of Smarter Food Safety

**Adam Friedlander, MS**

*Manager, Food Safety and Technical Services, FMI, Washington, D.C., United States*

## Introduction

*Cannabis sativa* L. (hereinafter referred to as "cannabis") is a flowering plant species within the Cannabaceae family that can produce "hemp" or "marihuana." Throughout American history, hemp was cultivated to produce a variety of goods and services for industrial and horticultural industries (7 CFR Part 990). In 1970, the federal government prohibited the cultivation, distribution, and possession of cannabis and cannabis-derived products, such as hemp and marihuana (Pub. L. No. 91-513). In 2018, hemp's federal restrictions were lifted under the 2018 Farm Bill, but marihuana and hemp-derived compounds, such as cannabidiol (CBD), remain illegal when used in food (FDA, 2020b).

Cannabis plants are known to have over 100 phytocannabinoids compounds, which contain then predominate chemical compounds, delta-9-tetrahydrocannabinol ($\Delta^9$-THC) and CBD (Thomas and ElSohly, 2015). In female cannabis flowers, $\Delta^9$-THC is the foremost psychoactive chemical causing intoxicating and euphoric effects (known as a "high") and is approved to treat specific medical conditions (NIDA, 2019; FDA, 2020b). CBD is a nonpsychoactive chemical that does not produce a "high" but is also approved to treat specific medical conditions (WHO, 2017; FDA, 2020b).

Marihuana, by far, is the most used illicit drug in the United States. Nearly 125 million American adults have reported using cannabis in their lifetime, and 40 million adults have reported using cannabis within the past year (SAMHSA, 2019). The Federal Bureau of Investigations released 2018 data that showed approximately 610,000 Americans were incarcerated for illegally possessing cannabis and approximately 53,000 Americans were incarcerated for illegally selling or manufacturing cannabis (FBI, 2020). Put another way, out of all 2018 cannabis incarcerations (which comprised 40% of total U.S. drug arrests), 92% resulted from illegal possession and 8% resulted from illegal sale or manufacturing (FBI, 2020).

Despite the drug's illicit federal classification, numerous state and local jurisdictions have decriminalized or legalized cannabis for personal or medical use. In a recent Pew Research Center survey, approximately 66% of American adults support federal decriminalization or legalization of cannabis (Daniller, 2019). Currently, 33

**Building the Future of Food Safety Technology. https://doi.org/10.1016/B978-0-12-818956-6.00009-9**

states, the District of Columbia, Puerto Rico, Guam and the US Virgin Islands have enacted medical cannabis legislation, and 11 states and the District of Columbia have legalized cannabis use for recreational purposes (NCSL, 2019a, 2019b). Each regulatory and enforcement official, whether federal, state, or local, aims to protect the public health and well-being of all citizens and to ensure all stakeholders comply with pertinent jurisdiction requirements.

This chapter will examine the potential modernization of cannabis in federal statutes and marketplaces and envision the role that citizens, patients, consumers, industry, and regulatory officials have in shaping industry frameworks throughout the next decade and beyond.

## How the classification of cannabis impacts congressional and executive branch actions

Growing interest in the cannabis food marketplace requires significant collaborative efforts to safeguard public health and to ensure compliance with all applicable regulatory requirements. This section aims to identify key regulatory, legal, and political frameworks to enhance understanding of where cannabis and cannabis-derived products belong in federal marketplaces.

Cannabis is classified as a highly restricted Schedule I substance under the **Federal Comprehensive Drug Abuse Prevention and Control Act of 1970** (Pub.L. 91−513), also known as the Controlled Substance Act (CSA). All persons in the United States are prohibited from cultivating, distributing, and possessing cannabis (21 U.S.C. § 801 et seq.). This act, signed by President Richard Nixon, grants the Drug Enforcement Administration (DEA)-an agency within the Department of Justice (DOJ)-authority to enforce controlled substance laws in the country.

The CSA organizes all drugs, substances or other chemicals into five schedules, based upon their acceptable medical use, potential for abuse and potential for dependency (21 U.S.C. § 801). As a Schedule I substance, cannabis is classified as having (1) no acceptable medical use; (2) a high potential for abuse; and (3) a high potential for dependency. Other examples of Schedule I substances include heroin, lysergic acid diethylamide, and psilocybin ("magic mushrooms").

To add, reclassify, or remove drugs from this list, Congress or the Executive Branch must act. Below are examples of recent Congressional and DOJ actions that aim to guide food businesses in providing consumer protections.

The Agricultural Improvement Act of 2018 (Pub.L. 115-334), also known as the 2018 Farm Bill (7 CFR Part 990), removed hemp and hemp derivatives from the list of controlled substances under the CSA. With strong support from US Senate Majority Leader Mitch McConnell (R-KY) and US Senate Minority Leader Charles Schumer (D-NY), President Donald Trump enacted S. 2667, the 2018 Farm Bill, into law on December 20, 2018. This bill redefined hemp as

*Cannabis sativa* L. *and any part of that plant, including the seeds thereof and all derivatives, extracts, cannabinoids, isomers, acids, salts, and salts of isomers, whether growing or not, with a delta-9 tetrahydrocannabinol concentration of not more than 0.3% on a dry weight basis*

This significant development legalized the production and commercialization of hemp and hemp derivatives, including CBD, which has subsequently generated immense consumer interest in recent years (FMI, 2019). While the **US Department of Agriculture** (USDA) was granted authority to regulate hemp cultivation, the Farm Bill explicitly preserved the US Food and Drug Administration's (FDA's) authority over FDA-regulated products, including food, drugs, dietary supplements, and cosmetics (FDA, 2020a). Furthermore, all food products that contain, or claim to contain, CBD or $\Delta^9$-THC-and are derived from the *C. sativa* L. plant with more than 0.3% $\Delta^9$-THC-are considered marihuana (a controlled substance) and thus are not permitted in interstate marketplaces (FDA, 2020b).

The **116th Congress** (2019–20) introduced numerous bills to amend current US law surrounding cannabis enforcement. These bills include

- **Marijuana Opportunity, Reinvestment, and Expungement Act** (H.R. 3884/S. 2227): Rep. Jerrold Nadler (D-NY) and Sen. Kamala Harris (D-CA) introduced this bill to "decriminalize and deschedule cannabis, to provide for reinvestment in certain persons adversely impacted by the War on Drugs, to provide for expungement of certain cannabis offenses, and for other purposes." This bill also seeks to strike the word "Marihuana" or "Marijuana" from all federal statutes and replace it with the word "Cannabis." Neither the House of Representatives nor the Senate has voted on this bill.
- **Marijuana Justice Act of 2019** (H.R. 1456/S. 597): Rep. Barbara Lee (D-CA) and Sen. Cory Booker (D-NJ) introduced this bill to "amend the Controlled Substances Act to provide for a new rule regarding the application of the Act to marihuana, and for other purposes." Neither the House of Representatives nor the Senate has voted on this bill.
- **Veterans Medical Marijuana Safe Harbor Act** (H.R. 1151/S. 445): Rep. Barbara Lee (D-CA) and Sen. Brian Schatz (D-NH) introduced this bill to "allow veterans to use, possess, or transport medical marijuana and to discuss the use of medical marijuana with a physician of the Department of Veterans Affairs as authorized by a State or Indian Tribe, and for other purposes." Neither the House of Representatives nor the Senate has voted on this bill.
- **VA Medicinal Cannabis Research Act of 2019** (H.R. 712/S. 179): Rep. Luis Correa (D-CA) and Sen. Jon Tester (D-MT) introduced this bill to "direct the Secretary of Veterans Affairs to carry out a clinical trial of the effects of cannabis on certain health outcomes of adults with chronic pain and post-traumatic stress disorder, and for other purposes." Neither the House of Representatives nor the Senate has voted on this bill.

- **Ending Federal Marijuana Prohibition Act of 2019** (H.R. 1588): Rep. Tulsi Gabbard (D-HI) introduced this bill to "limit the application of Federal laws to the distribution and consumption of marihuana, and for other purposes." The House of Representatives has not voted on this bill and the Senate has not introduced this bill.
- **Secure and Fair Enforcement Banking Act of 2019** (H.R. 1595/S. 1200): Rep. Ed Perlmutter (D-CO) and Sen. Jeff Merkley (D-OR) introduced this bill to "create protections for depository institutions that provide financial services to cannabis-related legitimate businesses and service providers for such businesses, and for other purposes." This legislation passed in the House of Representatives on September 25, 2019, with a roll call vote of 321-103. The Senate has not voted on this bill.
- **To amend the Federal Food, Drug, and Cosmetic Act with respect to the regulation of hemp-derived cannabidiol and hemp-derived cannabidiol containing substances** (H.R. 5587): Rep. Collin Peterson (D-MN) introduced this bill to "amend the Federal Food, Drug, and Cosmetic Act with respect to the regulation of hemp-derived cannabidiol and hemp-derived cannabidiol containing substances." The House of Representatives has not voted on this bill and the Senate has not introduced this bill.

**The Attorney General of the United States** has authority to add, reclassify, or remove drugs or substances from the CSA list (21 U.S.C. §811). This Executive Branch official shall consider the following:

1. Its actual or relative potential for abuse.
2. Scientific evidence of its pharmacological effect, if known.
3. The state of current scientific knowledge regarding the drug or other substance.
4. Its history and current pattern of abuse.
5. The scope, duration, and significance of abuse.
6. What, if any, risk there is to the public health.
7. Its psychic or physiological dependence liability.
8. Whether the substance is an immediate precursor of a substance already controlled under this title.

President Barack Obama's Justice Department generally used enforcement discretion for state or local jurisdictions that legalized cannabis for personal or medical use, except for specific criminal instances (DOJ, 2013). On August 29, 2013, Deputy Attorney General James Cole released a memorandum for all US attorney's that discussed enforcement priorities, which stated

*In jurisdictions that have enacted laws legalizing marijuana in some form and that have also implemented strong and effective regulatory and enforcement systems to control the cultivation, distribution, sale, and possession of marijuana, conduct in compliance with those laws and regulations is less likely to threaten the federal priorities [set forth above].*

President Trump's Justice Department reversed this policy (DOJ, 2018). On January 4, 2018, Attorney General Jeff Sessions released a memorandum for all US attorneys that discussed enforcement priorities, which stated

> *Given the Department's well-established general principles, previous nationwide guidance specific to marijuana enforcement is unnecessary and is rescinded, effective immediately.*

## Why cannabis is currently prohibited in food

As the Legislative Branch and Executive Branch consider possible changes to cannabis' status under federal statutes, it is critical to recognize that these actions do not necessarily legalize the use of cannabis or cannabis-derived products in the nation's food supply.

The **US FDA**-an agency within the Department of Health and Human Services— works to ensure food, drug, cosmetic, medical device, and dietary supplement products that enter instate commerce are safe as intended for human and animal use (FDA, 2020b). The FDA's authority derives from the **US Food, Drug, and Cosmetic (FD&C) Act of 1938** (Pub.L. 75−717), an act signed by President Franklin Roosevelt, to grant the agency authority in protecting consumers from deleterious food, drug, or cosmetic products.

As noted previously, while the 2018 Farm Bill removed hemp and hemp derivatives from the CSA, the FDA's authority to protect public health and enforce federal statutes was preserved in the Farm Bill, specifically Section 351 of the **Public Health Services Act** under the FD&C Act, governing biological product licenses (FDA, 2020a). In other words, cannabis and hemp products are still subject to the same authorities and requirements as other FDA-regulated products, regardless of classification under the CSA (FDA, 2020a).

Under Section 505 of the FD&C Act, the FDA has authority to approve new drugs for introduction into interstate commerce (21 U.S.C.§ 355). To date, the FDA has approved one "cannabis-derived" and three "cannabis-related" drugs, which contain CBD and $\Delta^9$-THC, respectively. These drugs include (Schedule V), Syndros (Schedule II), Cesamet (Schedule II), and Marinol (Schedule III) (FDA, 2020a). The FDA explains

> *FDA has approved Epidiolex, which contains a purified form of the drug substance CBD for the treatment of seizures associated with Lennox-Gastaut syndrome or Dravet syndrome in patients 2 years of age and older. That means FDA has concluded that this particular drug product is safe and effective for its intended use … The agency also has approved Marinol and Syndros for therapeutic uses in the United States, including for the treatment of anorexia associated with weight loss in AIDS patients. Marinol and Syndros include the active ingredient dronabinol, a synthetic delta-9-tetrahydrocannabinol which is considered the psychoactive component of cannabis. Another FDA-approved drug,*

*Cesamet, contains the active ingredient nabilone, which has a chemical structure similar to THC and is synthetically derived. Cesamet, like dronabinol-containing products, is indicated for nausea associated with cancer chemotherapy.*

While FDA-approved cannabis drugs may be administered by registered physicians and prescribed to their patients, all other food, drug, cosmetic, or dietary supplements that contain CBD or $\Delta^9$-THC compounds remain subject to FDA authority. According to the FDA,

*Under section 301(ll) of the FD&C Act [21 U.S.C. § 331(ll)], it is prohibited to introduce or deliver for introduction into interstate commerce any food (including any animal food or feed) to which has been added a substance which is an active ingredient in a drug product that has been approved under section 505 of the FD&C Act [21 U.S.C. § 355], or a drug for which substantial clinical investigations have been instituted and for which the existence of such investigations has been made public.*

As far as the federal government is concerned, industry stakeholders may only introduce cannabis food products into interstate commerce, permitted under Section 301(ll) of the FD&C Act, under two conditions. First, FDA could commence notice and comment rulemaking, as directed under the **Administrative Procedure Act** (5 U.S.C. Subchapter II), to establish a pathway forward to cannabis and cannabis-derived products. Second, the FDA may allow these products into market if the "article was marketed in food before the drug was approved or before the substantial clinical investigations involving the drug had been authorized" (FDA, 2020a). According to the agency, regarding the latter condition, "no available evidence" could assert cannabis-derived compounds were used in food before clinical investigations began, thus prohibiting the introduction of cannabis and cannabis-containing foods or supplements into interstate commerce (FDA, 2020a). However, FDA, in the future, may still introduce notice and comment rulemaking to define a regulatory pathway for the lawful marketing of cannabis-derived food and dietary supplement products (FDA, 2020a). As stated by then FDA Commissioner Scott Gottlieb, MD, "the FDA may also provide potential regulatory pathways for products containing cannabis and cannabis-derived compounds [into interstate commerce]" (FDA, 2019c).

On May 31, 2019, the FDA hosted a public meeting on **Scientific Data and Information about Products Containing Cannabis or Cannabis-Derived Compounds**. This meeting sought to inform the agency of current scientific data knowledge or gaps within the research community to establish a possible regulatory pathway for cannabis or cannabis-derived food products, with an emphasis on CBD (FDA, 2019d). More than 4000 comments were submitted into the public docket by July 16, 2019, and the FDA reviewed each comment (FDA, 2020a). Many of the comments at this public meeting centered around health and safety risks, manufacturing and product quality, and marketing, labeling, and sales risks (FDA, 2020a). In a later agency notice, the FDA identified missing data elements, which restricted the agency from establishing a clear regulatory pathway forward, including

- Safety of CBD for uses other than the FDA-approved drug.
- Use by vulnerable populations, such as pregnant/nursing women, children, adolescents, elderly, etc.
- Cumulative exposure/appropriateness of safe threshold levels.
- Appropriate labeling.

Until data can establish the safety of cannabis in the food supply, the FDA may use its authority to remove cannabis products from the market. Since 2015, the FDA has sent dozens of warning letters to a variety of firms that were unlawfully marketing "unapproved new drugs" and also making "unsubstantiated therapeutic or disease claims" (FDA, 2019b). The agency has also sent warning letters to firms that were committing fraud by marketing products claiming to contain specific amounts of CBD when subsequent testing revealed these levels to be false (FDA, 2019b).

Shortly following that public meeting, on July 25, 2019, the Senate Committee on Agriculture, Nutrition, and Forestry held a related hearing on **Hemp Production and the 2018 Farm Bill**, where USDA and FDA officials, as well as industry stakeholders, testified. Peter Matz, Director, Food and Health Policy, on behalf of FMI, submitted for the Congressional record:

*FMI respectfully requests both USDA and FDA to move expeditiously to provide additional clarity and establish a pathway forward for the growth, distribution, sale and use of hemp-derived ingredients in regulated products. The safety concerns and marketplace confusion surrounding hemp and hemp-derived products will continue until guidance is provided governing the production, sale, quality and marketing of these products. Therefore, we urge USDA to develop a hemp production framework and FDA to develop thoughtful guidance around the sale of products containing hemp-derivatives, in order to meet consumer expectations and demands while also ensuring the safe marketing of these products for appropriate intended uses. This guidance would also be a tool to help facilitate consistent enforcement and oversight. More specifically, clarity regarding the saleability, labeling and quality standards for these products would promote consistency in enforcement regardless of the distribution channel through which these products are marketed.*

To establish a modern and legal pathway for cannabis-derived food products, industry stakeholders must work with regulatory partners to ensure compliance with all applicable local, state, and federal requirements (i.e., DOJ, USDA, FDA, etc.), while preparing to build the future of food safety for the global supply chain.

## Building the future of cannabis food safety

Alongside regulatory and legislative partners, the food industry has a duty to protect consumer health. Yet, each year, a suspected 48 million Americans are sickened, 118,000 are hospitalized, and 3000 die from foodborne illness (CDC, 2018). While young children, the elderly, and persons with weakened immune systems are most susceptible to illness, all consumers risk the possibility of eating products with harmful biological, chemical, or physical agents (CDC, 2018). Although significant progress was made in the previous 2010 decade to improve food safety, industry professionals will continue to face novel and emerging food safety threats throughout the new decade. As the food industry enters the 2020s, technology, data management, and collaboration will become increasingly critical to ensure all food products remain safe for human consumption, including for cannabis-derived food products.

On April 30, 2019, then Acting FDA Commissioner Dr. Ned Sharpless and Deputy Commissioner Frank Yiannas proposed a conceptual regulatory framework, entitled the "**New Era of Smarter Food Safety,**" to more effectively utilize technology and human resources that build a "more digital, traceable, and safer food system" (FDA, 2019a). Through a series of public meetings, public comments, and educational campaigns, the agency provided industry stakeholders numerous opportunities to guide FDA in drafting guidance for the upcoming decade that builds upon the **FDA Food Safety Modernization Act** ("FSMA") **of 2011** (Pub.L. 111−353, 124 STAT 3885), a significant law enacted by President Obama to prevent product contamination and reduce foodborne illness (FDA, 2017). Unlike FSMA, the FDA's "New Era of Smarter Food Safety" aims to focus on response and prediction by engaging all food industry stakeholders in four key categories (FDA, 2020a):

- Tech-Enabled Traceability and Foodborne Outbreak Response.
- Smarter Tools and Approaches for Prevention.
- Adapting to New Business Models and Retail Food Safety Modernization.
- Food Safety Culture.

To be successful, food safety professionals must apply equivalent efforts in safeguarding cannabis-derived food products as they would do for any other agricultural commodity. Therefore, gaining expertise in each of the FDA's "New Era of Smarter Food Safety" categories will require significant work by all consumers, food businesses, and food regulators throughout the 2020 decade. Utilizing **whole genome sequencing** data may enhance traceability efforts during outbreak investigations by more rapidly and accurately identifying potentially contaminated food products and linking genetically similar environmental data with clinical data (Friedlander, 2017). Developing practical and cost-effective **artificial intelligence** and **machine learning** capabilities may provide meaningful food safety data for industry stakeholders to predict high-risk CCPs (Friedlander and Zoellner, 2020). Promoting consistent adoption of the model **FDA Food Code** may help modernize the evolving food retail industry by standardizing inspections and food safety training (FDA, 2019E). Finally, fostering nationwide food safety culture will require strategic **consumer food safety education** campaigns to highlight the importance of safe, at-home, food handling practices (PFSE, 2019) (Hint: Clean, Separate, Cook, and Chill!).

Considering the vital role food safety plays in the global supply chain, food safety professionals may be called upon to develop inclusive and science-based strategies that can help raise cannabis food safety standards if, and when, the federal government begins to regulate these products as food. Throughout the next decade, the Institute of Food Technologists, Association of Food and Drug Officials, International Association for Food Protection, and a variety of other professional organizations will continue to play a significant role in educating and inspiring the next generation of cannabis food safety professionals. While more data are needed before the federal government can determine how to move forward, cultivating strong food safety leadership across the supply chain and constructing an interoperable database system to enhance traceability can help pave a meaningful path forward to lawfully market cannabis-derived food products in the United States.

## Disclaimer

The views and opinions expressed in this chapter are those of the author.

## References

*Administrative Procedure Act, 5 U.S.C. Subchapter II..*(2017).

*Agricultural Improvement Act of 2018, Pub. L. No. 115-334. 7 CFR Part 990.*(2018).

*Comprehensive Drug Abuse Prevention and Control Act of 1970, Pub. L. No. 91-513.*(2018).

*Controlled Substance Act of 1970, 21 U.S.C. §801.*(2018).

*Controlled Substance Act of 1970, 21 U.S.C. §811.*(2018).

Daniller, A. (2019, November 14). *Two-thirds of Americans support marijuana legalization.* Retrieved from https://www.pewresearch.org/fact-tank/2019/11/14/americans-support-marijuana-legalization/.

*Ending Federal Marijuana Prohibition Act of 2019, H.R. 1588, 116th cong..*(2016).

Farm Bill, S. (2018). *2667, 115th cong.*

Federal Bureau of Investigation. (2020). *2018 crime in the United States.* Retrieved from https://ucr.fbi.gov/crime-in-the-u.s/2018/crime-in-the-u.s.-2018/topic-pages/persons-arrested.

FMI. (2019, May 31). *FDA public hearing about products containing cannabis or cannabis-derived compounds; public comment.* Retrieved from https://www.fmi.org/docs/default-source/regulatory/fmi-comment——fda-cannabis-public-hearing-5-31-19.pdf?sfvrsn=159d576e_0.

*Food, Drug, and Cosmetic Act of 1938, 21 U.S. Code § 355.*(2011).

Friedlander, A. (2017, June 6). *The new food safety testing gold standard: Whole genome sequencing.* Retrieved from https://www.fmi.org/blog/view/fmi-blog/2017/06/06/the-new-food-safety-testing-gold-standard-whole-genome-sequencing.

Friedlander, A., & Zoellner, C. (2020, July-August). *Artificial intelligence opportunities to improve food safety at retail.* Food Protection Trends, 40 (4), in press.

*Marijuana Justice Act of 2019, H.R. 1456, 116th cong.* (2019).

*Marijuana Justice Act of 2019, S. 597, 116th cong.* (2019).

*Marijuana Opportunity Reinvestment and Expungement Act of 2019, H.R. 3884, 116th cong.*(2019).

*MORE Act of 2019, S. 2227, 116th cong.* (2019).

National Conference of State Legislators. (2019, October 16a). *State medical marijuana laws*. Retrieved from http://www.ncsl.org/research/health/state-medical-marijuana-laws.aspx.

National Conference of State Legislatures. (2019, October 17b). *Marijuana overview*. Retrieved from https://www.ncsl.org/research/civil-and-criminal-justice/marijuana-overview.aspx.

National Institute on Drug Abuse. (2019, December). *Marijuana*. Retrieved from https://www.drugabuse.gov/node/pdf/1380/marijuana.

Partnership for Food Safety Education. (2019, February). *Safe style recipe guide*. Retrieved from http://www.saferecipeguide.org/wp-content/uploads/2019/02/SafeRecipe-Styleguide-Print.pdf.

*Secure and Fair Enforcement Banking Act of 2019, H.R. 1595, 116th cong.* (2019).

*Secure and Fair Enforcement Banking Act of 2019, S. 1200, 116th cong.* (2019).

Substance Abuse and Mental Health Services Administration. (2019, August 20). *2018 NSDUH detailed tables*. Retrieved from https://www.samhsa.gov/data/report/2018-nsduh-detailed-tables.

Thomas, B., & ElSohly, M. (2015, December 8). *"The analytical chemistry of cannabis." Botany of* Cannabis sativa *L.* Cambridge, Massachusetts: Elsevier Academic Press. https://doi.org/10.1016/C2014-0-03861-0

*To amend the Federal Food, Drug, and Cosmetic Act with respect to the regulation of hemp-derived cannabidiol and hemp-derived cannabidiol containing substances, H.R. 5587, 116th Cong.* (2020).

U.S. Department of Justice. (2013, August 29). *Guidance regarding marijuana enforcement*. Retrieved from https://www.justice.gov/iso/opa/resources/3052013829132756857467.pdf.

U.S. Department of Justice. (2018, January 4). *Marijuana enforcement*. Retrieved from https://www.justice.gov/opa/press-release/file/1022196/download.

U.S. Food and Drug Administration. (2017, December 13). *Full Text of the Food Safety Modernization Act (FSMA)*. Retrieved from https://www.fda.gov/Food/GuidanceRegulation/FSMA/ucm247548.htm.

U.S. Food and Drug Administration. (2019a). *New Era of smarter food safety*. Retrieved from https://www.fda.gov/food/food-industry/new-era-smarter-food-safety.

U.S. Food and Drug Administration. (2019b). *Warning letters and test results for cannabidiol-related products*. Retrieved from https://www.fda.gov/news-events/public-health-focus/warning-letters-and-test-results-cannabidiol-related-products.

U.S. Food and Drug Administration. (2019c). *Statement from FDA Commissioner Scott Gottlieb, M.D., on new steps to advance agency's continued evaluation of potential regulatory pathways for cannabis-containing and cannabis-derived products*. Retrieved from https://www.fda.gov/news-events/press-announcements/statement-fda-commissioner-scott-gottlieb-md-new-steps-advance-agencys-continued-evaluation.

U.S. Food and Drug Administration. (2019d). *Scientific data and information about products containing cannabis or cannabis-derived compounds*. Retrieved from https://www.fda.gov/media/128592/download.

U.S. Food and Drug Administration. (2019e). *Benefits associated with complete adoption and implementation of the FDA food Code*. Retrieved from https://www.fda.gov/food/fda-food-code/benefits-associated-complete-adoption-and-implementation-fda-food-code.

U.S. Food and Drug Administration. (2020a). *FDA's regulation of cannabis products, including hemp-CBD*. Retrieved from webinar https://www.registercheck.com/website/international-aloe-science-council/.

U.S. Food and Drug Administration. (2020b). *FDA regulation of cannabis and cannabis-derived products, including cannabidiol (CBD)*. Retrieved from https://www.fda.gov/news-events/public-health-focus/fda-regulation-cannabis-and-cannabis-derived-products-including-cannabidiol-cbd.

U.S. Senate Committee on Agriculture, Nutrition, and Forestry. (2019, July 25). *Hemp production and the 2018 farm bill*. Retrieved from https://www.agriculture.senate.gov/hearings/hemp-production-and-the-2018-farm-bill.

*VA Medicinal Cannabis Research Act of 2019, S. 179, 116th cong.* (2019).

*Veterans Medical Marijuana Safe Harbor Act, S. 445, 116th cong.* (2019).

World Health Organization. (2017, November 6). *Cannabidiol (CBD)*. Retrieved from https://www.who.int/medicines/access/controlled-substances/5.2_CBD.pdf.

# Food defense and technology

# Food defense-"Back to the basics"

**Jason P. Bashura, MPH, RS**

*Food Defense Subject Matter Expert, New York, United States*

*For the life of me, I cannot understand why the terrorists have not attacked our food supply because it is so easy to do.*

**Tommy G. Thompson, former Secretary, Health and Human Services (2001—05)**

**(Pear, 2004)**

## Prologue

I can recall when, as a public health undergraduate student at Southern Connecticut State University in the early 1990s, I learned of "compulsory vaccination" and *Jacobson v. Massachusetts*, 197 U.S. 11 (1905), as well as how mandatory quarantine orders (CDC, 2012) have been used to protect, preserve, and promote health and well-being in the face of imminent threats to public health. Additional basic elements of any public health mitigating investigation would include the epidemiological contact tracing (WHO, 2017). Looking at these basic public health protecting measures through the lens of the FDA's "New Era of Smarter Food Safety" (FDA, 2019e) that is quickly coming in to focus, and being in the throes of the coronavirus pandemic (COVID-19) of early 2020, I now find myself considering the traceability of our food supply-but using an example of contact tracing of an individual who was or might have been in contact with others during a period of infectivity.

Take for example Ottilie Lundgren, from Oxford, Connecticut, who, in late 2001, died from inhalational anthrax exposure suspected to have been cross-contaminated in the US mail-although anthrax was never found in her home. Investigators found spores on an envelope several miles from her home in Seymour, CT (Roos, 2001). Imagine the daunting task of sorting through or having to random sample test 85,000,000 pieces of mail to determine where they were sent from and where they went.

Consider as well the ever famous "father of epidemiology"-John Snow-with the infamous Broad Street well pump handle investigation that stemmed the cholera outbreaks in England during the mid-1800s (Buechner, Constantine, & Gjelsvik, 2004). Snow went out and identified on a map where every sick person lived to determine the common activity or source of contamination, eventually deducing that they all obtained water from the same well.

What does this have to do with where we are today? Well, nothing, directly, but EVERYTHING, indirectly. To quote Leonardo de Vinci, "Everything is connected

**Building the Future of Food Safety Technology. https://doi.org/10.1016/B978-0-12-818956-6.00010-5**

to everything else." Our ability to see and realize these connections is the challenge. The movement of data such as pieces of mail, of people, and of ingredients in our food system is "theoretically" trackable. The challenges are in the HOW it is traced and in the recording of each of those trackable moments.

Having lived in the northeast for most of my life, we endured ice storms, nor'-easters, and even an occasional hurricane. When my family and I moved to the mid-Atlantic area in late 2008, we thought that we had "addressed" all of the logistics of our big move, until the first time the power went out-and it was out for more than 6 hrs. This was early 2009 and we were 300 miles from our friends and family of southern Connecticut, when the power went out in the townhouse we were renting in Maryland. I can remember our neighbor at the time-Mr. Cesar, a police officer for the Howard County Police Department-telling me that power outages happen "all the time" as we tried to figure out dealing with the power outage. I can count on one hand how many times we lost power for more than 5 minutes in Connecticut, and for that, we are grateful. It seems the RISK of losing power is greater in Maryland, than it is in Connecticut-at least in our experience. Is it the infrastructure? Is it the preplanning? Is it the proportion of above ground versus underground supply lines? Or, is it just a matter of perspective?

Fast forward to a few years later, we bought our home and settled into a great neighborhood where our neighbors quickly became our family-as most everyone that lives here is not "from" here. In a 7-year period, we probably have lost power three times a year, some of those events spanning multiple days. In early 2018, with the news of a looming ice storm on the horizon, I reached out to a couple of tree trimmers to help trim the tops of some of the spindly pines that dot our backyard and the tops dangle peerlessly close to the power lines when they are wet or topped with snow or ice. So, out of an abundance of concern of losing power with frigid temperatures on the horizon, we opted to have the trees aggressively trimmed, which ultimately led to one of them being cut down altogether. What does this have to do with food defense? Nothing, directly, but everything, indirectly. But how? It all has to do with risk, vulnerability, and threat.

Take a moment and review this last paragraph again, slowly, and think of these questions to yourself:

- What is the **RISK** being described?
- What is (are) the **VULNERABILITY (ies)**?
- What is the **THREAT**?

This chapter will focus on food defense activities and reducing the risk of food terrorism. Additionally, I will provide a glimpse "back" on the journey that the art of what we refer to as food defense today has taken to get to where it is today-this will include some historical perspectives of food defense and a review of a "hypothetical" intentional adulteration event that could result in public health harm. Later in this chapter, I will review some of the potential research needs and elements that are critical to addressing and minimizing the likelihood of acts of food terrorism from occurring in the future. Finally, some key partnerships and collaborations will be identified and discussed.

Answers to the three questions above:

The **_RISK_** of losing power due to the **_THREAT_** of an ice storm led us to trim/cut back the **_VULNERABLE_** tree tops/branches. This mitigation strategy-ultimately-mitigated the RISK of losing power by eliminating the vulnerability: branches coming down on the power lines and taking out our power. Perhaps Donald Rumsfeld (then the Secretary of Defense) summed this up best when he stated in a February 12, 2002, DOD news briefing:

> _Reports that say that something hasn't happened are always interesting to me, because as we know, there are known knowns; there are things we know we know. We also know there are known unknowns; that is to say we know there are some things we do not know. But there are also unknown unknowns-the ones we don't know we don't know. And if one looks throughout the history of our country and other free countries, it is the latter category that tend to be the difficult ones._

**(Profita, 2006)**

# Defining food defense terms

Terms like **food security**, **food biosecurity**, and **food terrorism** have circled the globe since the early 2000s. We need to "level set" on some definitions for the remainder of this chapter. While the content below might be new to you or cause your eyebrows to furl when you read it-that is ok. That means that there is either new information or a different angle being described that youhad not thought of before.

Agriculture (Agro) Defense-protecting US agriculture-crops, livestock, and food-from global biothreats, while safeguarding people from zoonotic animal diseases and foodborne pathogens (Kansas State University, 2020).

**_Food Safety_** addresses the accidental or unintentional contamination of food products (USDA, 2009).

**_Food Security_** accesses to an ample, nutritious food supply (WHO, 2002).

**_Food defense_**

1. The **USDA**'s Food Safety and Inspection Service (FSIS) defines "Food Defense" as "… the protection of food products from contamination or adulteration intended to cause public health harm or economic disruption" (USDA, 2019).
2. The **FDA**'s definition of "Food Defense" is found in 21 CFR 121 as "… the effort to protect food from intentional acts of adulteration where there is an intent to cause wide scale public health harm" (FDA, 2020b).
3. The **Department of Homeland Security** (DHS) adds to the definition of "Food Defense" by including a discussion of their focus on the "farm-to-table" continuum with "Pre-harvest elements … include crops and animals in the field, as well as fertilizers and animal feed" and how "The harvesting or slaughter of agricultural products marks the beginning of the post-harvest food sector," which also includes "processing, storage, transportation, retail, and food service" (DHS, 2007).

4. **The Food Safety System Certification's FSSC 22000-0-005.2** defines "Food Defense" as a process to prevent "… food and feed supply chains from all forms of ideologically or behaviorally motivated, intentional adulteration that might impact consumer health."

5. **The National Center for Food Protection and Defense** (NCFDP) (2011) defines "Food Defense" in terms of three different risks:

   a. **Industrial Sabotage: "**Intentional contamination by an insider or competitor to damage the company, causing financial problems/recall but not necessarily to cause public harm."

   b. **Terrorism**: "The reach and complexity of the food system has caused concern for its potential as a terrorist target."

   c. **Economically Motivated Adulteration**: "Acts against a product for the purpose of increasing the apparent value of the product or reducing the cost of its production, i.e., for economic gain."

*Food Protection* a concept that leverages the outputs of food safety and food defense activities (FDA, 2007).

*Food Terrorism* is defined as an act or threat of deliberate contamination of food for human consumption with chemical, biological, or radionuclear agents for the purpose of causing injury or death to civilian populations and/or disrupting social, economic, or political stability (WHO, 2002).

*Food Fraud* is a collective term used to encompass the deliberate and intentional substitution, addition, tampering, or misrepresentation of food, food ingredients, or food packaging, or false or misleading statements made about a product for economic gain (Congressional Research Service, 2014).

*Vulnerability* has been defined as a physical feature or operational attribute that renders an entity open to exploitation or susceptible to a given hazard (DHS, 2008).

*Threat* has been defined as something that can cause loss or harm, which arises from the ill intent of people (BSI, 2017) as well as "natural or man-made occurrence, individual, entity, or action that has or indicates the potential to harm life, information, operations, the environment and/or property" (DHS, 2008).

*Risk* is defined as "potential for an unwanted outcome resulting from an incident, event, or occurrence, as determined by its likelihood [a function of threats and vulnerabilities] and the associated consequences" (FDA, 2007).

*Intentional adulteration*

1. The term "intentional" is defined by Merriam-Webster (n.d.) as "done by intention or design: INTENDED-intentional damage-DELIBERATE."

2. The term "**food**" is defined in 21 US Code § 342 as

   a. articles used for food or drink for man or other animals,

   b. chewing gum, and

   c. articles used for components of any such article.

3. In terms of food, the term "**adulterated**," based on 21 US Code § 342, gains the following definition elements:

"A food shall be deemed to be adulterated-

**a.** Poisonous, insanitary, etc., ingredients. If it bears or contains any poisonous or deleterious substance which may render it injurious to health;

**b.** Absence, substitution, or addition of constituents

    i. If any valuable constituent has been in whole or in part omitted or abstracted there from; or

    ii. if any substance has been substituted wholly or in part therefore; or

    iii. if damage or inferiority has been concealed in any manner; or

    iv. if any substance has been added thereto or mixed or packed therewith so as to increase its bulk or weight, or reduce its quality or strength, or make it appear better or of greater value than it is."

**4.** Therefore the term **"intentional adulteration"** could be defined as "The willful addition of an adulterant or removal of a key component of an ingredient or food to cause public health or economic harm."

The concept of getting *"back to the basics"* on food defense-*in essence*-is a non-technological approach to addressing a problem-*intentional adulteration*-that requires a HUMAN aggressor with intent (motivation) for the intended outcome to be realized. There are technologies available today to detect nonconformities in food matrices, detect motion, capture video, and analyze ingredient composition and yet other technologies can facilitate restricting access to certain "vulnerable" areas of a food manufacturing, storage, or production areas. However, at the end of the day, **Food Defense** is about a steady state culture of conscious awareness-a suite of behaviors exhibited by individuals that can hinder, minimize, or prevent an act of intentional adulteration from occurring.

## Food defense-a historical perspective

Within the United States, food defense "activities" can be likened to the concept of "Homeland Security meets food safety"-as they involve food safety policies and procedures being leveraged, refined, and updated to protect food manufacturing environments from those individuals seeking to do harm via the food supply-the very definition of **"Food Terrorism."**

The tragic events of September 11, 2001, forced us all to rethink how we took certain aspects of safety and security for granted. While concerns over the safety of air travel captured much attention, the US government did not ignore concerns over the safety of the American food supply. Even those in key federal government positions questioned the ease with which terrorist organizations might seek to contaminate parts of our food supply and distribution systems, such as (then) Health and Human Services Secretary Tommy G. Thompson, who stated in 2004 "For the life of me, I cannot understand why the terrorists have not attacked our food supply because it is so easy to do" (Pear, 2004). By the end of 2001, the FDA and the USDA sought to determine the current state of the American food system's readiness against an intentional attack.

The United States is not alone in this perception, as the World Health Organization (WHO) stated in their post-9/11 document "Food Safety Issues: Terrorist Threats to Food-Guidance for Establishing and Strengthening Prevention and Response Systems": "The key to preventing food terrorism is establishment and enhancement of existing food safety management programmes and implementation of reasonable security measures" (WHO, 2002).

The Food and Agriculture "sector" was designated one of the United States' critical infrastructure and key resources (CIKR) (DHS, 2009) within Presidential Policy Directive 21 (Obama White House, 2013). The DHS formed the Food and Agriculture Sector Coordinating Council in 2004 (FDA, 2007). As a result of these activities, the US government assembled experts from across the government, private sector owners and operators, academic communities, and nongovernment organizations-henceforth the food and agriculture "system"-to identify critical elements within the CIKR and to devise the Food and Agriculture Sector's Sector Specific Plan (SSP) (CISA, 2015).

## Education and training resources

In early 2000s, under the direction of (then) Associate Commissioner for Foods, David Acheson, the FDA convened a series of meetings with the Council of Association Presidents (CAP) (FDA, 2019a) of the various associations of representing the membership of regulatory agencies of varying capacities across the United States (FDA, 2019d) to help with developing and refining some fundamental food defense resources which are still in use today: the Employees *FIRST* and the *ALERT* initiatives. I was fortunate to have been able to represent the National Environmental Health Association on the CAP and presented the perspective of the state/local regulatory health official. During one of these last meetings, we participated in a "live" town hall meeting that was seeking to educate the regulatory community about what food defense was all about and some of the activities that the FDA would be working on. Again, in getting back to the basics, Employees **FIRST** and the **ALERT** initiatives were focused on educating personnel **at the front lines (FIRST)** and **management (ALERT)** (Barringer, 2007) as to what they could do to help develop that "culture" of Food Defense.

| Employees FIRST (front line food workers) | The ALERT initiatives (Management) |
| --- | --- |
| **F**ollow company food defense plan and procedures. **I**nspect your work area and surrounding areas. **R**ecognize anything out of the ordinary. | **A**ssure ingredients and supplies are from safe sources. **L**ook after the security of products in your facility. **E**mployees-what do you know about personnel coming and going from your facility? |

| Employees FIRST (front line food workers) | The ALERT initiatives (Management) |
|---|---|
| **S**ecure all ingredients, supplies, and finished product. | **R**eport-can you provide reports for ingredients/products under your control? |
| **T**ell management if you notice anything unusual or suspicious. | **T**hreat-what do you do and who do you notify if you have a THREAT at your facility? |

In 2008, as a direct hire to the FDA, I was humbled, thrilled, scared, nervous, and proud-I was being offered a position to work on the FDA's Food Defense Team, to help build and inform the direction of the Food Defense strategy for the United States-not bad for a culinary school dropout who worked in local and state public health in Connecticut and never lost sight of the BIG picture. The opportunity to work for the FDA would mean additional responsibilities and the opportunity to help provide state/local public health perspective into the Federal "strategy." I had been working at the FDA for maybe 3 months when the Peanut Corporation of American outbreak hit. This incident was an eye-opener to me. I worked down the hall from the Emergency Coordination and Response Team when I received a phone call from a colleague who asked me what I knew about *Salmonella* in peanut butter. I remember the conversation like it was yesterday because I knew that was going to be a BIG deal, especially as we were working on the Food Safety Enhancement Act, H.R.2749, 111th Cong. (2010) (precursor to FSMA) contents pertaining to a "Food Defense rule."

One of my first projects based on education and training was to work on finishing a task order that the Institute of Food Technologists (IFT) was working on, at that time led by Jennifer McEntire and Tejas Bhatt. The Food Related Emergency Exercise Bundle (FREE-B) was a series of tabletop exercises that were designed and intended to be used to help facilitate the development of or to test existing food emergency response plans for regulatory and industry partners. While most of the scenarios were intentional adulteration based, the storylines would lead a participant to believe that the scenarios could have gone either way, depending on the information that was shared with the participants. The FREE-B was literally a "Federal project" in the boundaries and limits of government consternation; between legal approval of the use of logos and endorsements from various other Federal partners, the project seemed to be redefining its scope as we neared completion. However, we held firm and launched the FREE-B at the IFT annual conference in 2011, and it continues to have new scenarios added to it, to this day.

As described above, the FREE-B (FDA, 2017) is a suite of exercises intended to help drive improvements based on focusing on getting back to the basics-**communication** is ALWAYS a key finding and takeaway from any exercise that is completed; how we communicate, not just when or what is communicated, continues to be a challenge. Developing characteristics and skill sets of **leadership** and being able to demonstrate those in times of crises, these build capacity and the ability to "clear the room" of the smoke and fog that often accompanies the process of making big decisions. Having the confidence in your knowledge and the ability to articulate your position are key to your success-and the success of the organization-these are critical in executing against the plan. By participating in exercises as described above, industry stakeholders gain the ability and opportunity to "sharpen their edge."

Another project related to **education and training** pertinent to Food Defense was the Innovative Food Defense Program-a grant funding opportunity to help develop, predictably, "INNOVATIVE" approaches to food defense. Concepts have leveraged technology to measure/track the distribution of contaminated food (in Wisconsin), while others focused on the use of comic strip-like illustrations to "tell a story," such as in Somerset County, NJ ("Food Safety", 2020). Others examined the ability for an appropriately credentialed regulatory official to "penetrate a facility"-get as far as they could within a retail food setting without being challenged to produce identification-and/or proof of identity/affiliation, such as in Cuyahoga County (OH) Board of Health (Armstrong, 2020).

While those Innovative Food Defense Program examples shared above are just a few of the programs that the FDA funded, they are shining examples of what COULD happen if the we were to really get *back to basics* and rethink some of the current approaches to Food Defense in the United States. Inherent challenges have existed within Federal government as they relate to the issuance of grants to state and local regulatory agencies. If there is a NEED for state, local, tribal, and territorial entities to apply for and for the federal government to be able to fund those requests, there is really no telling how much "new" or improved foundational resources could be generated to bolster the consciousness and awareness of a food defense culture within the regulatory community. The last example (Cuyahoga County) focused on imposter health inspectors, but this is an example of a program that COULD be used if applied at the state/federal levels, as well.

Ironically, the Cuyahoga County project was based on "real-life" incidents that were (*and still do today*) occurring involving imposter health inspectors not just domestically in the United States but globally as well. Those unauthorized personnel illegitimately seek access to the facility or simply try to "scam" the operator for some cash so that they do not have to endure an inspection happen more frequently than we would care to admit. These unauthorized personnel do not limit their scope to retail or food manufacturers, either-there are reports of other critical infrastructure sites being targeted as well. The need for diligence and recognizing WHO should be permitted in to your facility, ensuring that there is a mechanism to verify the credentials of the "inspector" and training your personnel to not be "fooled" in to paying off a scammer inspector (City of Monroe, 2018; Government of USVI, 2020). These are just a few examples of *getting back to the basics*-limiting access to only those that should/have a legitimate reason to be there.

# Foundational approaches to critical infrastructure and food defense

The Food and Agriculture Sector's (SSP) rewrite for 2010 started shortly after I arrived at the FDA in late 2008. In partnership with a colleague who quickly became a friend at the USDA's FSIS, Michael Bailey and I worked tirelessly to combine a previous "separated" SSP (a USDA section and an FDA section) into one, unified document. Michael and I worked with tremendous secretarial support from the US DHS, and Mariella and Scott were beyond fantastic to work with but always on task with (a) what needed to be done and (b) by when-it was essentially project management 101. Within the 2010 SSP, Michael and I had even proposed some potential workgroups to help reduce risk within the food and agriculture sector. The five working groups that we had suggested were the

**1)** Education and training working group,
**2)** Partnership working group,
**3)** Communications/IT working group,
**4)** Transportation/shipping working group, and
**5)** Laboratory capacity working group.

Within the SSP was a section on the Joint Committee on Research (JCR)-an opportunity whereas the private sector and government leadership within the Food and Agriculture Sector had identified a series of food defense related activities or research that were identified as being needed. The JCR "is a body through which the SCC and GCC can collaborate and identify sector research needs" (SSP, 2010). The JCR, unfortunately, is not functional at this time (2020). Some of the work that the JCR had indicated for select agent research/declassification of material that can help industry to prioritize their R&D efforts only stands to benefit all of the food and agriculture sector owners and operators.

In their October 2017 Blue Ribbon Study Panel Report titled Special Focus: Defense of Animal Agriculture, the Bipartisan Commission on Biodefense stated "Although the nation has made great strides, it still falls critically short in rapid biodetection, diagnosis, and integrated biosurveillance of outbreaks" (Bipartisan, 2017). As a "gap" that can be seen and has been described, getting BACK to the BASICS through open dialogue and identifying strengths and opportunities in research can and will help to protect the food supply. That collaboration comes with a cost though-and it is **knowledge**-which can be a powerful tool, and it can be hard for agencies/departments to share information if the focus or objective of the information sharing is not addressing an aligned goal.

The JCR recommended the development of an academic entity developing a resource that could enable an open search of research in an area of focus or concern. The Food Protection and Defense Institute (FPDI) developed the Food Defense Research Database (FDRD) in 2009. Additionally, the FDRD was capable of sorting and archiving open source news, presentations, and peer-reviewed articles of content pertaining to food and agriculture defense (FDA, DHS, & USDA, 2011). Unfortunately, along with other funding cuts and resource reprioritization, the FDRD was not sustained by the FPDI.

The FDA developed the Food Protection Task Force (FPTF) grant program as a means to "create an effective nationwide infrastructure for enhancing outreach, response, integration and information sharing in state, local, and tribal governments" (FDA, 2019b). Shortly after establishing the FPTF grants, the FDA expanded a novel concept known as the Food Protection Rapid Response Teams (RRT)-spearheaded by committed FDA personnel that continually seek to develop, grow, and share best practices via the RRT playbook (FDA, 2019c).

The FDA funds their Division of Food Defense Targeting (DFDT)-formerly known as the Prior Notice Center (FDA, 2020a)-that leverages a Predictive Risk-based Evaluation for Dynamic Import Compliance Targeting (PREDICT) program. PREDICT assists entry reviewers in targeting higher-risk shipments for examination. This **TECHNOLOGY** behind the essential work that the DFDT does could be amplified if there was an opportunity for the private sector to be able to inform and fine-tune the focus of the work that is being done. This is "future" thinking, but the progress realized tomorrow has to be sewn through the seeds of ideas in the fields of hope today. The FDA's DFDT also "coordinates a broad range of activities that focus on protecting the food supply" (Spink, 2013).

Some of the collaborations that I was fortunate to be associated with while I was with the FDA include the US FBI's Agroterrorism Workshops (FBI, 2014) and the Early Warning Infectious Disease Surveillance (EWIDS) (GlobalSecurity, 2011). EWIDS included "the Great Lakes Border Health Initiative," which was an amazing interaction with dedicated professionals that actually resulted in the birth of another FREE-B exercise, based on specific issues that some of the regulatory officials that were present there were experiencing. The Multi-State Partnerships for Security in Agriculture (MSPAS) and the Southern Agriculture and Animal Disaster Response Alliance (SAADRA) were "state stakeholder"-based groups that were focusing on trying to comply with the DHS Homeland Infrastructure Threat and Risk Analysis Center data calls, intending to identify/protect CIKR within the states, but the data call always seemed to produce a lot of work and not a lot of return on investment— illustration of tier 1 or 2 critical infrastructure within the states. Both the MSPAS and SAADRA convened regular meetings and drove information sharing through to the private sector owners and operators within their respective states and jurisdictions. Other amazing collaborations that helped to drive and improve our knowledge base in the food defense arena include the NCFDP, which is currently known as the Food Protection and Defense Institute (FPDI), and the Association of Food and Drug Officials (AFDO) Food Protection and Defense working group.

After leaving the federal government and joining industry in 2014, I quickly learned that there were disparate groups that were working on similar concepts related to food defense-namely the development of comments in advance of the Intentional Adulteration Rule (IA Rule) (FDA, 2016) embedded within the Food Safety Modernization Act (FSMA)-but these groups were not "coordinated." On

June 8, 2016, I convened the first Food Defense Consortium call-a loosely coordinated call to bring together private sector owners and operators to focus on a variety of elements embedded within FSMA's IA Rule. As of March 2020, the Food Defense Consortium developed and submitted comments on FSMA's IA Rule, related guidance, sought an extension for compliance date, and is currently working to engage with membership on a suite of food defense "best practices" that will encourage and focus on getting "***back to the basics***" related to foundational programs and existing measures that decrease vulnerability through accessibility restriction and/or feasibility reduction for an act of intentional adulteration to occur.

Working through the Food Defense Consortium, we have developed an "updated" pneumonic to help get back to the basics about food defense: helping to ensure that industry Knows the Food Defense *FACTS* and that front-line personnel are being Food Defense *AWARE*:

| Know the food defense FACTS | Be food defense AWARE |
|---|---|
| *F*ood defense plan: The facility has a food defense team and developed a plan that includes the outcomes of RISK assessment (that includes vulnerability and threat contributions) | Pay *A*ttention to your workplace and know who you should report unusual findings to<br>*W*atch out for unauthorized personnel in areas they should not be in |
| *A*ccess control is limited/controlled<br>*C*ommit to helping develop a CULTURE of food defense<br>*T*raining has been completed<br>*S*ay something if you SEE or HEAR something out of place or unusual | *A*ccess control matters-follow physical security best practices<br>*R*espond and tell management or a supervisor if something is out of the ordinary.<br>*E*veryone, all the time … no exceptions! |

## Information sharing

Recognizing that there is not a formal mechanism for information sharing within the food and agriculture sector as there is for other critical infrastructure sectors, the concept of the *Food Defense TRUST* was conceived within the Food Defense Consortium. The *TRUST* is a double entendre for the term used to describe a group with similar intentions or objectives, but, more importantly, that it is about actually developing trusted relationships. While the need for an information sharing and analysis center (ISAC) has been a challenging issue to share among the food and agriculture sector, in the midst of the COVID-19 pandemic, an ISAC would certainly have made information sharing simpler, clearer, and easier.

## Case studies

### Salmonella attack in Oregon (1984)

The "reality" of a food terrorism event is even clearer in the "infamous" salmonellosis outbreak that transpired in The Dalles, OR, in 1984. Some of the followers of the Bagwan Shree Rajneesh attempted to influence a local zoning election by sickening greater than 750 people by intentionally contaminating salad bars and selfserve areas in several restaurants with *Salmonella* (Török et al., 1997), which was not actually "solved" until a year later-though many of the clues that are listed above had indeed been visible as well. After the outbreak had subsided, and life had returned to "normal"-there was an investigation in to the Rajneesh compound that resulted in an "admission" to local/federal officials-affirming what was believed to be true but could not be proven-that the outbreak indeed had a direct connection to the Ranjesspuram. Moreover, officials "found glass vials containing *Salmonella* 'bactrol disks' in the laboratory of a Rajneeshpuram medical clinic"-the epitome of the "smoking gun."

### EHEC 0104:H4 outbreak in Germany (2011)

Germany experienced one of their largest outbreaks of a foodborne infection in 2011. Recorded illnesses caused by enterohaemorrhagic *Escherichia coli* (EHEC) with the serotype O104:H4 numbered at 2987 (nearly triple Germany's annual average) with 18 deaths. Further, the number of recorded illnesses caused by hemolytic uremic syndrome (HUS) numbered at 855 (more than 13 times Germany's annual average of 65 cases) with 35 deaths (Berger, 2012).

Several "unknowns" plagued investigators as they sought to determine the source of the outbreak. According to some sources, Egyptian fenugreek sprouts are the suspected food vehicle for the outbreak (Neuman & Sayare, 2011; Radosavljevic, Finke, & Belojevic, 2014). According to other sources, the "… sudden and unexplainable emerging of a fast-increasing number of cases and deaths from bloody diarrhea and HUS might have been caused naturally, accidently, or intentionally" ("Deliberate act," 2012). We have seen this time and time again whereas "armchair" quarterbacks seem to forget that, while hindsight is 20/20, maintaining an open mind can help to see the BIG picture in the midst of the investigation.

Teams investigating the fenugreek seeds in the 2011 outbreak noted many clues. As described in the Medical Aspects of Biological Warfare (Dembek, Pavlin, Siwek, & Kortepeter, 2018), these include

Clue 1: A highly unusual event with large numbers of casualties.
Clue 2: Higher morbidity or mortality than is expected.
Clue 3: Uncommon disease.
Clue 4: Point source outbreak.
Clue 5: Multiple epidemics.
Clue 6: Lower attack rates in protected individuals.

Clue 7: Dead animals.

Clue 8: Reverse or simultaneous spread.

Clue 9: Unusual disease manifestation.

Clue 10: Downwind plume pattern.

Clue 11: Direct evidence.

If these "clues" are to be followed, then, the road map can help to guide decisions that are being made. Going **back to the basics** of the investigation-leveraging an open-minded approach-could help to inform the investigation, while not focusing explicitly on the anticipated path forward.

## Global "reactions" after intentional adulteration events

The United Kingdom's response to the 2013 "horse meat scandal" included the establishment of the UK's National Food Crime Unit, headed by Andy Morling ("First assessment of food crime in the UK published," 2015). Similarly, Australia revised their food protection regulations based on intentional adulteration incidents in 2018 when acts of sabotage involved needles inserted into strawberry in all six Australian states (Siddique, 2018). This pushed law enforcement entities in Australia and beyond into unfamiliar territory. Specifically, leaders introduced new laws and policies pertaining to differentiating a tampering event where someone was seeking retaliatory action against another person, or a firm, or if the actions equate with terrorism.

The conclusions and recommendations section of these food protection regulations identified several specific goals, including the need to improve communication, collaboration elements, traceability, and industry preparedness and response (Food Standards Australia New Zealand, 2018; "Recommendations made in strawberry tampering report," 2019).

As Category B of the New Era of Smarter Food Safety (FDA, 2019e) calls out "To fully realize a preventive controls system that rapidly incorporates new knowledge, we must also ask if we can make processes and communications more effective, efficient, and in some cases, simpler" (FDA, 2019e).

This section on *Food Defense: Getting Back to Basics* has stressed the point that we must embrace the opportunity to identify improvements to facilitate access to Food Defense research, tools, technologies, and resources developed over the last 20 years. We must also prioritize those solutions-the future of food safety technology-that can be developed to support the greatest return on investment of time and financial need to actually minimize the likelihood of an act of intentional adulteration.

With current examples of devices, software, and platforms, along with the hype around IOT, AI, machine learning, and digital end-to-end traceability solutions and their roles in Food Safety-including Food Defense-leaders must remember that technology alone cannot solve all the challenges our modern food supply systems face.

Some suggestions to support future efforts and technology include

- The need for an **Information Sharing and Analysis Center** or **Organization** in order to facilitate the exchange of information in a non attributable manner.

- More **collaborative environments** where threat intelligence information can be freely shared between and among the food and beverage industry are needed. Examples like the Food Defense Consortium described above are "grass root" solutions where challenges previously existed. As included within the FDA's Food Protection Plan (FDA, 2007b), the key elements of prevention, intervention, and response are plainly evident in the approach that was taking in the crafting of the FSMA language, as well.
- **Research needs** should be reassessed and practical solutions to these knowledge gaps can be identified, predictive analytical tools. If the University of Minnesota's FPDI and the Texas A&M University's National Center for Foreign Animal and Zoonotic Disease (FAZD) were FULLY funded within the last decade, these gaps wouldn't exist today. If a hybrid government and industry approach to support the FPDI and FAZD could support, coordinate, and synthesize these research needs, gaps in education and training could be identified, and risk assessment-based resources could be developed to illustrate where limited resources need to be focused to minimize impacts to the system.
- **Access to tools and resources-**The FDA's New Era of Smarter Food Safety (FDA, 2019e) asks industry to consider and evaluate all available and innovative solutions that can increase access to tools and resources that have been developed to reduce risks within the Food and Agriculture sector. We must acknowledge that while some are presently at arms length, will the "connection" to these tools and resources become greater challenges over time? If the US government is able to fund the development of these resources, it should be able to make these resources freely available across the Food and Agriculture sector.
- **Streamlining the terms and definitions** used-in a GLOBAL landscape-will directly benefit the **education and training** needs described herein. The ability to align on terminology, concepts, and requirements-like what the Global Food Safety Initiative seeks to accomplish-will help to ensure that we are all speaking one language, not saying something, but meaning something else.

With the establishment of new policies designed to protect the critical infrastructure within the United States, industry experts continue to ask if they are being leveraged to the extent possible. Enforcement of laws to the maximum extent could help to decrease the likelihood of other, copycat incidents, but only time will tell.

## Summary

One of the questions embedded within the New Era of Smarter Food Safety (FDA, 2019e) is "What are the most significant actions FDA could undertake to promote and support the use of smarter tools for prevention?"

I would offer we consider getting **Back to the Basics**:

(1) Leveraging risk-based approaches to developing tools and resources targeted at education and training of an "all of industry" approach to aid in reducing the risk of intentional adulteration of the food supply.

**(2)** Ensure adequate access to adequate modular-based education and training opportunities for personnel within the food and agriculture system.

**(3)** FOCUS on the outcome-not the solution.

**(4)** COLLABORATE with and listen to feedback from industry and LISTEN to aid in understanding the comments, questions, and concerns that are raised.

**(5)** Leverage existing or indicate the need for new TECHNOLOGY to "fill gaps" that might exist.

The art of what we refer to today as food defense is predicated on the shared experiences, collective expertise and research that has evolved in the last 20+ years, This chapter did not cover what needs to be done in order to develop a food defense plan as per government or for GFSI scheme compliance; it was intended to be an "overview" of the foundation and history of food defense activities, research and collaborations that have occurred and to emphasize the need to ensure clear lines of information sharing in order to get ***BACK TO THE BASICS***. Reducing the risk of an act of Food Terrorism is not a responsibility to be taken lightly. This author is currently working on a future publication to aid in clarifying the nuances of various government-based regulations and GFSI scheme compliance requirements.

## References

21 U.S. Code § 342 . 21 U.S. Code § 342.

Armstrong, J. (2020). *"Food defense." Cuyahoga county (OH) board of health*. Retrieved from https://www.ccbh.net/food-defense/.

Barringer, A. (2007, March). Staying ALERT about food defense. *Food Safety Magazine*. Retrieved from https://www.foodsafetymagazine.com/magazine-archive1/february-march-2007/staying-alert-about-food-defense/.

Bipartisan Commission on Biodefense. (2017, October). *Bipartisan report of the Blue Ribbon Study Panel on Biodefense. Special focus: Defense of animal agriculture*. Retrieved from https://biodefensecommission.org/wp-content/uploads/2017/10/Defense-of-Animal-Agriculture-04.pdf.

Buechner, J., Constantine, H., & Gjelsvik, A. (2004). John snow and the broad Street pump: 150 years of epidemiology. *Medicine and Health, Rhode Island, 87*(10), 314–315. Retrieved from https://pdfs.semanticscholar.org/8e27/f9190ce14ab0d27609f5f1cfe577b 23c2dce.pdf?_ga=2.57048938.1174845908.1584485689-1822336766.1584485689.

"EHEC O104:H4 In Germany 2011: Large Outbreak of Bloody Diarrhea and Haemolytic Uremic Syndrome by Shiga Toxin-Producing E.coli via Contaminated Food" In Institute of Medicine Burger, R. (2012). *Improving food safety through a one health approach: Workshop summary*. Washington, DC: The National Academies Press. https://doi.org/10.17226/13423.

CDC. (2012, January 10). *History of quarantine*. Retrieved from https://www.cdc.gov/quarantine/historyquarantine.html.

City of Monroe, MI. (2018, May 22). *Water department utility imposters*. Retrieved from https://www.monroemi.gov/news/what_s_new/city_of_monroe_water_department_utility_imposters.

Congressional Research Service. (2014, January 10). *Food fraud and "economically motivated adulteration" of food and food ingredients.* Retrieved from https://crsreports.congress.gov/product/pdf/R/R43358/4.

Cybersecurity and Infrastructure Security Agency. (2015). *Food and agriculture sector's 2010 sector specific plan.* FDA, USDA, DHS. Retrieved from https://www.cisa.gov/sites/default/files/publications/nipp-ssp-food-ag-2015-508.pdf.

*Deliberate act cannot be ruled out for Germany's 2011 outbreak.* (2016, March 22). Retrieved from https://www.foodsafetynews.com/2016/03/deliberate-act-cannot-be-rule-out-for-germanys-2011-outbreak/.

Dembek, Z., Pavlin, J., Siwek, M., & Kortepeter, M. (2018). Epidemiology of biowarfare and bioterrorism. In J. Bozue, C. Cote, & P. Glass (Eds.), *Medical aspects of biological Warfare.* Fort Sam Houston, Texas: Office of the Surgeon General Borden Institute US Army Medical Department Center and School Health Readiness Center of Excellence. Retrieved from https://www.cs.amedd.army.mil/borden/FileDownloadpublic.aspx?docid=ca8b9390-4b19-4e75-bb4e-49364ddd61af.

DHS. (2007, February 3). The department of Homeland security's role in food defense and critical infrastructure protection. *Office of Inspector General.* Retrieved from https://www.oig.dhs.gov/assets/Mgmt/OIG_07-33_Feb07.pdf.

DHS. (2008, September). *"DHS risk lexicon." risk steering committee.* Retrieved from https://www.dhs.gov/xlibrary/assets/dhs_risk_lexicon.pdf.

DHS. (2009, November 19). *Critical infrastructure and key resources (CIKR).* Retrieved from https://www.dhs.gov/blog/2009/11/19/cikr.

FBI. (2014, June). Commercial facilities: Food defense awareness and outreach. In *Infrastructure countermeasures unit.* Retrieved from https://www.fbi.gov/file-repository/commercial-facilities-food-defense.pdf/view.

FDA. (2020a). *Prior Notice of imported foods.* Retrieved from https://www.fda.gov/food/importing-food-products-united-states/prior-notice-imported-foods.

FDA. (2007a). *National infrastructure protection plan.* Retrieved from https://www.fda.gov/food/food-defense-programs/national-infrastructure- protection-plan.

FDA. (2007b). *Food protection plan: An integrated strategy for protecting the nation's food supply.* Retrieved from https://www.fda.gov/media/75264/download.

FDA. (2016, May 7). *Mitigation strategies to protect food against intentional adulteration.* Retrieved from https://www.federalregister.gov/documents/2016/05/27/2016-12373/mitigation-strategies-to-protect-food-against-intentional-adulteration.

FDA. (2017, November 28). *Food related emergency exercise Bundle (FREE-B).* Retrieved from https://www.fda.gov/food/food-defense-tools-educational-materials/food-related-emergency-exercise-bundle-free-b.

FDA. (2019a). *Mitigation strategies to protect food against intentional adulteration: Guidance for industry* [Revised Draft Guidance]. Retrieved from https://www.fda.gov/media/113684/download.

FDA. (2019b). *Food protection task force (FPTF).* Retrieved from https://www.fda.gov/federal-state-local-tribal-and-territorial-officials/national-integrated-food-safety-system-ifss-programs-and-initiatives/food-protection-task-force-fptf.

FDA. (2019c). *Rapid response teams (RRTs).* Retrieved from https://www.fda.gov/federal-state-local-tribal-and-territorial-officials/national-integrated-food-safety-system-ifss-programs-and-initiatives/rapid-response-teams-rrts.

FDA. (2019d). *Regulatory associations.* Retrieved from https://www.fda.gov/federal-state-local-tribal-and-territorial-officials/communications-outreach/regulatory-associations.

FDA. (2019e). *New era of smarter food safety*. Retrieved from https://www.fda.gov/food/new-era-smarter-food-safety.

FDA. (2020b). *Food defense*. Retrieved from https://www.fda.gov/food/food-defense.

FDA, DHS, & USDA. (2011). *2011 sector annual report: Food and agriculture*. Retrieved from https://www.fda.gov/media/85846/download.

First assessment of food crime in the UK published. *New Food Magazine*, (2016, March 23). Retrieved from https://www.newfoodmagazine.com/news/23396/food-crime-in-the-uk/.

Food Standards Australia New Zealand. (2018, October). *Report to government: Strawberry tampering incident*. Retrieved from https://www.foodstandards.gov.au/publications/SiteAssets/Pages/Strawberry-tampering-    incident/FSANZ%20Strawberry%20Report%20doc.pdf.

*Food safety enhancement act, H.R.2749, 111th Cong.*(2010).

GlobalSecurityorg. (2011, July 13). *Homeland security: Early warning infectious disease surveillance (EWIDS)*. Retrieved from https://www.globalsecurity.org/security/systems/ewids.htm.

Government of the U.S. Virgin Islands. (2020, January 28). *Beware: Health Inspector Imposters. Individuals posing as health inspectors are targeting restaurants and retail operators in the territory*. Dept. of Health/Division of Environmental Health [Press Release]. Retrieved from https://doh.vi.gov/sites/default/files/Press%20Release%20-%20DEH%20-%20Beware%20Health%20Inspector%20Imposters.pdf.

Jacobson v. Massachusetts, *197 U.S. 11*.(1905).

Kansas State University. (2020, March 26). About the facility and U.S. bio/agrodefense policy. *National Bio and Agro-defense Facility*. Retrieved from https://www.k-state.edu/nbaf/about/.

Merriam-Webster. (n.d.). *Intentional*. Retrieved from http://www.learnersdictionary.com/definition/intentionally.

National Center for Food Protection and Defense. (2011, April 30). *Backgrounder: Defining the public health threat of food Fraud*. St. Paul, Minneapolis. Retrieved from http://foodfraud.msu.edu/wp-    content/uploads/2014/07/food-fraud-ffg-backgrounder-v11-Final.pdf.

Neuman, W., & Sayare, S. (2011, June 29). Egyptian seeds are linked to *E. coli* in Germany and France. *The New York Times*. Retrieved from https://www.nytimes.com/2011/06/30/world/middleeast/30ecoli.html.

Pear, R. (2004, December 4). U.S. Health chief, stepping down, issues warning. *The New York Times*. Retrieved from https://www.nytimes.com/2004/12/04/politics/us-    health-chief-stepping-down-issues-warning.html.

Profita, H. (2006, November 9). Known knowns, known unknowns and unknown unknowns: A retrospective. *CBS News*. Retrieved from https://www.cbsnews.com/news/known-knowns-known-unknowns-and-unknown-unknowns-a-retrospective/.

Radosavljevic, V., Finke, E., & Belojevic, G. (2014). *Escherichia coli* O104:H4 outbreak in Germany-clarification of the origin of the epidemic. *The European Journal of Public Health, 25*(1), 125−129. Retrieved from https://academic.oup.com/eurpub/article/25/1/125/497381.

*Recommendations made in strawberry tampering report*. (2019, February 18). Food Safety News. Retrieved from https://www.foodsafetynews.com/2019/02/recommendations-made-in-strawberry-tampering-report/.

Roos, R. (2001, December 6). *85 million mail items processed at anthrax-contaminated facilities, CDC reports*. University of Minnesota, Center for Infectious Disease Research and

Policy. Retrieved from http://www.cidrap.umn.edu/news-perspective/2001/12/85-million-mail-items-processed-anthrax-contaminated-facilities-cdc-reports.

Siddique, H. (2018, September 17). Strawberry needle sabotage scare spreads to all six Australian states. *The Guardian*. Retrieved from https://www.theguardian.com/australia-news/2018/sep/17/australian-police-say-needle-found-in-banana-as-strawberry-sabotage-spreads.

Somerset, N. J. (2020). *Food safety*. Retrieved from https://www.co.somerset.nj.us/government/public-health-safety/health-department/services/health-education-promotion-wellness/food-safety.

Spink, J. (2013, October). "Economically motivated adulteration: Another dimension of the "expanding umbrella of food defense.". *Food Safety Magazine*. Retrieved from https://www.foodsafetymagazine.com/magazine-archive1/octobernovember-2013/economically-motivated-   adulteration-another-dimension-of-the-e2809cexpanding-umbrella-of-food-defensee2809d/.

The British Standards Institution. (2017, November). *PAS 96:2017 Guide to protecting and defending food and drink from deliberate attack*. Sponsored by the Department for Environment, Food & Rural Affairs (Defra) and the (UK) Food Standards Agency (FSA). Retrieved from https://www.food.gov.uk/sites/default/files/media/document/pas962017_0.pdf.

Török, T., et al. (1997, August 6). A large community outbreak of salmonellosis caused by intentional contamination of restaurant salad bars. *Journal of the American Medical Association, 278*(5). Retrieved from https://www.cdc.gov/phlp/docs/forensic_epidemiology/Additional%20Materials/Articles/Torok%20et%20al.pdf.

USDA. (2009, October). *Food defense guidelines for slaughter and processing establishments*. Retrieved from https://www.fsis.usda.gov/wps/wcm/connect/cd18dfb5-9443-42f8-b8c5-cadf862fcbc4/SecurityGuide.pdf?MOD=AJPERES.

USDA. (2019, December 12). *Food defense overview*. Retrieved from https://www.fsis.usda.gov/wps/portal/fsis/topics/food-defense-and-emergency-response/food-defense-overview.

WHO. (2002). *Food safety issues: Terrorist threats to food — guidance for establishing and strengthening prevention and response systems*. Food Safety Department. Retrieved from https://apps.who.int/iris/bitstream/handle/10665/42619/9241545844.pdf;jsessionid=E81C27869CBDE829D5386C0835 CD5282?sequence=1.

WHO. (2017, May). *Contact tracing*. Retrieved from https://www.who.int/features/qa/contact-tracing/en/.

# Food security and technology

# Food deserts and food insecurity: in tribal lands and from coast to coast

**Darin Detwiler, LP.D**

*Assistant Dean and Associate Teaching Professor, Northeastern University, Founder and CEO of Detwiler Consulting Group, LLC., Boston, MA, United States*

## Introduction

Some who live on the Navajo Nation in northeastern Arizona consider themselves lucky to be living only 25 to 35 miles away from an off-reservation grocery store, as it is not uncommon for others to travel 75 miles (one way) to reach one. On the Navajo Nation, only 13 full-service grocery stores serve its 300,000 inhabitants across its 27,413 square mile land base (Echo Hawk Consulting, 2015)-equivalent to the land size that almost entirely covers the same amount of square miles as in the states of Massachusetts (10,565), New Hampshire (9350), and Vermont (9623) combined (Kreider, 2019).

The USDA's Economic Research Service defines a "Food Desert" as "Low-income census tracts with a substantial number or share of residents with low levels of access to retail outlets selling healthy and affordable foods are defined as food deserts" (Ver Ploeg, Nulph, & Williams, 2011). The USDA also defines how census tracts (small, subdivision of a county inhabited by an average of around 4000 people) qualify as food deserts if they meet low-income and low-access thresholds:

- **Low-income:** "a poverty rate of 20 percent or greater, or a median family income at or below 80 percent of the statewide or metropolitan area median family income";
- **Low-access:** "at least 500 persons and/or at least 33 percent of the population lives more than 1 mile from a supermarket or large grocery store (10 miles, in the case of rural census tracts)" (Ver Ploeg, Nulph, & Williams, 2011).

At least 23.5 million Americans live in food deserts, meaning that they live over one mile from a supermarket and do not own a car (Food Deserts in America, 2018). Food insecurity (aside from simply residing in a food desert) is also of concern as the USDA estimates that 37.2 million people lived in food-insecure households. Some 11.1% of US households without children were food secure throughout 2018, whereas 13.9% of US households with children under age 18 were food secure throughout 2018 (Coleman-Jensen, Gregory, and Rabbitt, 2019).

Building the Future of Food Safety Technology. https://doi.org/10.1016/B978-0-12-818956-6.00011-7

In contrast, national data on indigenous food insecurity indicate that 23% of Native Americans living on reservations in the United States are food insecure, with some of the poorest reservations experiencing levels of 50% or more. Virtually all reservations in the United States qualify as rural food deserts, as defined by the USDA. Further, one survey found that, between 2000 and 2010, 25% of American Indians and Alaskan Natives remained consistently food insecure and they were twice as likely to be food insecure compared to white populations (Jernigan, Huyser, Valdes, and Simonds, 2016).

Food insecurity is strongly correlated with diet-related diseases such as obesity, heart disease, and diabetes. Currently, obesity, diabetes, and heart disease rates in Native American populations are more than double the national average (Kuhnlein & Receveur, 1996; O'Connell, Buchwald, & Duncan, 2011). These issues position the hybrid retail outlet in a vital space where definitions matter. If they are to be defined as restaurants, what are the implications for food safety policies? Targeting food insecurity is a great concern across reservations. If establishments that are serving the populations cannot be clearly defined, then they can neither be adequately regulated nor be measured to get accurate data. The result may be a gap between policy and realistic conditions within communities.

Due to this lack of options, many often stop at convenience "hybrid" stores with seating areas, where they can purchase some staples and eat a quick meal during commutes to and from work. These hybrid retail outlets have grown in environments characterized by high rates of poverty, low economic development, and weak infrastructure. In the absence of supermarkets, they are often the only food outlets within communities.

However, a 2014 study by the Diné Policy Institute found that 70 to 80% of the foods offered in these stores are processed (Diné Policy Institute, 2014). More prevalent than grocery stores, these types of food establishments typically offer a disproportionate amount of processed foods high in sugar, sodium, and saturated fats.

The National Restaurant Association calls these hybrids "retail-host restaurants"- and labels them as one of the fastest growing segments for restaurant food. In contrast, most "traditional" grocery stores, convenience marts, etc., only sell food items, thus are considered "point-of-sale" businesses, while restaurants prepare and serve food items and are, thus, considered "point-of-service" businesses (Flynn, 2016).

Hybrid stores existed earlier in the 20th century (think Woolworth Department Store's lunch counters made famous by the 1960's Civil Rights sit-ins). That trend had died off until now.

Today, the National Restaurant Association's definition of hybrids includes

• Health and personal care store restaurants
• General merchandise/variety store restaurants
• Food store and grocery store restaurants-including deli and salad bars
• Gasoline service station restaurants

Examples include

- Whole Foods Markets with restaurants that offer hot meals, as well as beer and wine service
- Wegmans with full-service pubs

At the same time, these also include

- Corner convenience stores, such as 7-Eleven
- Gas station convenience marts

How big is this trend? Sales by these in-store restaurants in 2015 topped $40 billion. In 2016, hybrids took in about $3 out of every $4 in revenue generated by the retailer. In terms of future development, hybrids are growing at a rate of near 6% per year (Flynn, 2016). Some experts offer that the hybridization of retail/restaurant/and technology can provide "a multi-sensorial experience that goes much further than a mere retail transaction," but also a means to avoid becoming trapped into a sea of store closures (Delgado, 2019).

The gas station convenience marts and even the larger, retail-pub supermarkets offer many challenges in terms of food reputations. Hybrid retail establishments represent a gray area in regulation and policy. As they may be categorized as restaurants or as retail, they therefore fall into different sets of codes and standards, thus the relationship between the government's regulatory roles may cause food safety to slip through the cracks. Another challenge is how these hybrid configurations weaken food defense barriers. In a Native American context, hybrid establishments raise a number of historical, cultural, and political concerns pertaining to food safety and food security-specifically their impacts on food insecurity and indigenous political independence.

Many hybrid retail facilities, however,-especially gas station convenience marts-carry less than one-quarter of the items listed in the USDA's Thrifty Food Plan, which lists the nutritious foods that can be acquired on a budget to make healthy meals (USDA, 2007). Worse, the largest percentages of foods available at these stores fall into the sugar/sweets group.

The unique nature and context of these establishments raise important questions regarding food safety and regulation standards, as well as tribal and US governments' roles. Native American groups are legally designated as sovereign, meaning that they possess the right to operate their own legal, economic, and political systems and deal with other governments in nation-to-nation relationships. These rights, however, need to be viewed as transcending tribal, state, and federal levels.

The Food and Agriculture Organization of the United Nations defined "Food Security" in its 2009 Declaration of the World Food Summit on Food Security as "Food security exists when all people, at all times, have physical, social and economic access to sufficient, safe and nutritious food which meets their dietary needs and food preferences for an active and healthy life" (UN FAO, 2009).

Food security can be viewed through four dimensions:

| | |
|---|---|
| **Access** | The affordability and allocation of food, as well as the preferences of individuals and households. |
| **Availability** | The supply of food through production, distribution, and exchange. |
| **Stability** | The ability to obtain food over time, as food insecurity can be transitory, seasonal, or chronic. Can be impacted by failures in food sustainability, defense, etc. |
| **Utilization** | The metabolism of food by individuals-can be affected by food safety, nutritional values, food choice, and cultural preferences. |

The "Utilization" component of food security very much depends on food safety, quality, and authenticity-including nutritional values, food choice, and cultural preferences. Foods pertaining to modern diets, such as vegan, vegetarian, allergy conscious, impacted immune status, etc., require food authenticity from retailers and their suppliers.

Food deserts and food insecurity exist throughout the United States and are even more prevalent across rural indigenous communities in the United States. Causes are rooted in the intersection of history, politics, economics, culture, and geography, which form a unique environment that has thus far proven minimally responsive to mainstream programmatic and policy solutions. Regulating these hybrid retail outlets while cooperating with local governments and respecting culture will be of the utmost importance because it can potentially open up a new space for collaboration to address issues.

Successful use of RegTech can produce the conditions needed to alleviate food insecurity and food deserts. These technologies can reduce food waste and have the potential to protect populations from foodborne illness through standards compliance. Further, they can help stakeholders ensure that the most accurate data about food security is available to policymakers. Data collection and analytics are only one part of the solution, as food regulation in order to protect people living on reservations needs to place a high priority on respecting their sovereign legal rights and their right to consume traditional foods.

# References

B. Brown, C. Noonan, M. Nord, Prevalence of food insecurity and health-associated outcomes and food characteristics of northern plains Indian households, Journal of Hunger & Environmental Nutrition 1 (4) (2007) 37–53.

A. Coleman-Jensen, C. Gregory, M. Rabbitt, Food security in the U.S, USDA Economic Research Service, 2019, September 4. Retrieved from, https://www.ers.usda.gov/topics/food-nutrition-assistance/food-security-in-the-us/.

J. Delgado, How a hybrid model can help retailers survive the online-shopping trend, Global Trade Magazine (2019, November 29). Retrieved from, https://www.globaltrademag.com/how-a-hybrid-model-can-help-retailers-survive-the-online-shopping-trend/.

Diné Policy Institute, Dine food sovereignty, Diné Policy Institute, Tsaile, AZ, 2014. Retrieved from, https://www.dinecollege.edu/wp-content/uploads/2018/04/dpi-food-sovereignty-report.pdf.

Echo Hawk Consulting, Feeding ourselves: Food access, health disparities, and the pathways to healthy native American communities, Echo Hawk Consulting, Longmont, CO, 2015.

D. Flynn, Retail-host restaurant trend is not without food safety concerns, Food Safety News (2016, April 11). Retrieved from, http://www.foodsafetynews.com/2016/04/retail-host-restaurant-trend-is-not-without-food-safety-concerns/#.Vwun_PkrLIV.

Food Deserts in America, 2018, May 10. Tulane university school of social work. Retrieved from, https://socialwork.tulane.edu/blog/food-deserts-in-america.

V. Jernigan, K. Huyser, J. Valdes, V. Simonds, Food insecurity among American Indians and Alaska Natives: A national profile using the current population survey—food security supplement, Journal of Hunger and Environmental Nutrition. 2017 12 (1) (2016, October 25) 1—10. Retrieved from, https://www.ncbi.nlm.nih.gov/pmc/articles/PMC5422031/.

M. Kreider, 13 grocery stores: The Navajo Nation is a food desert, Planet Forward (2019, December 10). Retrieved from, https://www.planetforward.org/idea/13-grocery-stores-the-navajo-nation-is-a-food-desert.

H.V. Kuhnlein, O. Receveur, Dietary change and traditional food systems of indigenous people, Annual Review of Nutrition 16 (1996) 417—442.

M. O'Connell, D.S. Buchwald, G.E. Duncan, Food access and cost in American Indian communities in Washington state, Journal of the American Dietetic Association 111 (9) (2011) 1375—1379.

United Nations (UN) Food and Agriculture Organization (FAO), Declaration of the world food Summit on food security, 2009. Retrieved from, http://www.fao.org/fileadmin/templates/wsfs/Summit/Docs/Final_Declaration/WSFS09_Declaration.pdf.

U.S. Department of Agriculture, Thrifty Food Plan, 2006, Center for Nutrition Policy and Promotion, 2007, April. Retrieved from, https://fns-prod.azureedge.net/sites/default/files/usda_food_plans_cost_of_food/TFP2006Report.pdf.

M. Ver Ploeg, D. Nulph, R. Williams, Mapping food deserts in the United States, USDA Economic Research Service, 2011, December 1. Retrieved from, https://www.ers.usda.gov/amber-waves/2011/december/data-feature-mapping-food-deserts-in-the-us/.

# The future of nutrition and food security

# 12

**Karen Jensen, MBA, RD**

*Senior Manager of Regulatory & Sustainability, Reily Foods Company, Knoxville, TN, United States*

As we look to the future for food security and technology, specifically within the realm of nutrition, it is first important to define Food Insecurity. According to the United States Department of Agriculture (USDA), **Food Insecurity** is the limited or uncertain ability to acquire acceptable foods in socially acceptable ways. Historically, nutrition has contributed to food security with breakthrough discoveries around vitamins and appropriate fortification of the food supply.

## Dietary guidelines role in public health

Nutrition, in comparison with the other sciences, is relatively young. Our understanding of digestion and macro- and micronutrients continues to evolve. This is evidenced in the fact that potassium and vitamin D were elevated to nutrients of concern and became required inclusions on the nutrition fact panels of US packaged foods as of 2020 while at the same time, vitamins A and C were determined to no longer be nutrients of concern and were pulled from the required nutrients on food labels. Nutrition research is shifting away from single nutrient trials to more comprehensive full diet studies. One way in which nutrition research is translated into public awareness is via the Dietary Guidelines, which are revised every 5 years. Before the Department of Health and Human Services (HHS) and the USDA release each new edition of the Dietary Guidelines, the departments convene an Advisory Committee to review the body of nutrition science. The Advisory Committee is composed of nationally recognized nutrition and medical researchers, academics, and practitioners.

The Committee develops an Advisory Report that is intended to synthesize current scientific and medical evidence in nutrition. HHS and USDA use information in the Advisory Report, along with comments from the public, to inform the new edition of the Dietary Guidelines. As with many government processes, politics plays a role, with the administration in power influencing the regulations. Lobbyists ranging from the National Cattlemen's Meat Board to the Natural Products Association also act to advance their agendas. The Guidelines are used to shape the Food Labeling Requirements and Public Assistance Food Choices and to inform Consumer Nutrition Education campaigns.

Building the Future of Food Safety Technology. https://doi.org/10.1016/B978-0-12-818956-6.00012-9

## The nutrition agenda

Looking to the future, we can expect plant-based foods, sustainable foods, bioengineered foods, nanotechnology foods, and 3D printed foods to be among the key topics on the Nutrition Agenda.

## Plant-based foods

Plant-based foods have broken through to the mainstream in recent years. Not to be confused with vegetarian foods per se, the plant-based movement has focused on replacements for meats, butter, milk, and eggs. For example, the Impossible Burger uses textured wheat protein, coconut oil, potato protein, yeast, soy protein, and gums to achieve a taste and texture similar to that of a ground beef patty. Milk replacements have exploded on the scene with variations of nuts, fruits, and grains as their source. At the same time, dairy milk consumption has dropped off precipitously, leading to bankruptcies within the dairy industry.

The emergence of plant-based products has led to significant litigation activity as the viability of traditional meats and dairy products are challenged. Meat and dairy industry groups have argued that names such as "burger" and "milk" should not be allowed for these replacement products and have called for the Food and Drug Association (FDA) to intervene. With soy milk having been commercially available for over 50 years, it would seem unlikely that the FDA will step forward to defend the use of "milk" or "meat" naming in any meaningful way. Dairy and meat companies that have embraced the plant-based wave rather than fighting it through litigation are now prospering. Danone North America, for example, has a portfolio that includes dairy yogurt as well as plant-based milks and desserts.

While plant-based foods tend to have a positive health halo in the minds of consumers, not all of them have solid nutrition credentials. The inclusion of negative nutrients such as saturated fats, sodium, and simple sugars is, in many cases, higher than that of the product it is intended to replace. *Caveat emptor* applies in this case, with the burden being placed on the consumer to read the label and make an informed decision.

From a public health point of view, the affordability of plant-based foods is initially poor, but improves as market share increases. As the cost of dairy and beef production increases, it is very possible that plant-based foods will become more affordable and provide a meaningful source of protein across all demographics.

## Sustainable food

Sustainable food is a somewhat nebulous term in that society has defined it very broadly across spheres of economics, environment, ethics, culture, and more. Some products purport to be sustainable based on their claim to support a social cause. Others may claim sustainability based on the ethical work conditions employed during manufacturing.

For a more scientific and comprehensive definition of sustainable food, we turn to the United Nations 2030 Agenda for Sustainable Development (UNGA, 2015). This Agenda, adopted in 2015, includes 17 very specific **Sustainable Development Goals** (SDGs). The Agenda was designed to guide the actions of the international community particularly as it relates to addressing poverty and hunger and shifting toward sustainable development by 2030. A focus on rural development and investment in agriculture-crops, livestock, forestry, fisheries, and aquaculture-are considered powerful tools in this Agenda. Specific to food security, the Agenda includes Goal #2: ending World Hunger. According to the USDA, hunger is defined as an individual-level physiological condition that may result from food insecurity (Coleman-Jensen, Gregory, and Rabbitt, 2019).

Amid this concern over world hunger, one might assume that there is not enough food produced today to feed our global population. Many experts hold that there is, in fact, enough food to feed the world population (Erdman, 2018). This highlights the fact that food security is driven by availability, access, and utilization of food. Approximately 98% of people experiencing food insecurity live outside the United States and other developed nations. While the United Nation's Food and Agriculture Organization estimates the number of undernourished people in the world at about 925 million, the largest percentage of those live in Asia and the Pacific Islands, as well as in sub-Saharan Africa (FAO, IFAD, UNICEF, WFP and WHO, 2019).

The World Health Organization holds that, on a global scale, more than 2 billion adults, adolescents, and children are now obese or overweight (WHO, 2018). While some might consider obesity a signal that we are turning the tide of world hunger, the consequences are an enormous drain on economic resources and public health.

Resolving the issue of availability, access, and utilization of food is further complicated by environmental issues of the diminishing availability of arable land; increasing soil degradation; lack of agricultural biodiversity; and more frequent and severe weather events.

Peter Drucker's statement that "you can't improve what you can't measure" applies to this situation. To that end, the UN ties the target of ending Hunger with the specific indicator 2.1.2, Prevalence of moderate or severe food insecurity in the population, based on the Food Insecurity Experience Scale. This scale uses direct interviews to objectively quantify the number of people facing food insecurity as well as the severity.

The food products that score well against the SDGs are those that include crops with excellent pesticide and fertilizer management. Optimized irrigation will become even more important as will the crop's ability to sequester carbon in the soil. Soybeans, for example, have a far greater ability to sequester carbon dioxide than corn or wheat. This allows for the offset of greenhouse gases such as those created in the burning of fossil fuels.

Legislation around carbon is expected to influence the cost and availability of food if and when they are placed into law. A number of Carbon Tax proposals have been put forward in the US Congress-in fact, eight different proposals were introduced in the 116th Congress (2019–20) (Ye, 2019). All provide rebates for emissions that are captured or sequestered. As it relates to the food supply, meat and dairy products have larger carbon footprints per calorie than grains or vegetables. This is largely due to the need for significant cropland to support the animals and the methane produced by their digestive process and manure management. If a carbon tax was applied to the food system, it would potentially increase the cost of meats and dairy products and reduce the costs of grains and vegetables. Meat companies would likely turn to companies that grow high carbon-sequestering crops such as soybeans or grasses to purchase carbon credits. Ideally, this would drive innovation around methane management, animal feed optimization, and other elements of the greenhouse gas equation. For the low-income demographic, this will likely mean that a vegan diet, heavy on the legumes, will continue to be the least expensive option.

It will be interesting to watch the consumption trends of both plant-based and sustainable foods. Science has argued again and again for the merits of a Mediterranean-style diet. The principal aspects of this diet include proportionally high consumption of olive oil, legumes, unrefined cereals, fruits, and vegetables, moderate consumption of fish and dairy products, moderate wine consumption, and low consumption of meat products. Of course, if science were the primary determinant of the human diet, obesity, type II diabetes, and other public health issues would be greatly reduced. Instead, our diets are affected by social media, culture, and other nonscientific factors. It will be up to plant-based food companies to change the consumer perception of a juicy steak or burger versus a plant-based offering on a holistic level. Touting its health benefits will not be enough and may even affect its perception negatively.

## Bioengineered foods

Bioengineered foods will continue to play a key role in food security and nutrition. While bioengineered papaya plants are credited with averting the potential wipeout of the species, consumer perception remains very negative. Golden rice, which is bioengineered to include the precursor of vitamin A could avert childhood blindness in developing countries, yet it continues to meet resistance from rice growers. Critics of bioengineered crops assert that they have led to the widespread use of Monsanto's Roundup product. Roundup has been tied to poor soil health, honeybee die-offs, and some human cancers. In the United States, Non-GMO Project Verified "butterfly" icons pepper the grocery aisles in response to the negative perception of bioengineered foods. In 2019, the USDA established labeling standards that require disclosure for any food product that contains even a trace of recombinant DNA. The threshold is 0%. In Europe, by contrast, the threshold is 0.9% bioengineered content. The US and European production of bioengineered crops vary starkly. In the United States, the majority of corn, soy, and canola produced are bioengineered. In Europe, bioengineered crops have met with significant resistance and remain at less than 10%. Interestingly, the European Union imports more than 30 million tons of bioengineered grain annually.

The disconnect between the need to boost production and overcome plant diseases versus the antibioengineering consumer perception and safety concerns will continue to be a challenge. There is conjecture that bioengineering may be poised to rescue the orange crop from citrus greening and the banana crop from the devastating fungal diseases that it faces. Will the possibility of facing extinction of our beloved oranges or bananas be the event that shifts consumer perception of bioengineered crops?

## Nanotechnology food

Nanotechnology food sounds very "space age" but is actually used within the food industry in limited applications today. Nanomaterials are typically defined as materials smaller than 100 nm (a human hair is approximately 75,000 nm) and have unique properties due to the high surface-to-volume ratio and novel physiochemical properties such as color, solubility, and thermodynamics. An example of nanomaterials being used today is titanium dioxide, which is included in dried coconut and frosting to make them appear more bright white. A number of nanosensors are currently under development with the intention of sensing the gases created when foods spoil so that a sensor strip on the food packaging will change color and alert the consumer to this food safety risk. Zinc and silver nanoparticles are being used in food packaging for their antimicrobial characteristics.

As with any new innovation, there is concern that the science will get ahead of the regulation and consumer safety will be compromised. Specific concerns with nanotechnology are centered around their accumulation within the human body and the elevated use of organic solvents and emulsifiers used to prepare nanocarriers (Yu et al., 2018). If we are able to find the balance between innovation and regulation, nanotechnology may improve food safety and reduce food waste. Companies that plan to include nanotechnology in their products would be wise to get out ahead of consumer perception so that they do not face the backlash seen by bioengineering.

As nanomaterials are designed and tested, the costs will likely remain high. Once economies of scale are reached, cost would be reduced and availability would increase. With that, nanomaterials could begin to have an impact on the reduction of food waste and ultimately contribute to food security. So, while consumers may not see a label that states "Now with nanomaterials!" it is likely that nanomaterials will be incorporated in the food system with an emphasis on their function rather than their name.

## 3D printed foods

3D printed foods have come a long way and are poised to break through to the mainstream. Not surprisingly, NASA has been at the forefront, using 3D printers to make more appealing food for astronauts, such as pizza. The premise of a 3D food printer is similar to that of printers used to create elaborate plastic forms. The extruder is replaced with a syringe system that contains food ingredients. The system is driven by computer-assisted design to create 3D designs more precisely than one could complete by hand (Carlotta, 2019).

The implications for nutrition are vast. Vitamins and minerals can be engineered into foods at optimum levels and with optimum absorption, particularly in the hospital setting. Vegetables can be stealthily included in foods for children. The texture and taste of a single entrée could be personalized for the toddler, diabetic teen, and senior citizen in the family. Fewer preservatives would be incorporated into the food supply as food is printed on demand.

Even more impressive is the potential to reduce food waste with the use of 3D printed foods and thus its contribution to food security. Nontraditional protein sources such as mealworms and crickets could be blended in with more traditional flours to make nutrient-dense, inexpensive doughs. Scraps of fish that are not perfect fillets could become ingredients for other entrées, taking the concept of fish sticks to a whole new level. Perhaps, 3D food printers will be the catalyst that allows sustainable foods to flourish. Lentils and soybean, which have low carbon footprints, could be elevated by the 3D printer to gourmet fare. Algae, which has not found widespread popularity in its current form, could be transformed. Leftovers could be eliminated or curtailed, also reducing food waste.

Currently, the cost of a 3D food printer is cost prohibitive for individuals, but is becoming within reach for high-end bakery operations seeking the perfect cake decor. A lack of understanding of the technology stands in the way of widespread adoption even as prices drop. Of course, the microwave faced the same skepticism and lack of understanding of the technology and today the microwave is ubiquitous.

Despite the dire warnings of Global Hunger, advances in science can be expected to contribute solutions specifically for Food Insecurity. The science of nutrition will continue to evolve, clarifying the optimal macro- and micronutrients and their delivery. Beyond data collection and analysis technologies, those related to plant-based foods, sustainable foods, bioengineered foods, nanotechnology foods, and 3D printed foods are expected to proliferate and increase the food supply and reduce food waste, thus improving food security. It will be critical for regulations to keep up with these new technologies so that consumer safety can be ensured while still fostering innovation. Synergies between these emerging technologies may multiply their benefits, when used effectively.

## References

Carlotta, V. (2019, February 4)). A guide to 3D printed food − revolution in the kitchen? *3D Natives*. Retrieved from https://www.3dnatives.com/en/3d-printing-food-a-new-revolution-in-cooking/.

Coleman-Jensen, A., Gregory, C., & Rabbitt, M. (2019, September 4). Food security in the U.S. *USDA Economic Research Service*. Retrieved from https://www.ers.usda.gov/topics/food-nutrition-assistance/food-security-in-the-us/.

Erdman, J. (2018, February 1). We produce enough food to feed 10 billion people. So why does hunger still exist? *The Medium.* Retrieved from https://medium.com/@jeremyerdman/we-produce-enough-food-to-feed-10-billion-people-so-why-does-hunger-still-exist-8086d2657539.

FAO, IFAD, UNICEF, WFP, & WHO. (2019). The state of food security and nutrition in the world 2019. In *Safeguarding against economic slowdowns and downturns.* Retrieved from http://www.fao.org/3/ca5162en/ca5162en.pdf.

UNGA. (2015, October 21). *Transforming our world: The 2030 Agenda for sustainable development, UNGAOR, 70th Sess, UN doc A/RES/70/1.* Retrieved from https://www.un.org/ga/search/view_doc.asp?symbol=A/RES/70/1&Lang=E.

WHO. (2018, February 16). *Fact sheet: Obesity and overweight.* World Health Organization. Retrieved from https://www.who.int/news-room/fact-sheets/detail/obesity-and-overweight.

Ye, J. (2019, September). Carbon pricing proposals in the 116th congress. *Center for Climate and Energy Solutions.* Retrieved from https://www.c2es.org/document/carbon-pricing-proposals-in-the-116th-congress/.

Yu, et al. (2018). An overview of nanotechnology in food science: Preparative methods, practical applications and safety. *Journal of Chemistry, 2018.* https://doi.org/10.11155/2018/5427978. Article ID 542978.

# Food security's impact from food safety technology and beyond

# 13

**Bridget Sweet, LPD, MS, REHS/RS, CP-FS**

*Executive Director of Food Safety at Johnson & Wales University, President and CEO of Sweet Safe, LLC., Providence, RI, United States*

Within the United States, an overabundance of produced food exists each year. Approximately 40% of food that is produced is not consumed, as the majority of this food is still edible and safe to eat. Concurrently, millions of Americans are food insecure and are unsure of where they might find their next meal. The USDA defined food-insecure households as those that may not be able to guarantee enough food for all members of their household. "Recognizing these facts, efforts to recover and redirect surplus food are on the rise, and businesses, nonprofits, and government agencies are joining the movement to reduce the waste of wholesome food" (Broad Leib et al., 2018). Reducing this waste and recovering the food can potentially feed the hungry as well as reduce the negative effects on the environment. The face of hunger has changed drastically as the American landscape has changed.

Hunger is no longer affiliated with only those who are homeless or unemployed; the face of hunger incorporates millions of working Americans-people who are uncertain as to where they might find their next meal.

> *In the United States, the most prosperous nation on the planet, hunger figures continue to climb as we waste billions of pounds of food annually. More than 50 million Americans-roughly one in six-lived in food-households in 2011. Wasted food prevents needed calories from reaching the mouths of the needy*
>
> **Finn, 2014**

This is not a challenge that is restricted to the United States, as this is a global challenge. The United Nations created 17 SDGs as a plan to address global challenges, with hunger identified in SDG 2 ("Zero Hunger") and food waste identified in SDG 12 ("Responsible Consumption and Production"). The USDA and the EPA announced in September 2015 the crafting of a domestic goal to mirror SDG 12's Target 12.3 in an effort to reduce domestic food loss and waste by half by the year 2030 (EPA, 2019a). This goal would help feed the hungry, save money for businesses, and offer a number of environmental protections.

The reduction of food insecurity has gained significant momentum through increased food donations from a variety of sources. Unfortunately, food operators, who want to implement a food donation program, are often concerned with liability

Building the Future of Food Safety Technology. https://doi.org/10.1016/B978-0-12-818956-6.00013-0

risks, food safety concerns, and/or lack of infrastructure. Technology offers hope as a tool to bridge this gap and increase the access of prepared foods to donation agencies and food banks.

The EPA has long been a leader in the sustainable management of food and, in October 2019, signed a Memorandum of Understanding with FDA, the USDA, and the Food Waste Reduction Alliance (FWRA)-a collaborative effort of the Grocery Manufacturers Association, the Food Marketing Institute (now going by "FMI"), and the National Restaurant Association (Grocery Manufacturers Association, 2019; EPA, 2019c)-to encourage collaboration, outreach, and education regarding food waste within the various sectors of the food system. The EPA demonstrated an innovative use of technology when the agency created an interactive Excess Food Opportunities Map (EPA, 2019b). This interactive map shows the locations of 1.2 million potential generators as well as provides the locations of 4000 potential recipients of excess foods. Food banks and other food donation programs are included as potential recipients, creating a platform for information sharing between generators and recipients.

Prepared food donations are often shrouded in confusion at both the generator level and the recipient level. A study commissioned by the FWRA spanned across three industry segments in the food system-manufacturing, wholesale and retail, and restaurants-to identify potential barriers to food donation and diversion. Across these segments, the commonly identified barriers related to food safety concerns, logistics and storage, liability concerns, regulatory limitations, and transportation of the excess food to the recipient agency. At the food service level, additional concerns about organizational capacity were observed, both internally and externally.

Technology is not a magic bullet that can solve the food donation gap in donating excess foods to food banks and other recipient agencies; however, it has had a profound impact on food donation as a whole. The evolution of automated temperature control systems for cold holding allows for the integrity of the cold chain to be upheld before potential temperature abuse could arise. The ability for these temperature monitoring systems to upload data directly into the cloud allows for greater food safety controls. Agencies are more likely to accept food that has been prepared if they have the proper food safety logs in place to assure that the food has been handled properly. Regulatory concerns related to safe food handling can also be addressed through this type of temperature logging system. Coupled with the food safety risks, the perception of liability is a constant fear for many operators while making the decision to donate prepared foods.

In 1996, President Clinton signed the Bill Emerson Good Samaritan Food Donation Act (2 USC 1791) into law, to protect good faith food donors from civil and criminal liability in the event that the recipient fell ill after consuming the product. This federal law also provides protection to donors that crossed state lines. In theory, this law would negate the concerns of liability; however, many operators are still hesitant. The Harvard Food Law and Policy Innovation Clinic created state-specific food waste fact sheets to address these concerns, and they are excellent resources while navigating and implementing a food donation program. While not derived from technology, the ease of access to these fact sheets through technology is a net positive to increasing food diversion and donation.

Access to this information is critical in creating a food donation program, whether to a food bank or other recipient organization. Food safety must be a pillar in crafting a program; however, logistical challenges must also be addressed. Storage of surplus and excess foods is a challenge within operations. Space is a valuable commodity in the restaurant industry, and there is simply never enough. Storage concerns also transcend cold holding, or dry storage; quality also comes into play. Food that is intended for donation should still be wholesome and treated within the parameters of the FDA Model Food Code. While the use of technology to address logistical challenges related to incorporating a food donation program is in its infancy, the returns are high, both for food banks and operators. According to the "The Business Case for Reducing Food Loss and Waste" (Hanson and Mitchell, 2017), the return on investment is high. The nonfinancial net positives-corporate social responsibility, community engagement, environmental sustainability, and ethical responsibility-are coupled with the financial net positives creating a demand for safe food donation practices. Research has demonstrated that every single dollar a firm spends on food waste reduction creates a potential for a 14 dollar return on investment (Hanson & Mitchell, 2017).

Technology is vital in bridging the gap between surplus food and those who are food insecure. The operational challenge of not wanting to store food for an extended period of time has been addressed through a variety of applications and web-based systems, designed to connect the generator with a recipient agency. The EPA's Excess Food Opportunities Map is a great first step in identifying stakeholders and partners, to be enhanced by additional technological advances.

At the operator level, technology programs exist to track food waste. These programs are instrumental in educating the staff in the awareness of food waste and surplus foods and allow for potential source reduction. These programs also have the ability to support food donation programs. **Lean Path** and **Phood Solutions** are technology-based programs that can be used to weigh and track food waste. Through the use of these metrics, culinarians can make more informed decisions, as well as redirect unwanted meals to those in need.

While Lean Path and Phood Solutions are "back of house" technology tools, a myriad of options exist for connecting operators to food banks, including

- **Spoiler Alert**
- **Food Donation Connection**
- **We Don't Waste**
- **Food For Free**
- **Matching Excess and Need for Stability Database**

These programs facilitate availing excess foods to a variety of programs, such as food banks, soup kitchens, and other emergency feeding agencies. Donors are now able to list their excess food items on various platforms and connect with local soup kitchens, pantries, and food banks in the area. Through these platforms, the donor agencies are notified in real time and have the capability to claim the food and arrange for the food to be picked up.

**Spoiler Alert** is a business to business platform that manages inventory and cross-functional performance metrics to increase efficiency. Through this platform, food donation is facilitated and data are tracked to optimize the potential tax incentive that may occur through food donation. **Food Cowboy** is another program that is rooted in technology and allows for efficient communication between food donors and recipient organizations. This platform links those working with large volumes of edible but rejected food items to recipient organizations, while tabulating the potential tax incentive. Programs such as Spoiler Alert and Food Cowboy allow operators to recoup the tax incentive and redistribute food in a timely manner allowing the operator to keep their focus on their customer base.

The use of technology can be found broadly throughout the food system from farm to fork, and freight management, satellite tracking, remote sensing of temperature, and global positioning systems are all common. Food banks and other recipient organizations, however, are not using technology in the same manner as they have a different bottom line: they are attempting to feed the hungry, not gain a competitive advantage. The technology that is already in place in the food systems is captured and supported through some of the previously mentioned platforms and web-based systems to bridge the data gap and ultimately increase donations. One of the main reasons why food goes to waste is due to insufficient space and refrigeration at recipient agencies. This challenge is addressed through the use of technology as recipient agencies may receive real-time notifications for what food is available. They can make an informed decision to contact the surplus food source and intend to receive the food or not. An additional reason for food waste is that the operator cannot justify the cost of transportation or onsite holding of the food products. This is also addressed through the various applications that enable real-time notifications from the operator to the recipient agencies.

**Food Rescue US** app provides an on-demand portal for various components of the food recovery system. The technology and ease of use allows for the donor to provide the information, making it possible for the available foods to go to those in need. Ease of use is extremely important from the operator's perspective due to the competing priorities that exist in a restaurant. Through the Food Rescue US app, volunteers can enter their scheduling preferences and schedule transfers of food bridging the logistical gap of transportation and onsite holding.

Technology is instrumental in allowing access to food banks and other recipient agencies. Food waste occurs due to capacity and storage limitations, transportation limitations, and recall limitations, all of which can be addressed through technology advances within the food system. Social media also plays a role in the technological realm of food donation to food banks. Social media refers to "a group of Internet-based applications which build on the ideological and technological foundations of Web 2.0, and which allow the creation and exchange of User Generated Content" (Kaplan and Haenlein, 2010). Feeding America, the largest hunger relief organization in the country, piloted surveys through social media in their efforts to understand gaps in the foods supplied to their clients. Feeding America continues to develop their platform and delivery models with social impacts and technology as driving forces. Feeding America's designed their **MealConnect program** with Google.org and created streamlined interactions, a free and intuitive online platform and has over 2500 hunger relief organizations onboard.

According to Abraham Maslow's "hierarchy of needs," people are motivated by certain needs and some needs take precedence over others. The physiological needs are based on the biological requirements for survival, of which food falls into this category. Maslow theorized that if these physiological needs are not met, the human body cannot function properly (Maslow, 1943). Millions of Americans are facing challenges of food security and run the risk of not functioning properly, all while 40% of food produced is discarded. Ethically, wasted food and food waste have a significant impact on businesses, and food insecurity has been identified as a national public health concern (Gundersen and Ziliak, 2015).

While food safety technology has proven its potential in reducing some food waste, more innovation is still needed to reduce food insecurity. Redirecting excess food will help bridge the gap of food security and better optimize the potential for the millions of Americans who are struggling with food insecurity. Technology and the desire for social impact will continue to refine and improve the food donation paradigm, delivering safe wholesome food to those in need.

## References

Broad Leib, E., Chan, A., Hua, A., Neilson, A., & Sanders, K. (2018, March). Food safety regulations and guidance for food donations. *Harvard Law School, Center for Health Law and Policy Innovation*. Retrieved from https://www.chlpi.org/wp-content/uploads/2013/12/50-State-Food-Regs_March-2018_V2.pdf.

EPA. (2019a). *United States 2030 food loss and waste reduction goal*. Retrieved from https://www.epa.gov/sustainable-management-food/united-states-2030-food-loss-and-waste-reduction-goal.

EPA. (2019b). Excess Food Opportunities Map. *Sustainable Management of Food*. Retrieved from https://www.epa.gov/sustainable-management-food/excess-food-opportunities-map.

EPA. (2019c). Memorandum of Understanding Among [EPA], [FDA], [USDA], and the Founding Partners of the Food Waste Reduction Alliance relative to a federal government and non-government Organization formal collaboration on industry education and engagement with respect to the importance of food waste reduction. Retrieved from https://www.epa.gov/sites/production/files/2019-10/documents/signed_food_waste_mou.pdf.

Finn, S. (2014). Valuing our food: minimizing waste and optimizing resources. *Zygon, 49*, 992−1008. https://doi.org/10.1111/zygo.12131

Grocery Manufacturers Association. (2019). *Food Waste Reduction Alliance*. Retrieved from https://foodwastealliance.org/.

Gundersen, C., & Ziliak, J. P. (2015). Food insecurity and health outcomes. *Health Affairs, 34*(11), 1830−1839. https://doi.org/10.1377/hlthaff.2015.0645

Hanson, C., & Mitchell, P. (2017). *The business case for reducing food loss and waste*. Washington, DC: Champions 12.3.

Kaplan, A., & Haenlein, M. (2010). Users of the world, unite! the challenges and opportunities of Social Media. *Business Horizons, 53*(1), 59—68. https://doi.org/10.1016/j.bushor.2009.09.003

Maslow, A. (1943). A theory of human motivation. *Psychological Review, 50*(4), 370—396. Retrieved from https://psycnet.apa.org/record/1943-03751-001.

## Further reading

*Food Cowboy*. https://www.foodcowboy.com/.

*Food Rescue US*. https://foodrescue.us/.

*Lean Path*. https://www.leanpath.com/.

*MealConnect. (Feeding America.)* https://mealconnect.org/.

*Matching Excess and Need for Stability (MEANS) Database*. https://www.meansdatabase.com/.

*Phood Solutions*. https://www.phoodsolutions.com/.

*Spoiler Alert*. https://www.spoileralert.com/.

# Food authenticity and technology

# Food safety starts with authenticity

# 14

**Darin Detwiler, LP.D**

*Assistant Dean and Associate Teaching Professor, Northeastern University, Founder and CEO of Detwiler Consulting Group, LLC., Boston, MA, United States*

While the investigation and reporting of foodborne illnesses by government agencies and health departments are critical in the prevention of foodborne disease, postincident investigation and reporting are, however, only *reactionary* steps, whereas authentication-the positive identification of authentic food ingredients-should be seen as a key *proactive* element of mitigating risks to public health.

Though our food supply has become global and though we benefit from advances in food manufacturing, food distribution, and food policies, the approach to keeping our food safe and abundant has been rather spotty. Different approaches have been developed at different times, although not enough has been done to coordinate these different approaches into one harmonized and standardized system for the entire world.

Consumers assume that food makers determine whether or not their ingredients are authentic. The ability to determine food authenticity starts with defining food. The approach to defining food must be consistent and emanate from one single, recognized, global source. Once the definitions for each different kind of food are published, then existing technologies can be applied and new technologies can be developed to detect inauthenticity.

With a definitive and agreed upon definition as to the composition of each different kind of food ingredient in the world, trade can be enhanced, new food sources can be developed, and demand can be satisfied. Food authenticity aims to provide assurance that foods are as they are advertised. Food authenticity does not focus on the ethical, economic gains, or intents behind the act. Further, the construct of an authenticity approach is attached to a much earlier point in time from farm to fork.

Building the Future of Food Safety Technology. https://doi.org/10.1016/B978-0-12-818956-6.00014-2

## Food Fraud (as it pertains to authenticity)

Food Fraud includes economically motivated, intentional criminal activities associated with food authenticity.

- According to FSSC-0-005.1, **"Food Fraud Prevention"** is defined as "The process to prevent food and feed supply chains from all forms of economically motivated, intentional adulteration that might impact consumer health" (Spink 2016).
- The 2011 FDA Food Safety Modernization Act ("FSMA") (Pub.L. 111–353, 124 STAT 3885), final rule for **Mitigation Strategies to Protect Food Against Intentional Adulteration** (2020) discusses Mitigation Strategies to Protect Food Against Intentional Adulteration as being

> *… aimed at preventing **intentional adulteration** from acts intended to cause wide-scale harm to public health, including acts of terrorism targeting the food supply. Such acts, while not likely to occur, could cause illness, death, economic disruption of the food supply absent mitigation strategies.*

- The National Center for Food Protection and Defense defines seven different dimensions of "Food Fraud" (National Center, 2011; Spink, 2009):
  - **Adulteration**: Mixing matter of an inferior and sometimes harmful quality with food intended to be sold. As a result, it becomes impure and unfit for human consumption. (A.K.A. Dilution.)
  - **Tampering**: Legitimate product and packaging are used in a fraudulent way. (A.K.A. Misbranding.)
  - **Overrun**: Legitimate product is made in excess of production agreements.
  - **Theft**: Legitimate product is stolen and passed off as legitimately procured.
  - **Diversion**: The sale or distribution of legitimate products outside of intended markets.
  - **Simulation**: One product is designed to look like a real, labeled product. (A.K.A. Substitution.)
  - **Counterfeiting**: Intellectual Property Rights infringement: fraudulent product/packaging.

Food Fraud risks demand vigilant actions to protect authenticity, and thus brand reputation. Impact on public health typically takes place long before any regulator or court will determine whether an act is intentional, economically motivated, or worse. The FDA's (now former) Deputy Commissioner for Foods and Veterinary Medicine, Stephen Ostroff, M.D., stated at a 2016 food industry conference, that the FDA will only focus on Food Fraud when it affects food safety (Ostroff, 2106). Unfortunately, before any fraudulent or other intentional act gains classification is when such acts are identified-typically after public health threats have become a reality. As a result, regulators must focus on authenticity to (as FSMA's mission states) "reduce risk of illness attributed to food from facilities subject to preventive controls rule under the act" (Milazzo, 2015).

Specific sections of FSMA focus on improving "capacity to detect and respond to food safety problems," and "the safety of imported foods," but, perhaps more importantly, the "capacity to prevent food safety problems." Authenticity is a key component of FSMA's mission beyond the intentional adulteration rule, including both preventive controls rules and even the foreign supplier verification rules.

The future of food safety technology-in terms of food authenticity-includes the need to provide for a technology-enabled workforce that is able to more effectively detect, prevent, and respond to all concerns regardless of their label. As many food authenticity matters are initially identified as a food safety issues, the role of technology in any form must not be considered in a silo for any one food concern.

# References

FDA. (2020, February 13). *FSMA final rule for mitigation strategies to protect food against intentional adulteration.* Retrieved from https://www.fda.gov/food/food-safety-modernization-act-fsma/fsma-final-rule-mitigation-strategies-protect-food-against-intentional-adulteration.

Milazzo, D. (2015, April 23). Report from preventive controls team for FSMA implementation. In *The FDA Food Safety Modernization Act: Focus on implementation for prevention-oriented food safety standards public meeting. Presentation for FDA, Washington, DC.*

National Center for Food Protection and Defense. (2011, April 30). *Backgrounder: Defining the public health threat of food fraud.* Retrieved from http://foodfraud.msu.edu/wp-content/uploads/2014/07/food-fraud-ffg-backgrounder-v11-Final.pdf.

Ostroff, S. (2016, November). FDA's take on criminal liability. In *Plenary session and town meeting conducted at the food safety consortium, Schaumburg, IL.*

Spink, J. (2009). Defining food fraud & the chemistry of the crime. In *Presented at FDA public meeting: Economically motivated adulteration. College Park, MD.* Retrieved from http://www.fda.gov/NewsEvents/MeetingsConferencesWorkshops/ucm163619.htm.

Spink, J. (2016, December 23). *FFI report: Review − new FSCC 22000 version 4 regarding food fraud and food defense.* Michigan State University Food Fraud Initiative. Retrieved from http://foodfraud.msu.edu/wp-content/uploads/2016/12/MSU-FFTT-FFIR-FSSC-22000-update-Edition-4-2017-v8-b.pdf.

# Food authenticity in the wine industry

**Mira Rodgers, MS**

*Enologist at Courtside Cellars, LLC., San Luis Obispo, California, United States*

## Introduction

When looking back on the food and beverage industry, the origin of the first alcohol is a common argument. Was it wine, Tapai, beer, vodka? Although studies indicate that it was Tapai, many of these alcoholic alternatives seem to have been around forever. The oldest winery was found by a University of California Davis research team dating back to 4100 B.C. in an Ancient Armenian cave with evidence of a wine press, storage vessels, and grape residue (Owen, 2011). Wine has been a prevalent part of the food and beverage industry and authenticity is a common concern.

Since the US Constitution's 21st Amendment 1933 repeal of Prohibition in the United States (brought about through the 18th Amendment, 1919), wine regulations have evolved to protect consumers and prevent deception. The evolution of premium wine, as opposed to wines commonly referred to as "Two-buck Chucks," further affirmed the need for renewed regulations to protect the authenticity of wines as depicted on the label. Several instances have occurred with people attempting to take advantage of the regulatory system by falsifying information to increase revenue by either cutting costs or claiming higher value wines. Along with other segments of the food and beverage industry, it is impossible to verify every ingredient, claim, and/or percent in every finished wine product in the market. Although the Food and Drug Administration (FDA), The US Department of the Treasury's Alcohol and Tobacco Tax and Trade Bureau (TTB), United States Department of Agriculture (USDA), and other regulatory bodies would like to stand behind the labels, claims, and source verification of every product distributed in the United States, food quality incidents indicate that there is still a gap to bridge.

The quality of the wines we bring home are usually linked to the appellation of vineyards, production site of the wine, grape varieties used, and claims made on the label. The laws that regulate the production, importation, wholesale business, labeling, and advertising of alcohol all fall under the TTB. These regulations are based on United States Code: Federal Alcohol Administration Act, 27 U.S.C. §§ 201-211 (Suppl. 1 1934). The importance of regulating these claims is most easily seen when we step into the wine aisle at our local grocery store. When selecting a bottle

*Building the Future of Food Safety Technology.* https://doi.org/10.1016/B978-0-12-818956-6.00015-4

**147**

of wine, many people look for names on the label that they recognize such as Napa Valley, Dry Creek Valley, and Monterey County. These names instill a sense of quality and luxury in a brand and are dependent on certain appellations as defined either by the TTB or county lines that denote an expectation when handling the grapes and the ultimate finished wine product.

The federal government has struggled to prosecute wine fraud with incidents dating back to the 1970s in cases such as those involving Almaden Winery, Bavaro Brothers, Louis A Feliciano's Chateau Mouton Rothschild, and Jeffery Hill. Almaden Winery claims their vineyards are the first planted in California when their founder came over from France in 1852. In 1974, the winery was fined the largest ever-recorded sum of $250,000 up until that point in time for falsifying the wine labels on 28,000 cases of wine sold to airlines (Dinkelspiel, 2015b). In the 1980s, the Bavaro brothers played an active role in a scheme to take advantage of the heavily demanded yet diminishing supply of Chardonnay and Zinfandel in the San Joaquin Valley in 1987 (Berger, 1989). Working with Michael Liccardi, a wine broker, they harvested Carignane and Valdepena grapes and sold them as zinfandel grapes (Dinkelspiel, 2015b). During the same time, another man, Fred Franzia, decided to capitalize on the expanding market by also selling "zinfandel" grapes by using zinfandel grape leaves to cover incoming lots and falsifying field tags, which are filled out by growers to provide information for certification from the California Department of Food and Agriculture. In the end, the California Department of Food and Agriculture and TTB worked together and built a case with over "twenty civil and criminal lawsuits against Delicato, its president, Anthony Indelicato, the Bavaro brothers, Michael Licciardi, Fred Franzia, Bronco Wines, D. Papagni Fruit Co., and others" (Dinkelspiel, 2015b).

In 1982, Louis A. Feliciano commissioned Chateau Mouton Rothschild label wallpaper, then cut labels to relabel 40 cases of wine. Instances like these have emerged various times throughout the short history of the wine industry in the United States ranging from falsifying grape varieties, alcohol content, and label information. One of the most recent scandals to hit the market occurred in Napa, California, when Mr. Jeffrey James Hill, a winemaker and vineyard manager was charged with eight counts of fraud in 2015 including falsifying labels and vineyard tags and mail fraud (Goel, 2015a,b). With incidents like these in the local news, consumers may question the allure of buying expensive bottles of wine from areas like Sonoma's Dry Creek and Napa Valley when cheaper alternatives are readily available from their local grocery store and not care as much about the label claims. Why spend extra money on a product that may not be as exclusive and personal as it may seem? As an impacted industry with over 500 wineries in Napa alone and more competition from beer, spirits, and most recently, marijuana, it is critical to identify sources of unease and provide a product that is reliable, eye-catching, and matches price-quality expectations of the consumer.

## Background

Many regulations have helped shape the wine industry today with many of them stemming from United States Code: Federal Alcohol Administration Act, 27 U.S.C. §§ 201-211 (Suppl. 1 1934) signed into law by President Roosevelt to regulate alcohol production post The Prohibition. The overall mission of the FAA Act is to ensure the integrity of the industry, protect the consumers, and prevent unfair trade. Today, the Alcohol and Tobacco Tax and Trade Bureau (TTB), created in January of 2003 after the reorganization of the Bureau of Alcohol, Tobacco, and Firearms under The Homeland Security Act of 2002, 6 U.S.C. ch. 1 § 101 116 Stat. 2135 (2002) now oversees the act of ensuring the provisions of the FAA Act (TTB, 2018). With regulations surrounding Certificate of Label Approval/Exemption or COLAs, American grape variety names, fact review methods, production specification, and more, there have been greater strides toward better regulations to protect both consumers and the wine industry (TTB, 2017).

In 1976, premium wines were recognized in the US wine market after the notorious Paris Tasting at the school L'Arcadé mie du Vin, where French and Napa wines were compared in a blind tasting by a panel of French wine experts (Lukacs, 1996). The US market, once dominated by table wines and imports, had its very own, internationally recognized winemaking gem: Napa Valley. With increased focus on the premium wine industry, the TTB issued the requirement for labels to include the appellation in 1978 (TTB, 2017). A typical wine label conveys four main pieces of information to the consumer: a producer or brand name, the grape variety, geographic origin of a majority of the grapes, and the vintage year (although this may not always be included in lower tiered wines). Wine consumers make purchase decisions based on a multitude of factors including three primary product identifiers: brand, origin, and grape variety or style, with an optional fourth as the points or ratings assigned by respected wine experts such as Robert Parker.

This issue certainly is not unique to California's Napa Valley, or even the United States. Within Europe, wine is produced in many countries including Spain, Italy, and, the most prominent of all, France. The Bordeaux region of France is world renowned for its prominent and exclusive wines. With a much older history in wine than California, France and the other European nations have been fighting this battle since the beginning of the 18th century. Starting with defining grape growing boundaries and preventing the use of the names of these growing regions on any grapes grown outside of the designated lines. By the early 1900s, of course, people began trying to take advantage of these regulations and Europe was faced with fraudulence in the industry. Since then, France has passed several laws starting in 1905 for labeling wine bottles and subsequent laws in 1919, 1927, and 1935 to designate the well-known French appellations (Maher, 2001). These laws are critical to wineries in France, Napa, and across the globe for two main reasons according to Maher (2001): "the creation of a distinctive product identifier and the assurance to the consumer of the authenticity of products bearing that identifier" (Maher, 2001, p. 3).

As mentioned earlier, improper labeling in the United States occurred as early as the 1980s with the Bavaro brothers when they took part in a scheme to take advantage of the heavily demanded yet diminishing supply of Chardonnay and Zinfandel in the San Joaquin Valley in 1987 (Berger, 1989). A major portion of this demand came from the introduction of white zinfandel for which sales skyrocketed when entered into the market thereby bolstering California wine sales. This was a result of Bob Trinchero's accidental blush wine in 1975 when the normal fermentation process took an unexpected turn that he decided to bottle anyway (Dinkelspiel, 2015b). By 1987, Trinchero was selling two million cases of what was called "White Zin," and the wine industry quickly followed with almost 125 other wineries in California introducing their own version of the new phenomenon into the market (Dinkelspiel, 2015b). As expected, the demand for the zinfandel grape caused rapid inflation of the zinfandel grape prices. It did not take long for one gentleman to set up a grape selling scheme. Michael Liccardi, a wine broker, recruited two grape growing brothers to harvest Carignane and Valdepena grapes and sell them as zinfandel grapes.

The red grape varieties with tight clusters, small berries, and thick skins could easily be mistaken for one another, especially when arriving in the dark early hours of morning along with assurances from one of the most prominent wine brokers in the state (Dinkelspiel, 2015b). During the same period, Fred Franzia, decided to capitalize on the expanding market by also selling fake "zinfandel" grapes by using zinfandel grape leaves to cover incoming lots and falsifying field tags, which are filled out by growers to provide information to the California Department of Food and Agriculture and TTB, known at that time as the ATF. The bravado of Franzia and Liccardi, along with others, that openly bragged about it triggered many complaints from frustrated people to both the California Department of Food and Agriculture and TTB. Both agencies had to work together to crack the counterfeit ring. By the early 1990s, Steven Lapham, a US Attorney's Office employee, along with a team of agents working in the vineyards of the Central Valley and California state prosecutors, had built over "twenty civil and criminal lawsuits against Delicato (Napa Winery), its president, Anthony Indelicato, the Bavaro brothers, Michael Licciardi, Fred Franzia, Bronco Wines, D. Papagni Fruit Co., and others" (Dinkelspiel, 2015b). All persons charged were either convicted or plead guilty to the charge and paid fines as retribution for their crimes.

Wines can also see a dramatic variation in price based on appellation. Appellations can be defined by political boundaries, like county lines, or federally recognized regions known as American Viticultural Areas, or AVAs (Wine Institute, 2005—18). To make these appellation claims on wine labels wineries must follow the associated TTB regulations. For a winery to claim a wine under a certain AVA, at least 85% of the grapes must be from within that defined region. When claiming a county, the regulation requires at least 75% of the grapes originated within the politically established county lines. To make matters even more complicated, these percentages change based on estate claims or others that can be made as well. Within the wine industry there are certain AVAs and counties that elicit a more prestigious reaction than others. For instance, many consumers may recognize high-end bottles of wine based on appellation names like Sonoma County, Napa Valley, and Alexander Valley. A higher price tag for wines produced in these well-known appellations is justified by the higher quality of the grapes and finished products.

Based on claims related to appellation and variety, grapes can be sold at very different price points. Verification of the claims are mainly supported by the aforementioned field tags required by the regulation bodies. Although any system is vulnerable, especially in the hands of those willing to bend the rules, sometimes there is little that can be done by the regulators, except wait and watch for evidence as they did in some instances in the 1990s. Wines from more prestigious AVAs or those that utilize certain winemaking techniques usually fall into a higher price bracket. It is important to keep this in mind as these distinctions are what define wine classifications ranging from value products, or two-buck chucks, to luxury wines that are typically priced at 50 dollars or more per bottle with other pricing segments in between (See Table 1).

Since 1980, we have seen a dramatic increase in the consumption of wine in the United States (McMillan, 2018). The 2018 State of the Wine Industry Report indicated that in 1993, the United States hit a record high with the consumption of 370 million gallons of wine annually that gradually increased to the current 770 million gallons we see today. But this rapid growth is not translated across all pricing segments of wine. Specifically, in premium wine sales, a steady decrease has been seen within the industry with the changing market dynamics, sales practices, and direct-to-consumer experiences (McMillan, 2018). Market dynamics are influenced by changing consumers, consumer demands, and alternative beverage or similar options. Sale practices and direct-to-consumer experiences focus on winery sales and how-to best target certain consumers. Similar experiences can also be seen in the industry as a result of access to information and discussion platforms, like those we see in the food industry. For example, the Chipotlé outbreaks of 2015—17 almost destroyed the Chipotlé Mexican Grill franchise as well as affecting many other Mexican restaurants in the industry as people were instantly alerted of issues through social media, blogs, and other points of communication along the Internet. These changes in the market will be important to follow in order to monitor consumer trends and maintain a positive image in the public eye.

**Table 1** Wine segments and typical price ranges.

| Wine segment | Typical pricing |
| --- | --- |
| Value | <$10 |
| Popular | $10–$15 |
| Premium | $15–$20 |
| Super premium | $20–$30 |
| Ultra premium | $30–$50 |
| Luxury | >$50 |

Table by author, based on information from Puckette, M. (2016, April 29). Reality of wine prices (what you get for what you spend). Retrieved from: http://winefolly.com/update/reality-of-wine-prices-what-you-get-for-what-you-spend.

The importance of these key components of the wine industry can be demonstrated through the case of Jeffry James Hill. The Napa Valley winemaker and vineyard manager was charged with several allegations to include misrepresenting wines and grapes, such as Napa Valley Cabernet; falsifying documentation; diverting grapes; and falsifying labels. Mr. Hill's gross deception for the regulations illustrates the current gaps in the industry regulations that must be addressed. By claiming a more prestigious AVA, Hill was able to sell his grapes and wine at a much higher price point. He also stole grapes from a winery called Del Dotto in Napa's Oakville AVA and sold them to a winery called Don Sebastiani & Sons. Due to the misrepresentation of the grapes, the Don Sebastiani & Sons company was forced to recall its wine on account of mislabeling causing about three million dollars' worth of damage. Similar to the incidents reviewed from the 1990s, Hill falsified field tags and documentation to change not only grape regions but also the grape varieties themselves. He was finally charged with four counts of wire fraud and four counts of mail fraud (Goel, 2016). It is reassuring to see the law take action against people who try to take advantage of the system, but there is still much more to be done.

## Challenges

Many people believe the wine industry is lagging far behind the food industry in terms of quality and safety, but there are unique attributes to the wine industry that sets it apart. Napa Valley was put on the map in 1976 at a world-renowned Judgment of Paris when California wines competed at the same levels as French wines in a blind tasting. As a result of the case of falsifying wine labels, first and foremost it will have a direct effect on the wineries such as Del Dotto and Don Sebastiani & Sons who saw a direct hit to not only their wine production but also their brand image as a result of lost product and recalls. The devastation would have been greater for small family wineries, but there is something that the wine industry has come to depend on, especially in Napa Valley: teamwork.

Napa Valley wine industry members realized something in 1976 in France: wineries are more likely to succeed together. Although some of these incidents could have proved detrimental to the wineries themselves or the Napa reputation, through the camaraderie and support of fellow industry members wineries create their own control system. In every industry, people will always try to take advantage of the system like Hill or Liccardi did, but by supporting the Napa Valley name by supporting one another has bolstered the quality and authenticity of the wines from the region. Napa Valley, where the majority of California fraudulence occurred, is still recognized globally as a prestigious wine region. Wine producers have trust in the support networks they have created and therefore see the threat of authenticity and falsification in the industry as less impactful than consumers (Table 2, Bateman, 2010). This is not necessarily a bad thing, but a sign of the cooperative nature that the wine industry maintains.

**Table 2** When observing the impact based on producer versus consumer insight, we can see a difference in reactions. While consumers feel a moderate to considerable impact is present across the industry, producers seem to believe that there is little to no impact (19/08, 2010).

| Area of impact | Do not know | | No impact | | Very little impact | | Moderate impact | | Considerable impact | |
|---|---|---|---|---|---|---|---|---|---|---|
| | Prod | Cons | Prod | Cons | Prod | Cons | Prod | Cons | Prod | Cons |
| Profitability | 18% | 3% | 42% | 10% | 26% | 38% | 13% | 35% | 0% | 13% |
| Reputation | 18% | 2% | 24% | 5% | 18% | 12% | 11% | 47% | 29% | 35% |
| Liability issues | 21% | 8% | 32% | 12% | 16% | 27% | 13% | 32% | 18% | 22% |
| Ability to set prices | 18% | 7% | 45% | 20% | 21% | 33% | 11% | 25% | 5% | 15% |
| Demand for rare/cult wines | 18% | 5% | 29% | 20% | 26% | 28% | 21% | 30% | 5% | 17% |

*Prod, Producer findings; Cons, Consumer findings.*

Over time, wine fraud has the potential to impact both finished products and winery tasting rooms, especially in prestigious appellations such as Napa and even across the globe, but currently it seems to have minimal impact. The key to understanding why lies with how the wine industry is different from others within the food and beverage category in two main aspects: consumer knowledge varies drastically and recalls are typically not safety related. In the food market, foods are produced to promote consistency that consumers associate with the foods. For instance, consumers know exactly how milk is supposed to taste when purchased and if sour that is a clear indicator to consumers that something is wrong with the item purchased. Most items in the food industry must uphold certain consumer expectations, while wine on the other hand is different. Each wine is made to be different and different wines seem to personify different characters, so identifying something as defective becomes a little more difficult. Some winemaking styles utilize oxidation resulting in aldehydic wines that exhibit bruised apple, sherry, and nutty attributes others enjoy the impact of Brettanomyces in their wines which can translate to band-aid, meaty, and barnyard characteristics. Many winemakers and consumers may identify these attributes as negative in wine. There is such variation in style, vintage, and varietal that it is difficult to identify an outlier as a defect or just unappealing.

Most consumers in the industry seem to understand wine on a basic level. They like white wines or red wines or maybe even certain varietals but are indifferent to other attributes that distinguish premium wine from luxury wine. If they open a bottle of wine that they do not fully enjoy, they are likely to dump the bottle down the drain with a possible complaint to the local store and infrequently to the winery. Vivid wine drinkers are unlikely to differentiate if the grape came from Napa Valley or the Central Valley, for example. More importantly, it may or may not generalize that wine brand to a region as many other factors can affect the quality of the final product such as shipment and storage. The same is true for the casual wine consumer, which represents the majority, that their criteria for wine selection is based on the price, region, and attractiveness of the label. Consumers, regardless of their wine enthusiasm, have faith in the wine industry perhaps due to the limited occurrence of fraudulent activity, limited exposure, and most importantly, limited safety implications.

Thankfully, instances of wine authenticity failures or counterfeiting occur as of now have not been associated with any risk to the consumers. Therefore, public exposure to such activities remains contained within the industry. On the contrary, food safety events that result in illness or, in some instances, death will trigger national and even global attention. Events like these tend to affect not only the reputation of the restaurant or company implicated but sometimes extend to similar businesses. For instance, Peanut Corporation of America (PCA) that ultimately left 9 people dead, 714 people hospitalized, and over 3600 products recalled across 47 states was one of the most extensive recalls in US history (Detwiler, 2015). Especially since the FDA and Center of Disease control discovered the involvement of the CEO, Steve Parnell, and senior management to cover up the positive Salmonella results and authorized product release with falsified or no certificates of analysis (Goetz, 2013). Although PCA was the only producer identified responsible in the recall, producers like Jif, Peter Pan, Skippy, and Smuckers experienced an overall 24% loss in peanut butter sales with recalls amounting to approximately $1 billion (Mallove, 2010). Wineries or people involved in winery schemes never seem to bear that same reputational damage. Again, due to the supportive nature of the wine industry, companies that could have suffered sizable losses are still succeeding today. Del Dotto recently opened another wine tasting facility in the Napa Valley and Don Sebastiani & Sons still thrives in the Sonoma region of California.

## Use of technology for the sake of authenticity

In the alcohol industry, advanced techniques for laboratory analysis of alcoholic beverages include chromatographic methods (the separation and quantitative determination of a wide variety of organic and inorganic compounds) and the Fourier transform infrared spectroscopy technique (infrared spectrum analysis enabling quantification of the main compounds found in wine), to identify the authenticity and adulteration of beverages.

## The intersection of layer of transparency, traceability, technology, and regulation

Today, many companies' wine bottles now come with a smart label that includes a unique QR code for the buyer to scan. A QR code is a two-dimensional barcode that end users can read using their phone. This code allows users to open a website link with information about the company and the product.

Beyond telling the story of the company and their vineyards, the smart label offers a full account of the wine's journey based on data captured during each stage of the winemaking process: when and where the grapes were harvested, how the wine was treated, quality characteristics, the bottling date, lot number, and the updated status through each transaction between producers, brokers, importers, wholesalers, distributors, and retailers. To capture all this information, wine companies, such as this one, use a mix of traditional, manual records as well as new tools like drones and Internet of Things technology, and blockchain.

According to the Wine Compliance Alliance, TTB regulates any information "that appears on a wine label which describes the wine itself is directly regulated in its use" including "details about the wine's style, how it was made, where the grapes were grown, etc." A winery must maintain detailed records to backup all their claims. The same federal requirements hold true for any information which is provided to a customer who uses their smartphone to read a QR code-TTB regulations apply across the board. Whatever information about the wine that the consumer is led to by accessing a wine label's QR code is considered either labeling or advertising material by the TTB and so subject to their regulations.

## Conclusion

Although instances of wine authenticity have been called into question, incidents are usually very limited with no safety incidents. Usually, media attention and impact on consumers are minimal as compared to the food industry. As mentioned with the PCA incident, peanut products were in decline due to the recall and ensuing series of events for years. Napa was recently affected by wine authenticity issues and fraudulence yet saw a 5.8% increase in visitors from 2016 to 2018. As the second largest industry in Napa, tourism does not seem to be affected much by the incidents discussed especially with wine tasting as the most popular experience (VisitNapaValley, 2019). This is due to the communal nature and importance of support that Napa Valley has continued to foster. This dynamic extends beyond the Napa Valley as other wine regions in the United States continue to build in prevalence and popularity including the Willamette Valley in Oregon, the Finger Lakes region of New York, and Walla Walla in Washington.

Authenticity is critical to all industries within Food and Beverage. Consumers must trust the products they buy and the foods they consume. In the wine industry, there is a different aspect to this trust that consumers share with producers. Wine is a demonstration of creativity, patience, and talent that has the potential to match with any wine lover. With so many different winemaking styles and varietals, there is something for everyone and the story that wines share brings people together. There is authenticity in that alone that on some level provides consumers a sense of trust that encourages them and wine producers to continue supporting one another to strive for quality in each bottle. The future use of technology will only help to provide assurance for the many dimensions of authenticity and brand reputation needed in the long-standing relationship between wine producers and consumers.

## References

Bateman, N. (2010, March). *Master of wine dissertation: Counterfeit wine-its impact on the business of wine*. Retrieved from https://www.jancisrobinson.com/files/pdfs/Counterfeit_Wine_Dissertation.pdf.

Berger, B. (1989, June 10). *Grape-switching scandal rocks state wine industry*. The Los Angeles Times. Retrieved from http://articles.latimes.com/1989-06-10/news/mn-1211_1_wine-industry-grapes-premium-wine/2.

Detwiler, D. (2015, February 20). Cracking the case of a multi-state Salmonella outbreak: The victims' stories. *Food Quality and Safety Magazine*. Retrieved from http://www.foodqualityandsafety.com/article/cracking-the-case-of-a-multi-state-salmonella-outbreak/.

Dinkelspiel, F. (2015a). The tale of one of the largest cases of wine fraud in American history. *Vinepair*. Retrieved from https://vinepair.com/wine-blog/the-tale-of-one-of-the-largest-cases-of-wine-fraud-in-american-history.

Dinkelspiel, F. (2015b). *Tangled vines: Greed, murder, obsession, and an Arsonist in the vineyards of California*. Retrieved from https://books.google.com/books?

id=tc90CgAAQBAJ&pg=PA141&lpg=PA141&dq=almaden+winery+1974+fine+fro m+airlines&source=bl&ots=2lfsa02RQz&sig=W9bk3dAO_3Q-fdK2VvHTPWtbfU& hl=en&sa=X&ved=0ahUKEwjtr6Hrs-jZAh.

Goel, V. (2015a). *In Vino Veritas. In Napa, Deceit.* The New York Times. Retrieved from https://www.nytimes.com/2015/01/25/business/in-vino-veritas-in-napa-deceit.html.

Goel, V. (2015b). *In Vino Veritas. In Napa, Deceit.* The New York Times. Retrieved from https://www.nytimes.com/2015/01/25/business/in-vino-veritas-in-napa-deceit.html.

*The Homeland Security Act of 2002, 6 U.S.C. Ch. 1 § 101 116 Stat. 2135.*(2002).

Lukacs, P. (1996, December). *The rise of American wine.* http://www.americanheritage.com/ content/rise-american-wine.

Maher, M. (2001, December). *On vino veritas? Clarifying the use of geographic references on American wine labels.* Retrieved from https://scholarship.law.berkeley.edu/cgi/ viewcontent.cgi?article=1438&context=californialawreview.

Mallove, Z. (2010, February 4). *USDA releases study on peanut industry.* Food Safety News. Retrieved from https://www.foodsafetynews.com/2010/02/usda-releases-study-on-peanut-industry/.

McMillan, R. (2018). *State of the wine industry 2018.* Retrieved from https://www.svb.com/ uploadedFiles/Content/Trends_and_Insights/Reports/Wine_Report/SVB-2018-wine-repo rt.pdf.

Mullen, T. (2018, February 15). State of the wine industry 2018 highlights key trends. *Forbes Magazine.* Retrieved from https://www.forbes.com/sites/tmullen/2018/02/15/state-of-the-wine-industry-2018-highlights-key-trends/.

Owen, J. (2011, January 12). *Earliest known winery found in Armenian cave.* National Geographic News. Retrieved from https://www.nationalgeographic.com/news/2011/1/ 110111-oldest-wine-press-making-winery-armenia-science-ucla/#close.

1 Puckette, M. (2016, April 29). *Reality of wine prices (what you get for what you spend).* Retrieved from http://winefolly.com/update/reality-of-wine-prices-what-you-get-for-what-you-spend/.

UC Davis Foundation Plant Services Grapes. (n.d.). *Grape variety: Carignane.* Retrieved from Retrieved from http://fps.ucdavis.edu/fgrdetails.cfm?varietyid=373&bigpics=yes#24313.

United States Code: Federal Alcohol Administration Act, 27 U.S.C. §§ 201-211 (Suppl. 1 1934). U.S. Const. am. 18. U.S. Const. am. 21.

Visit Napa Valley. (2019, May 3). *Napa Valley's tourism industry continues to provide significant positive impact.* Retrieved from https://www.visitnapavalley.com/articles/post/napa-valleys-tourism-industry-continues-to-provide-a-significant-positive-impact/.

Wine Institute. (n.d.). *Appellation of origin & American viticultural areas.* Retrieved from Retrieved from https://www.wineinstitute.org/resources/avas.

Wine Labeling. (2017, November 2). *TTB: Alcohol Tobacco Tax and trade Bureau website.* Retrieved from https://www.ttb.gov/wine/wine-labeling.shtml.

Wine Statistics. (2018, February 2). *TTB: Alcohol Tobacco Tax and trade Bureau website.* Retrieved from https://www.ttb.gov/wine/wine-stats.shtml.

# The case for chocolate: lessons for food authenticity and big data

# 16

**Steven Sklare[1], Thodoris Kontogiannis[2], Giannis Stoitsis[3]**

[1]*President, Food Safety Academy, Chicago, IL, United States;* [2]*Researcher and Author, AgroKnow, Marousi, Attica, Greece;* [3]*CEO/Founder/Owner at FOODAKAI, Marousi, Attica, Greece*

## How global food safety intelligent digital tools can help keep food safe and protect a food company's brand

Almost everybody loves chocolate, an ancient, basic, almost universal and primal source of pleasure. The "once upon a time" tale of chocolate starts well before its purchase at a store.

> *The story of chocolate beings with cocoa trees that grew wild in the tropical rainforests of the Amazon basin and other areas in Central and South America for thousands of years …. Christopher Columbus is said to have brought the first cocoa beans back to Europe from his fourth visit to the New World between 1502 and 1504*

**Cadbury, 2020**

Unfortunately, the production of chocolate and chocolate products today is as complex as any other global food product with supply chains that reach from one end of the world to the other. The complexity of the supply chain and production, along with the universal demand for the finished product, exposes chocolate to increasing pressure from numerous hazards, both unintentional and intentional. For example, we know that more than 70% of cocoa production takes place in West African countries, particularly the Ivory Coast and Ghana (Industrial Franchise Association, 2020). These regions are politically unstable, and production is frequently disrupted by fighting. While production has started to expand into more stable regions, it has not yet become diversified enough to normalize the supply. About 17% of production takes place in the Americas (primarily South America) and 9% from Asia and Oceania (Industrial Franchise Association, 2020).

In today's world of global commerce these pressures are not unique to chocolate. Food quality and safety experts should be armed with tools and innovations that can help them examine specific hazards and fraud pertaining to chocolate and chocolate products. In fact, the global nature of the chocolate market requires fast reflexes that protect brand integrity and dynamic quality processes supported by informed decisions. Digital tools have become a necessity when a fast interpretation of dynamic

Building the Future of Food Safety Technology. https://doi.org/10.1016/B978-0-12-818956-6.00016-6

data is needed. If a food organization is going to effectively protect the public's health, protect their brand, and comply with various governmental regulations and nongovernmental standards such as GFSI, horizon scanning, along with the use of food safety intelligent digital tools, needs to be incorporated into food company's core Food Safety and Quality Assurance (FSQA) program.

This section pulls information from a 2019 Foodakai case study on chocolate products that presents an examination of the specific hazards and fraud pertaining to chocolate and chocolate products along with ways to utilize this information.

Cocoa and chocolate products rely on high-quality ingredients and raw materials, strict supplier partnership schemes, and conformity to clearly defined quality and safety standards. During the past 10 years, a significant number of food safety incidents have been associated with chocolate products. The presence of *Salmonella enterica*, *Listeria* monocytogenes, allergens, and foreign materials in cocoa/chocolate products have been reported on a global scale. Today, information on food safety incidents and potential risks is quickly and widely available by way of the Internet. However, because the pertinent data are frequently siloed, food safety professionals are unable to take full advantage of it.

## Top emerging hazards: chocolate products (2013–2018)

Publicly available data, from sources such as European Union RASFF, Australian Competition and Consumer Commission, UK Food Standards Agency, FDA, Food Standards Australia New Zealand (FSANZ), show a significant increase in identified food safety incidents for cocoa/chocolate products from 2013 to 2018. For this same time period, the top emerging hazards that were identified for chocolate products were the following:

- Allergens: 51.60%
- Biological: 16.49%
- Foreign bodies: 13.83%
- Chemical: 7.45%
- Fraud: 6.38%
- Food additives and flavorings: 4.26%
- Other hazards: 2.66%

By using such information to identify critical food safety protection trends, which we define to include food safety (unintentional adulteration) and food fraud (intentional adulteration, inclusive of authenticity/intentional misrepresentation), we can better construct our food protection systems to focus on the areas that present the greatest threats to public health, brand protection, and compliance.

# A data-driven approach

Assessment and identification of potential food protection issues, including food safety and fraud, at the stage of incoming raw materials is of vital importance for food manufacturers. Knowledge of the associated risks and vulnerabilities allows for timely actions and appropriate measures that may ultimately prevent an incident from occurring.

Specifically, the efficient utilization of global food safety and fraud information should allow for

- Identification of prevalent, increasing, and/or emerging risks and vulnerabilities associated with raw materials
- Comparative evaluation of the risk profile for different raw materials' origins
- Critical evaluation and risk-based selection of raw materials' suppliers

A comprehensive risk assessment must start with the consideration of the identified food safety incidents of the raw material, which include the inherent characteristics of the raw material. Next, the origin-related risks must be taken into account and then the supplier-related risks must be examined. The full risk assessment is driven by the appropriate food safety data, its analysis, and application of risk assessment scientific models on top of the data.

Using food safety intelligent digital tools to analyze almost 400 unique, chocolate product-related food safety incidents around the globe provides industry leaders with important, useful insights about cocoa as a raw material, as a raw material from a specific origin, and as a raw material being provided by specific suppliers. The graph below represents the results of the analysis illustrating the trend of incidents reported between 2002 and 2018. One can observe that, after a significant rise between 2009 and 2010, the number of incidents approximately doubled and remained at that level for the rest of the evaluated period (i.e., from 2010 to 2018), compared with the period from 2002 to 2005 (see Graph 1).

By further analyzing the data stemming from the 400 food safety incidents and breaking them down into more defined hazards, for incoming raw materials, we can clearly see that chemical hazards represent the major hazard category for cocoa.

- Chemical: 73.46%
- Biological: 16.49%
- Organoleptic aspects: 5.93%
- Other hazards: 4.38%
- Fraud: 2.32%
- Foreign bodies: 2.06%
- Food additives and flavorings: 0.77%
- Allergens: 0.52%
- Food contact materials: 0.52%

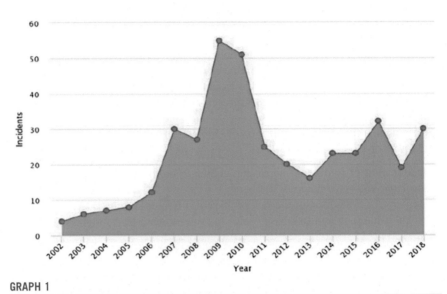

**GRAPH 1**

Chocolate product-related food safety incidents reported between 2002 and 2018.

*Graph from authors (2019).* Case Study: Chocolate products: Lessons learned from global food safety and fraud data and the guidance it can provide to the food industry. *Foodakai. Retrieved from https://reports.foodakai.com/ foodakai-chocolate-industry-report. Used with permission.*

Using the appropriate analytical tools, someone can drill down into the data and identify the specific incidents within the different hazard categories. For example, within the "chemical hazard" category specific hazards such as organophosphates, neonicotinoids, pyrethroids, and organochlorines were identified.

## Comparative evaluation of risk profiles for different origins of raw materials

The main regions of origin for cocoa globally are Africa, Asia, and South America. Collecting and analyzing all relevant data from recalls and border rejections and the frequency of pertinent incidents allows for an accurate identification of the top hazards for cocoa by region (see Table 1.)

**Table 1** The top five specific hazards for Africa, South America, and Asia.

|  | **Africa** | **South America** | **Asia** |
|---|---|---|---|
| 1 | Organophosphate | 2,4-Dinitrophenol (DNP) | 2,4-Dinitrophenol (DNP) |
| 2 | Molds | Pyrethroid | Poor or insufficient controls |
| 3 | Neonicotinoid | Aflatoxin | Aflatoxin |
| 4 | Pyrethroid | Cadmium | Spoilage |
| 5 | Organochlorine | Anilinopyrimidine | *Salmonella* |

*Top five hazards by region (Created by author)*

After the first level of analysis, a further interpretation of the data using the appropriate data intelligence tools can help to reach very specific information on the nature of the incidents. This provides additional detail that is helpful in understanding how the regional risk profiles compare. For example, the prevalence of chemical contamination, as either industrial contaminants or pesticides, has been a commonly observed pattern for all three of the regions in Table 1. However, beyond the general hazard category level, one can also identify different trends with regard to specific hazards for the three different regions. One such example is the increased presence of mold in cocoa beans coming from Africa.

The primary hazard categories for cocoa-as a raw ingredient-were identified and a comparison among the primary hazards for cocoa by region (origin-specific) should take place. The next step in a data-powered supplier assessment workflow would be to incorporate our use of global food safety data in evaluating the suppliers of the raw materials.

## The role of global food safety data

This focus on chocolate products has only touched the surface in terms of the information available in the complete report, which also includes specific information about key raw materials. To be clear, the techniques and tools used to generate this information are applicable to all food products and ingredients. Any efforts to produce food safely in the 21st century and beyond must include adapting of methods or some industry stakeholders will be left behind.

The regulatory environment in which the food industry must operate has never been more intense. The threats to an organization's brand have never been greater. This is not going to change. What must change is the way in which food companies confront these challenges.

Global food safety data can contribute to the establishment of an adaptive food safety/QA process that will provide time savings and improve a quality team's efficiency and performance.

Based on the continuous analysis of food recalls and rejections by key national and international food authorities, a food safety/quality assurance manager could establish an adaptive supplier verification process and risk assessment process by utilizing the knowledge provided by such data. In that way, QA, procurement, food safety, and quality departments can be empowered with critical supplier data that will inform the internal procedures for incoming materials and ingredients (e.g., raw materials, packaging materials) and allow for adaptive laboratory testing routines and compliance protocols. Moreover, food safety systems-and technologies-can become adaptive, enabling quality assurance and safety professionals to quickly update points of critical control when needed, and intervene in important stages of the manufacturing process for chocolate or any commodity.

## Big data and food fraud prediction

Future food safety information systems should be able to address the following critical questions that the FSQA experts need to answer:

- How can one monitor food fraud incidents around the world in almost real time?
- Can large-scale data analysis reveal patterns related to the way that people modify food products, ingredients, or packaging for economic gain?
- Is it possible to predict whether someone in the supply chain has substituted, misbranded, counterfeited, stolen, or enhanced food in an unapproved way?
- In which ways can big data help us detect if there is increased probability of food fraud?

Let us assume that we have in our hands the world's most comprehensive database of fraud-related incidents. This will include, among others,

- Food fraud incidents that have been officially announced by a governmental agency or inspection authority.
- Product or ingredient rejections at border customs because some type of adulteration has been found during an inspection.
- Laboratory test analyses that indicate that there has been a substitution or enhancement of a food for an economic purpose.

This would be a very large database about food fraud incidents that have already taken place. Interesting questions arise:

- Could an historical database of international food fraud be mined to successfully predict what will happen in the future?
- Can investigators look into product or ingredient categories and try to identify emerging fraud types before they actually occur?
- Can they foresee and calculate the probability of having fraud incidents within a particular supply chain?
- Is it even possible to predict the specific time period during which this probability is very high, so that preventive measures can be taken?
- What if more data are added into the mix?
- Is there a correlation between fraud incidents with price changes?
- Does the probability of fraud increase for suppliers based in countries with high corruption scores?
- Can a severe weather phenomenon be linked to an increase of food adulteration incidents in this area?

The food supply chain has many critical problems of this kind. People need to take decisions about whether risk exists. They need to know if a preventive action needs to be taken as early as possible. To do so, they rely on a large number and rich variety of data sources.

## The next frontier for food safety risk assessment

The economic importance of the food sector globally and domestically has put food safety as a national priority for many countries in Europe, America, and Asia.

Since the identification of food safety as a priority, countries have introduced modernized food safety approaches. This is evident not only by the update of food safety legislative framework along with organizational change but also by the increasing number of public and private initiatives fostering food safety modernization.

But the modernization of food safety and regulatory systems does not end up with having a robust risk assessment framework. The continuously evolving supply chains need adaptive frameworks that allow for timely response to food safety problems and moving from reaction to prevention.

What if live risk assessment could be performed, thus allowing the prediction of what the next critical incident in the supply chain will be?

A wide variety of tools is used today by FSQA professionals to assess risk ranging from literature-based classification of risks to Excel files and software tools such as the JIFSAN's iRisk Tool (FDA, 2017) and the University of Tasmania and USDA-ARS Combase (2020). Ingredients and raw materials are analyzed against biological, chemical, and physical hazards based on historical data and literature.

One of the main limitations of the existing approaches is that the estimated risk remains static. It is reviewed on an annual basis or every time that there is a significant change in the supply chain of each company. In our global and complex supply chain, emerging risks and increasing hazards are identified in most cases after the quality or food safety incidents have already affected consumers. This is far too late if we want to prevent risk and not just to react to incidents.

The next era of risk assessment should move to a live risk assessment approach that is based on live data streams and the risk prediction using supply chain data and machine learning (computational) models.

Thus far, a large number of computational models have been developed by the research community and can be found in catalogs such as Food Safety Model Repository-a community-driven search engine for predictive microbial models (OpenFSMR, 2020). The majority of models are hazard- and product-specific and can predict the growth of bacteria in specific conditions. Such models could be fed with incredible amounts of data and (most of the time) live data so they can support real-time risk prediction.

Besides live data stemming from sensors installed in different steps of the supply chain, there is a vast amount of data available from official national and international sources. The plethora of data that are available on a daily basis about food recalls and border rejections can be used to estimate the frequency of hazards and fraud cases in different types of food and beverages. This enables the live risk assessment allowing early highlighting of the increasing and the emerging risks. In that way, a food company will have a live risk for its ingredients, incoming raw materials, and product recipes. Moreover, any change in the risk trends will be tracked and all responsible departments are notified so as to deploy corrective actions.

Machine learning algorithms are being widely impacting industrial applications and platforms, including the food industry (Marvin et al., 2016). Beyond typical research experimentation scenarios, there is a need for food companies that wish to enhance their online data and analytics solutions to incorporate ways in which they can select, experiment, benchmark, parameterize, and choose the version of a machine learning algorithm that seems to be most appropriate for their specific application context. A big data platform that can support such tailor-made food data analytics and intelligence has been recently introduced (Polychronou et al., 2020). Machine learning algorithms that are adapted to the application context may be efficiently used for the prediction of risks in the supply chain and help food companies to move from reaction to prevention.

# References

Cadbury. (2020). *Discovering chocolate. The great chocolate discovery.* Cadbury website. Retrieved from https://www.cadbury.com.au/About-Chocolate/Discovering-Chocolate. aspx.

Foodakai. (2019). *Case study: Chocolate products (Lessons learned from global food safety and fraud data and the guidance it can provide to the food industry.).* Retrieved from https://reports.foodakai.com/foodakai-chocolate-industry-report.

FDA. (2017). FDA-iRISK® version 4.0. In *Center for Food Safety and Applied Nutrition (CFSAN), Joint Institute for Food Safety and Applied Nutrition (JIFSAN) and Risk Sciences International (RSI).* Retrieved from https://irisk.foodrisk.org/.

Industrial Franchise Association. (2020). *Chocolate industry analysis 2020 — cost & trends.* Franchise Help. Retrieved from https://www.franchisehelp.com/industry-reports/chocolate-industry-analysis-2020-cost-trends/.

Marvin, et al. (2016). A holistic approach to food safety risks: Food fraud as an example. *Food Research International, 89.* https://doi.org/10.1016/j.foodres.2016.08.028

OpenFSMR. (2020). *Bundesinstitut für Risikobewertung (BfR).* Retrieved from https://sites.google.com/site/openfsmr/.

Poluchronou, et al. (2020). Machine learning algorithms for food intelligence: Towards a method for more accurate predictions. In I. Athanasiadis, S. Frysinger, G. Schimak, & W. Knibbe (Eds.), *IFIP advances in information and communication technology: Vol. 554. Environmental software systems. Data science in action. ISESS 2020.* Cham: Springer.

University of Tasmania and the USDA Agricultural Research Service. (2020). *ComBase.* Retrieved from https://www.combase.cc/index.php/en/.

## Note:

# Data and food supply chain

# Optimizing global food supply chains: The case for blockchain and GSI standards

## 17

**John G. Keogh, MBA, MSc** [1], **Abderahman Rejeb**[2], **Nida Khan**[3], **Kevin Dean, MBA** [4],
**Karen J. Hand, PhD** [5]

[1]*Doctoral researcher, Henley Business School, University of Reading;* [2]*Doctoral Researcher, School of Regional Sciences and Business Administration, The Széchenyi István University, Győr, Hungary;* [3]*Doctoral researcher in blockchain and data analytics for traceability in finance, The Interdisciplinary Centre for Security, Reliability and Trust, University of Luxembourg, Luxembourg City, Luxembourg;* [4]*Technology Strategist, Dolphin Data Development Ltd., Toronto, ON, Canada;* [5]*Director, Research Data Strategy, Food for Thought, University of Guelph, Guelph, ON, Canada*

## Introduction

The globalization of food supply chains (FSCs) has added significant complexity to food systems and created an information asymmetry between food producers and food consumers. As a result, a growing demand exists for greater transparency into food origins, methods of cultivation, harvesting, and production as well as labor conditions and environmental impact (Autio et al., 2017; BildtgÅrd, 2008; Donnelly, Thakur, & Sakai, 2013). Moreover, the international debate on the integrity of FSCs has intensified due to recurring incidents and crises across the five pillars of the food system (earlier referred to as the five consumer reputations): food quality, food safety, food authenticity, food defense, and food security (Fig. 17.1).

Food-related incidents across all five pillars have been amplified through social media platforms (New, 2010), creating consumer distrust.

According to the most recent Edelman Trust Barometer (ETB), trust in the food and beverage industry has declined by two points since 2019 (Global Report: Edelman Trust Barometer 2020). This decrease is significant as the trust construct in the ETB encompasses both competence and ethics. Importantly, Edelman argued that ethics (e.g., comprised of integrity, dependability, and purpose) is "three times more important to company trust than competence" (Global Report: Edelman Trust Barometer 2020). A crucial argument is made in the ETB, suggesting that while business is considered competent, only nongovernment organizations (NGOs) are considered ethical. This claim may have a profound impact on FSCs and strongly suggests that in order to regain citizen-consumer trust, food businesses must be open to feedback and criticisms from NGOs. This point should be of particular

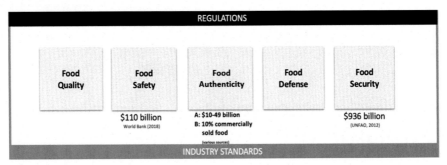

**FIGURE 17.1**

The five pillars of the food system.

significance to FSCs, considering that NGOs are tasked with monitoring and reporting on environmental stewardship, corruption, animal welfare, slavery, child labor, and worker rights and safety. Essentially, the journey toward food chain transparency means that food businesses must be prepared to take a proactive and continuous approach to find and reduce weaknesses in their FSCs. These weaknesses can impact all five pillars as outlined in Fig. 17.1, and monitoring and subsequent interventions will differ from pillar to pillar.

The economic costs and inefficiencies that are associated with the five pillars are significant. For instance, the World Bank (2018) estimated that **food safety**-related costs (e.g., lost productivity, medical costs) in low- to middle-income economies amount to USD 110 billion annually. Regarding **food security**, the United Nations Food and Agriculture Organization estimated that food security-related costs (e.g., wasted resources, economic losses) amount to USD 936 billion annually (UNFAO, 2018).

Regulatory authorities are increasingly concerned about **food security** (the adequate supply of safe, affordable, and nutritious foods that meet consumer preferences), **food defense**, and the risk of malicious attacks (terrorist acts on the food chain), as well as food fraud incidents (criminal acts related to **food authenticity**.) While the total impact of food fraud is impossible to quantify accurately, academics and industry sources suggest it ranges from USD 10–49 billion (Manning, 2016; Manning & Soon, 2016; PWC, 2016). The Canadian Food Inspection Agency website cites Grocery Manufacturing Association (rebranded in 2019 to Consumer Brands Association) that suggests food fraud is likely ten percent of all commercially sold foods (CFIA, 2019). Regulatory authorities must also address issues related to false information (fake news) or divisive information, which may include populist/nationalist ideals or other food sovereignty-related movements and objectives (Borras, 2020). These divisive issues have given rise to increased stakeholder distrust and a stronger emphasis on the need to improve food chain information transparency, reduce information asymmetry, and enhance trust.

FSCs are critical components of the broader food ecosystem because of their relevance to global and local populations, their role in economic prosperity, and the vulnerabilities arising from their operations and management (Voss, Closs, Calantone, Helferich, & Speier, 2009). An FSC is a network of highly interconnected stakeholders working together to ensure the delivery of safe food products (Schiefer & Deiters, 2013). FSC actors commit to implementing a set of processes and activities that help take the food from its raw material state to the finished product (Dani, 2015). Ensuring the delivery of safe food products is an utmost priority and a primary building block for a healthy and vibrant society. Over the years, FSCs have witnessed several structural changes and a shift toward the development of more unified, integrated, and coherent relationships between stakeholders (Bourlakis & Weightman, 2008). As such, an FSC has become a "chain of trust" that extends from suppliers, producers, distributors, wholesalers, retailers, and consumers (Choi & Hong, 2002; Johnston, McCutcheon, Stuart, & Kerwood, 2004). Although FSCs represent a metaphorical "chain of trust," the trustworthiness of the FSC is as fundamental to the integrity of our food systems as food traceability and transparency and is not without its own unique set of challenges.

## The vulnerability of FSCs

FSCs are vulnerable to natural disasters, malpractices, and exploitative behavior, leading to food security concerns, reputational damage, and significant financial losses. Due to the inherent complexities of global FSCs, it is almost impossible for stakeholders to police the entire flow of materials and products and identify all possible externalities. Recurring **disruptions** (e.g., natural disasters, avian flu, swine fever, COVID-19) and consecutive food **scandals** have increased the sense of urgency in the management of FSCs (Zhong, Xu, & Wang, 2017) and negatively impacted consumer trust.

The European "horsemeat scandal" in 2013 exemplified the vulnerabilities (Yamoah & Yawson, 2014), and legal scholars from Cambridge University posited

> *The ability of the EU's regulatory regime to prevent fraud on such a scale was shown to be inadequate. EU food law, with its (over) emphasis on food safety, failed to prevent the occurrence of fraud and may even have played an (unintentional) role in facilitating or enhancing it*

**(Barnard & O'Connor, 2017, p. 116).**

The Cambridge scholars further argued that the free movement of goods within the European Union created a sense of "blind trust" in the regulatory framework, which proved to be inadequate to protect businesses and consumers from unscrupulous actors. While natural disasters and political strife are outside of the control of FSC stakeholders, to preserve food quality and food safety and minimize the risk of food fraud or malicious attacks, FSC stakeholders need to establish and agree on foundational methods for analytical science, supply chain standards, technology tools, and food safety standards.

The redesign of the FSC is necessary in order to ensure unquestionable integrity in a resilient food ecosystem. This proposal would require a foundational approach to data management and data governance to ensure sources of accurate and trusted data to enable inventory management, order management, traceability, unsafe product recall, and measures to protect against food fraud. Failure to do so will result in continued consumer distrust and economic loss. Notably, a report by GS1 UK et al. (2009) reported that eighty percent of United Kingdom retailers had inconsistent product data, estimated to cost UKP 700 million in profit erosion over 5 years and a further UKP 300 million in lost sales.

## Blockchain Technology

The recent emergence of Blockchain technology has created significant interest among scholars and practitioners in numerous disciplines. Initially, Blockchain technology was heralded as a radical innovation laden with a strong appeal to the financial sector, particularly in the use of cryptocurrencies (Nakamoto, 2008, p. 9). The speculation on the true identity of the pseudonymous "Satoshi Nakamoto" gave rise to suspicion on the actual creators of Bitcoin and their motives (Lemieux, 2013). Moreover, Halaburda (2018) argued that there is a lack of consensus on the benefits of Blockchain and, importantly, how it may fail. Further, Rejeb, Sűle, & Keogh (2018, p. 81) argued "Ultimately, a Blockchain can be viewed as a configuration of multiple technologies, tools and methods that address a particular problem."

Beyond the sphere of finance, Blockchain technology is considered a foundational paradigm (Iansiti & Lakhani, 2017) with the potential for significant societal benefits and improve trust between FSC actors. Blockchain technology offers several capabilities and functionalities that can significantly reshape existing practices of managing FSCs and partnerships, regardless of location, and also offers opportunities to improve efficiency, transparency, trust, and security, across a broad spectrum of business and social transactions (Frizzo-Barker et al., 2019). The technological attributes of Blockchain can combine with smart contracts to enable decentralized and self-organization to create, execute, and manage business transactions (Schaffers, 2018), creating a landscape for innovative approaches to information and collaborative systems.

## Global supply chain standards

Innovations are not only merely a simple composition of technical changes in processes and procedures but also include new forms of social and organizational arrangements (Callon, Law, & Rip, 1986). The ubiquitous product bar code stands out as a significant innovation that has transformed business and society. Since the decision by US industry (GS1, 2020) to adopt the linear bar code on April 3,

1973, and the first scan of a 10-pack of Wrigley's Juicy Fruit chewing gum in Marsh's supermarket in Troy, Ohio, on June 26, 1974 (GS1, 2014), the bar code is scanned an estimated 5 billion times daily. GS1 is a not-for-profit organization tasked with managing industry-driven data and information standards (note, GS1 is not an acronym). The GS1 system of interoperable standards assigns and manages globally unique identification of firms, their locations, their products, and assets. They rely on several technology-enabled functions for data capture, data exchange, and data synchronization among FSC exchange partners. In FSCs, there is a growing need for interoperability standards to facilitate business-to-business integration. The adoption of GS1 standards-enabled Blockchain technology has the potential to enable FSC stakeholders to meet the fast-changing needs of the agri-food industry and the evolving regulatory requirements for enhanced traceability and rapid recall of unsafe goods.

Although there is a growing body of evidence concerning the benefits of Blockchain technology and its potential to align with GS1 standards for data and information (Fosso Wamba et al., 2019; Kamath, 2017; Lacity, 2018), the need remains for an extensive examination of the full potentials and limitations. The authors of this section, therefore, reviewed relevant academic literature to examine the full potential of Blockchain-enabled GS1 systems comprehensively, and therefore provide a significant contribution to the academic and practitioner literature. The diversity of Blockchain research in the food context is fragmented, and the potentials and limitations in combination with GS1 standards remain vaguely conceptualized. It is vitally essential to narrow this research gap.

This review will begin with an outline of the methodology applied to collect academic contributions to Blockchain and GS1 standards within a FSC context, followed by an in-depth analysis of the findings, concluding with potential areas for future research.

## Methodology

In order to explore the full potential of a system integrating Blockchain functionalities and GS1 standards, a systematic review method based on Tranfield, Denyer, & Smart (2003) guidelines was undertaken. The systematic review was considered as a suitable method to locate, analyze, and synthesize peer-reviewed publications. Research on Blockchain technology is broad and across disciplines; however, a paucity of research specific to food chains exists (Fosso Wamba et al., 2019). Similarly, existing research on Blockchain technology and GS1 standards is a patchwork of studies with no coherent or systematic body of knowledge. Therefore, the objective of this study was to draw on existing studies and leverage their findings using content analysis to extract insights and provide a deeper understanding of the opportunities for a GS1 standards-enabled Blockchain as an FSC management framework.

## Planning the review

As stated earlier, the literature on Blockchain technology and GS1 is neither well-developed nor conclusive, yet necessary to ensure successful future implementations. In order to facilitate the process of literature collection, a review protocol based on the "Preferred Reporting Items for Systematic Reviews and Meta-Analyzes" (PRISMA) was used (Liberati et al., 2009). The PRISMA approach consists of four processes: the use of various sources to locate previous studies, the fast screening of studies and removal of duplicates, the evaluation of studies for relevance and suitability, and the final analysis of relevant publications. Fig. 17.2 illustrates the PRISMA process. To ensure unbiased results, this phase of the study was completed by researchers with no previous knowledge or association with GS1.

## Conducting the review

Conducting the review began with a search for studies on Blockchain technology and GS1 standards. Reviewed publications originated from academic sources (peer-reviewed) and included journal articles, conference papers, and book chapters. Due to the nascent and limited literature on Blockchain technology and GS1 standards, we supplemented our analysis with other sources of information, including conference proceedings, gray sources, and reports.

The survey of the literature was conducted using four major scientific databases: Scopus, Web of Science, ScienceDirect, and Google Scholar. We used a combination of keywords that consisted of the following search string: "Blockchain*" AND "GS1" AND ("food chain*" OR "food supply*" OR agriculture OR agro. The Google Scholar search engine has limited functionality and allows only the full-text search field; therefore, only one search query "Blockchain* AND GS1 AND food" was used for the retrieval of relevant studies.

The titles and abstracts of publications were scanned to obtain a general overview of the study content and to assess the relevance of the material. As shown in Fig. 17.2, a total of 140 publications were found. Many of the publications were redundant due to the comprehensive coverage of Google Scholar; studies focused on Blockchain technology outside the context of food were removed. A fine-tuned selection of the publications was undertaken to ensure relevance to FSCs.

## Report of findings and knowledge dissemination

Table 17.1 contains a summary of the findings based on content analysis. The final 28 documents were classified, evaluated, and found to be sufficient in narrative detail to provide an overview of publications to date, specifically related to Blockchain technology and GS1 standards.

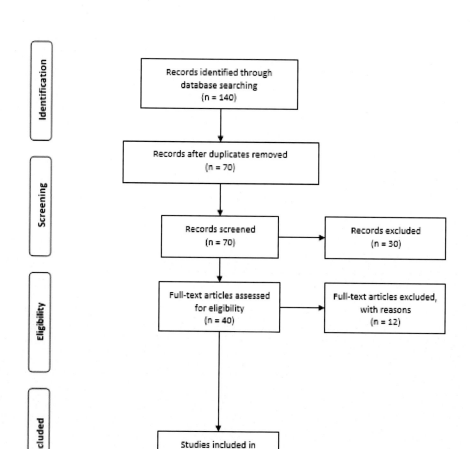

**FIGURE 17.2**

Graphic by authors.

*The PRISMA process adapted from Liberati, A., Altman, D. G., Tetzlaff, J., Mulrow, C., Gøtzsche, P. C., Ioannidis, J. P., et al (2009). The PRISMA statement for reporting systematic reviews and meta-analyses of studies that evaluate health care interventions: Explanation and elaboration.* Annals of Internal Medicine, 151*(4),* W–65.

# Findings

## Overview of Blockchain technology

The loss of trust in the conventional banking system following the 2008 global financial crisis laid the groundwork for the introduction of an alternative monetary system based on a novel digital currency and distributed ledger (Richter, Kraus, & Bouncken, 2015). "Satoshi Nakamoto" (a pseudonym for an unknown person,

**Table 17.1** Classification of literature according to the content analysis.

| Focus Publications | Traceability | Transparency | Interoperability | Standardization | Data Sharing | Security |
|---|---|---|---|---|---|---|
| (Augustin et al., 2020) | ✓ |  |  |  |  |  |
| (Ande et al., 2019) |  |  | ✓ |  |  | ✓ |
| (Bajwa et al., 2010) | ✓ | ✓ | ✓ |  | ✓ |  |
| (Behnke & Janssen, 2019) | ✓ |  |  |  | ✓ |  |
| (Biswas et al., 2017) | ✓ | ✓ |  | ✓ |  | ✓ |
| (Bouzdine-Chameeva et al., 2019) | ✓ | ✓ |  |  | ✓ |  |
| (Chanchaichujit et al., 2019) | ✓ | ✓ | ✓ |  |  |  |
| (Chemeltorit et al., 2018) | ✓ | ✓ | ✓ |  | ✓ |  |
| (Cho & Choi, 2019) |  |  | ✓ |  |  | ✓ |
| (Cousins et al., 2019) |  |  | ✓ |  | ✓ | ✓ |
| (Dasaklis et al., 2019) | ✓ |  |  |  |  |  |
| (dos Santos et al., 2019) | ✓ |  | ✓ |  |  | ✓ |
| (Figueroa et al., 2019) | ✓ | ✓ | ✓ |  |  |  |
| (Giusti et al., 2019) |  |  |  |  |  |  |
| (Helo & Shamsuzzoha, 2020) |  |  | ✓ |  |  |  |
| (Iida et al., 2019) | ✓ |  |  | ✓ | ✓ |  |
| (Kamble et al., 2019) | ✓ | ✓ | ✓ | ✓ | ✓ | ✓ |
| (Kim et al., 2018) | ✓ | ✓ | ✓ |  |  |  |
| (Olsen & Borit, 2018) |  |  | ✓ | ✓ |  |  |
| (Pigini & Conti, 2017) | ✓ | ✓ |  |  | ✓ | ✓ |
| (Ray et al., 2019) | ✓ |  | ✓ |  | ✓ |  |
| (Sander et al., 2018) |  | ✓ |  |  | ✓ |  |
| (Staples et al., 2017) | ✓ | ✓ | ✓ |  |  |  |
| (Toyoda et al., 2017) | ✓ |  | ✓ |  |  | ✓ |
| (Wang et al., 2019, pp. 512–523) | ✓ |  |  |  |  |  |
| (Xu et al., 2019) |  |  |  |  | ✓ | ✓ |
| (Yiannas, 2018) |  |  |  |  |  |  |
| (Yunfeng et al., 2018) | ✓ |  |  |  |  |  |

*Table, created by authors. Classification of literature according to the content analysis.*

group of people, organization, or other public or private body) introduced an electronic peer-to-peer cash system called Bitcoin (Nakamoto, 2008, p. 9). The proposed system allowed for payments in Bitcoin currency, securely and without the intermediation of a trusted third party (TTP) such as a bank. The Bitcoin protocol utilizes a Blockchain, which provides an ingenious and innovative solution to the double-spending problem (i.e., where digital currency or a token is spent more than once), eliminating the need for a TTP intervention to validate the transactions. Moreover, Lacity (2018, p. 219) argued "While TTPs provide important functions, they have some serious limitations, like high transaction fees, slow settlement times, low transaction transparency, multiple versions of the truth and security vulnerabilities."

The technology behind the Bitcoin application is known as a Blockchain. The Bitcoin Blockchain is a distributed database (or distributed ledger) implemented on public, untrusted networks (Kano & Nakajima, 2018) with a cryptographic signature (hash) that is resistant to falsification through repeated hashing and a consensus algorithm (Sylim, Liu, Marcelo, & Fontelo, 2018). Blockchain technology is engineered in a way that parties previously unknown to each other can jointly generate and maintain a database of records (information) and can correct and complete transactions, which are fully distributed across several nodes (i.e., computers), validated using consensus of independent verifiers (Tijan, Aksentijević, Ivanić, & Jardas, 2019). Blockchain is categorized under the distributed ledger technology family and is characterized by a peer-to-peer network and a decentralized distributed database, as depicted in Fig. 17.3.

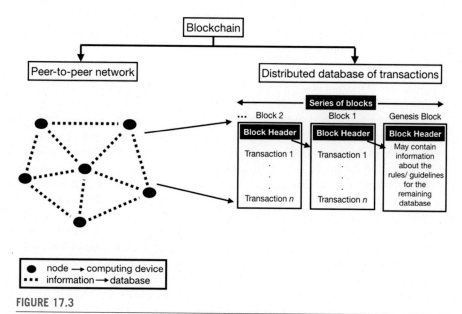

**FIGURE 17.3**

A diagrammatic representation of Blockchain technology.

*Graphic by authors.*

According to Lemieux (2016), the nodes within a Blockchain work collectively as one system to store encrypted sequences of transactional records as a single chained unit or block. Nodes in a Blockchain network can either be validator nodes (miners in Ethereum and Bitcoin) that participate in the consensus mechanism or nonvalidator nodes (referred to only as nodes). When any node wants to add a transaction to the ledger, the transaction of interest is broadcast to all nodes in the peer-to-peer network. Transactions are then collected into a block, where the addition to the Blockchain necessitates a consensus mechanism. Validators compete to have their local block to be the next addition to the Blockchain. The way blocks are constructed and propagated in the system enables the traceback of the whole chain of valid network activities back to the genesis block initiated in the Blockchain.

Furthermore, the consensus methodology employed by the underlying Blockchain platform designates the validator, whose block gets added to the Blockchain with the others remaining in the queue and participating in the next round of consensus. The validator node gains an incentive for updating the Blockchain database (Nakamoto, 2008, p. 9). The Blockchain may impose restrictions on reading the data and the flexibility to become a validator to write to the Blockchain, depending upon whether the Blockchain is permissioned or permission-less.

A consensus algorithm enables secure updating of the Blockchain data, which is governed by a set of rules specific to the Blockchain platform. This right to update the Blockchain data is distributed among the economic set (Buterin, 2014b), a group of users who can update the Blockchain based on a set of rules. The economic set is intended to be decentralized with no collusion within the set (a group of users) in order to form a majority, even though they might have a large amount of capital and financial incentives. The Blockchain platforms that have emerged employ one of the following decentralized economic sets; however, each example might utilize a different set of consensus algorithms:

**Owners of Computing Power**: This set employs Proof-of-Work (POW) as a consensus algorithm observed in Blockchain platforms like Bitcoin and Ethereum. Each block header in the Blockchain has a string of random data called a nonce attached to them (Nakamoto, 2008, p. 9). The miners (validators) need to search for this random string such that when attached to the block, the hash of the block has a certain number of leading zeros and the miner who can find the nonce is designated to add his local block to the Blockchain accompanied by the generation of a new cryptocurrency. This process is called mining. Mining involves expensive computations leading to (often massive) wastage of computational power and electricity, undesirable from an ecological point of view (O'Dwyer & Malone, 2014), and resulting in a small exclusive set of users for mining. This exclusivity, however, goes against the idea of having a decentralized set leading Blockchain platforms to employ other means of arriving at a consensus.

**Stakeholders**: This set employs the different variants of the Proof-of-Stake (POS) consensus mechanism. POS is a more just system than POW, as the computational resources required to accomplish mining or validation can be done through any computer. Ethereum POS requires the miner or the validator to lock a certain amount of their coins in the currency of the Blockchain platform to verify the block. This locked number of coins is called a stake. Computational power is required to verify whether a validator owns a certain percentage of the coins in the available currency or not. There are several proposals for POS, as POS enables an improved decentralized set, takes power out of the hands of a small exclusive group of validators, and distributes the work evenly across the Blockchain. In Ethereum POS, the probability of mining the block is proportional to the validator's stake (EthHub, 2020) just as in POW, and it is proportional to the computational hashing power. As long as a validator is mining, the stake owned by him remains locked. A downside of this consensus mechanism is that the richest validators are accorded a higher priority. The mechanism does, however, encourage more community participation than many other methods. Other consensus protocols include the traditional Byzantine Fault Tolerance theory (Sousa et al., 2018), where the economic set needs to be sampled for the total number of nodes. Here, the set most commonly used is stakeholders. Hence, such protocols can be considered as subcategories of POS.

**A User's Social Network**: This is used in Ripple and Stellar consensus protocols. The Ripple protocol, for example, requires a node to define a unique node list (UNL), which contains a list of other Ripple nodes that the defining node is confident would not work against it. A node consults other nodes in its UNL to achieve consensus. Consensus happens in multiple rounds with a node declaring a set of transactions in a "candidate set," which is sent to other nodes in the UNL. Nodes in the UNL validate the transactions, vote on them, and broadcast the votes. The initiating node then refines the "candidate set" based on the votes received to include the transactions getting the most significant number of votes for the next round. This process continues until a "candidate set" receives 80% votes from all the nodes in the UNL, and then it becomes a valid block in the Ripple Blockchain.

## Blockchain as a food supply chain disruptor

Blockchain technologies are considered a new type of disruptive Internet technology (Pan, Song, Ai, & Ming, 2019) and an essential enabler of large-scale societal and economic changes (Swan, 2015; Tapscott & Tapscott, 2017). The rationale for this argument is due to its complex technical constructs (Hughes et al., 2019), such as the immutability of transactions, security, confidentiality, consensual mechanisms, and the automation capabilities enabled by smart contracts. The latter is heralded as the most important application of Blockchain (the integrity of the code in smart contracts requires quality assurance and rigorous testing). By definition, a smart contract is a computer program that formalizes relationships over computer networks (Szabo, 1996, 1997). Although smart contracts predate Bitcoin/Blockchain by a decade and do not need a Blockchain to function (Halaburda, 2018), a Blockchain-based smart contract is executed on a Blockchain with a consensus mechanism determining its correct execution. A wide range of applications can be implemented using Smart contracts, including gaming, financial, notary, or computation (Bartoletti & Pompianu, 2017). The use of smart contracts in the FSC industry can help to verify digital documents (e.g., certificates such as organic or halal) as well as determine the provenance (source or origin) of specific data. In a cold chain scenario, Rejeb et al. (2019) argued that smart contracts connected to IoT devices could help to preserve the quality and safety of goods in transit. For example, temperature tolerances embedded into the smart contract can trigger in-transit alerts and facilitate shipment acceptance or rejection based on preset parameters in the smart contract. The first platform for implementing smart contracts was Ethereum (Buterin, 2014a, pp. 1−36), although most platforms today cater to smart contracts. Therefore, similar to the radical transformations brought by the Internet to individuals and corporate activities, the emergence of Blockchain provides opportunities that can broadly impact supply chain processes (Fosso Wamba et al., 2020; Queiroz, Telles, & Bonilla, 2019).

In order to understand the implications of Blockchain technology for food chains, it is essential to realize the potentials of its conjunction with GS1 standards. While the technology is still in a nascent stage of development and deployment, it is worthwhile to draw attention to the potential alignment of Blockchain technology with GS1 standards as proof of their success, and universal adoption is very likely to prevail in the future.

## Potentials of Blockchain-GS1 alignment in the FSC
### Defining traceability

Traceability is a multifaceted construct that is crucially important in FSCs and has received considerable attention through its application in the ISO 9000/BS 5750 quality standards (Cheng & Simmons, 1994). Scholars have stressed the importance and value of traceability in global FSCs (Charlier & Valceschini, 2008; Roth, Tsay, Pullman, & Gray, 2008). Broadly, traceability refers to the ability to track the flow of products and their attributes throughout the entire production process steps and supply chain (Golan et al., 2004). Furthermore, Olsen and Borit (2013) completed a comprehensive review of traceability across academic literature, industry standards, and regulations and argued that the various definitions of traceability are inconsistent and confusing, often with vague or recursive usage of terms such as "trace." They provide a comprehensive definition: "The ability to access any or all information relating to that which is under consideration, throughout its entire life cycle, by means of recorded identifications" (Olsen and Borit, 2013, p. 148).

The GS1 Global Traceability Standard (GS1, 2017c: 6) aligns with the ISO 9001: 2015 definition "Traceability is the ability to trace the history, application or location of an object [ISO 9001:2015]. When considering a product or a service, traceability can relate to origin of materials and parts; processing history; distribution and location of the product or service after delivery."

Traceability is also defined as "part of logistics management that capture, store, and transmit adequate information about a food, feed, food-producing animal or substance at all stages in the food supply chain so that the product can be checked for safety and quality control, traced upward, and tracked downward at any time required" (Bosona & Gebresenbet, 2013, p. 35).

## The role of technology

In the FSC context, a fundamental goal is to maintain a high level of food traceability to increase consumer trust and confidence in food products and to ensure proper documentation of the food for safety, regulatory, and financial purposes (Mahalik & Kim, 2016). Technology has played an increasingly critical role in food traceability over the past two decades (Hollands et al., 2018). For instance, radio frequency identification (RFID) has been adopted in some FSCs to enable non-line-of-sight identification of products to enhance end-to-end food traceability (Kelepouris et al., 2007). Walmart achieved significant efficiency gains by deploying drones in combination with RFID inside a warehouse for inventory control (Companik, Gravier, & Farris, 2018). However, technology applications for food traceability are fragmented, often proprietary and noninteroperable, and have enabled trading partners to capture only certain aspects of the FSC. As such, a holistic understanding of how agri-food businesses can better track the flow of food products and related information in extended, globalized FSCs is still in a nascent stage of development. For instance, Malhotra, Gosain, & El Sawy (2007) suggested it is imperative to adopt a more comprehensive approach of traceability that extends from source to final consumers in order to obtain a full understanding of information processing and sharing among supply chain stakeholders. In this regard, Blockchain technology brings substantial improvements in transparency and trust in food traceability (Behnke & Janssen, 2019; Biswas, Muthukkumarasamy, & Tan, 2017; Sander, Semeijn, & Mahr, 2018). However, arguments from many solution providers regarding traceability from "farm to fork" are a flawed concept as privacy law restricts tracking products forward to consumers. In this regard, tracking (to track forward) from farm to fork is impossible unless the consumer is a member of a retailers' loyalty program. However, tracing (to trace backward) from "fork to farm" is a feasible concept enabled by a consumer scanning a GS1-centric bar code or another code provided by the brand (e.g., proprietary QR code). Hence, farm-to-fork transparency is a more useful description of what is feasible (as opposed to farm-to-fork traceability). While a Blockchain is not necessarily needed for this function, depending on the complexity of the supply chain, a Blockchain that has immutable information (e.g., the original halal or organic certificate from the authoritative source) could improve the integrity of data and information provenance.

Blockchain is heralded as the new "Internet layer of value," providing the trinity of traceability, trust, and transparency to transactions involving data or physical goods and facilitating authentication, validation, traceability, and registration (Lima, 2018; Olsen & Borit, 2018). The application of GS1 standards with Blockchain technology integration enables global solutions linking identification standards for firms, locations, products, and assets with Blockchains transactional integrity. Thus, the combination of Blockchain and GS1 standards could respond to the emerging and more stringent regulatory requirements for enhanced forms of traceability in FSCs (Kim, Hilton, Burks, & Reyes, 2018).

A Blockchain can be configured to provide complete information on FSC processes, which is helpful to verify compliance to specifications and to trace a product to its source in adverse events (such as a consumer safety recall). This capability enables Blockchain-based applications to solve problems plaguing several domains, including the FSC, where verified and nonrepudiated data are vital across all segments to enable the functioning of the entire FSC as a unit. Within the GS1 standards framework, food traceability is industry-defined and industry-approved and includes categorizations of traceability attributes. These include the need to assign unique identifiers for each product or product class and group them to traceable resource unit (Behnke & Janssen, 2019).

FSC actors are both a **data creator** (i.e., they are the authoritative source of a data attribute) and a **data user** (i.e., a custodian of data created by other parties such as an upstream supplier). Data are created and used in the sequential order of farming, harvesting, production, packaging, distribution, and retailing. In an optimized FSC, the various exchange parties must be interconnected through a common set of interoperable data standards to ensure the data created and used provide a shared understanding of the data attributes and rules (rules on data creation and sharing are encompassed within GS1 standards).

A Blockchain can be configured to add value in FSCs by creating a platform with access and control of immutable data, which is not subject to egregious manipulation. Moreover, Blockchain technology can overcome the weaknesses created by the decades-old compliance to the minimum regulatory traceability requirements, such as registering the identity of the exchange party who is the source of inbound goods and registering the identity of the exchange party who is the recipient of outbound goods. This process is known as "one-up/one-down" traceability (Wang et al., 2019, pp. 512—523) and essentially means that exchange parties in an FSC have no visibility on products outside of their immediate exchange partners.

Blockchain technology enables FSC exchange partners to maintain food traceability by providing a secure, unfalsifiable, and complete history of food products from farm to retail (Molding, 2019). Unlike logistics-oriented traceability, the application of Blockchain and GS1 standards can create attribute-oriented traceability, which is not only concerned with the physical flow of food products but also tracks other crucial information, including product quality and safety-related information (Skilton & Robinson, 2009). On the latter point, food business operators always seek competitive advantage and premium pricing through the product (e.g., quality) or process differentiation claims (e.g., organically produced, cage-free eggs). This is in response to research indicating that an increasing segment of consumers will seek out food products best aligning with their lifestyle preferences such as vegetarian, vegan, or social and ethical values such as fair trade, organic, or cage-free (Beulens, Broens, Folstar, & Hofstede, 2005; Roe & Sheldon, 2007; Vellema, Loorbach, & Van Notten, 2006; Yoo, Parameswaran, & Kishore, 2015). In Fig. 17.4 below, Keogh (2018) outlines the essential traceability functions and distinguishes the supply chain flow of traceability event data versus the assurance flow of credence attributes such as food quality and food safety certification. For instance, in economic theory, goods are considered as comprising of ordinary, search, experience, or credence attributes (Darby & Karni, 1973; Nelson, 1970). Goods classified as ordinary (e.g., petrol or diesel) have well-known characteristics and known sources and locations to locate and purchase.

Regarding search, it refers to goods where the consumer can easily access trusted sources of information about the attributes of the product before purchase and at no cost. Search is "costless" per se and can vary from inspecting and trying on clothes before buying or going online to find out about a food product, including its ingredients, package size, recipes, or price. In the example of inspecting clothes before purchase, Dulleck, Kerschbamer, & Sutter (2009) differentiate this example as "search" from "experience" by arguing that experience entails unknown characteristics of the good that are revealed only after purchase (e.g., the actual quality of materials, whether it fades after washing).

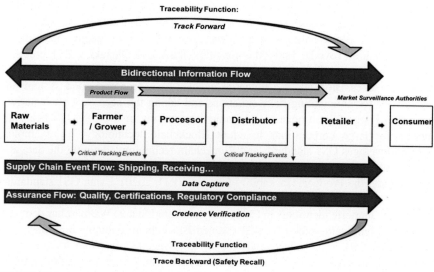

**FIGURE 17.4**

FSC product and information flows.

*Created by author in Keogh, J. G. (2018).* Blockchain, provenance, traceability & chain of custody. *Retrieved from https://www.linkedin.com/pulse/Blockchain-provenance-traceability-chain-custody-john-g-keogh/.*

Products classified as experience goods have attribute claims such as the product is tasty, flavorful, nutritious, or health-related such as lowers cholesterol and requires the product to be tasted or consumed to verify the claim, which may take time (e.g., lowers cholesterol). Verifying the experience attributes may be free if test driving a car or receiving a sample or taster of a food product in a store. Nevertheless, test driving or sampling will not confirm how the product will perform over time. Generally speaking, verifying experience attributes of food is not free, and it may take considerable time (and likely expense) to verify the claim.

Credence claims (Darby and Karni, 1973) are characterized by asymmetric information between food producers and food consumers. The reason for this is because credence attributes are either intrinsic to the product (e.g., food quality, food safety) or extrinsic methods of processing (e.g., organic, halal, kosher), and consumers cannot verify these claims before or after purchase (Dulleck et al., 2009). In this regard, a Blockchain offers a significant advancement in how credence claims flow (see Fig. 17.4) and are added to a product or batch/lot # record. For instance, the immutability of the data means that a brand owner can add a record such as a third-party certificate (e.g., laboratory analysis verifying a vegan claim or a USDA Organic certificate), but they cannot edit or change it. This feature adds much-needed integrity to FSCs and enhances transparency and consumer trust, especially if the third-party data are made available for consumers to query. In this context, the combination of GS1 standards and a Blockchain provides a consumer with the capability to scan a food product and query its digital record to verify credence claims.

At a more detailed level, the fragmentation of FSCs and their geographic dispersion illustrates the need for Blockchain and GS1 for achieving an optimal granularity level of traceability units (Dasaklis, Casino, & Patsakis., 2019). As such, the combination of Blockchain can help in the assurance of food quality and safety, providing secure (Toyoda, Takis Mathiopoulos, Sasase, & Ohtsuki, 2017), precise, and real-time traceability of products. Moreover, the speed of food authentication processes makes Blockchain a potential enabler of a proactive food system—a key catalyst for anticipating risky situations and taking the necessary preventative measures. Triggering automatic and immediate actions in the FSC has been an impetus for large corporations to adopt Blockchain technology; for example, Walmart leverages GS1 standards and Blockchain technology, defining the data attributes to be entered into their preferred Blockchain system, such as the attributes defined under the Produce Traceability Initiative (PTI, 2020). Using GS1 standards as a foundational layer, Walmart tracks pork meat and pallets of mangoes, tagged with unique numeric identifiers in China and the United States. Walmart has demonstrated the significant value of a GS1-enabled Blockchain, reducing both business and consumer risk in a product safety recall. More specifically, Walmart simulated a product safety recall for mangoes, and this exercise suggested a reduction in time to execute the product safety recall from 7 days pre-Blockchain to 2.2 s using a Blockchain (Kamath, 2017).

The contribution of GS1 to the de facto individualization of food products has motivated the study of dos Santos, Torrisi, Yamada, & Pantoni (2019), who examine the traceability requirements in recipe-based foods and propose whole-chain traceability with a focus on ingredient certification. With the use of Blockchain technology, it is possible to verify the source of any batch or a lot number of ingredients. Kim et al. (2018) developed an application called "Food Bytes" using Blockchain technology and enabling consumers to validate and verify specific quality attributes of their foods (e.g., organic) by accessing curated GS1 standard data from mobile devices, thereby increasing ease of consumer usability and ultimately trust. Blockchain technology can help FSC partners develop best practices for traceability and to curb fraudulent and deceptive actions as well as the adulteration of food products. To solve these issues, Staples et al. (2017) develop a traceability system based on HACCP, GS1, and Blockchain technology in order to guarantee reliable traceability of the swine supply chain. In their proposed system, GS1 aids in the coordination of supply chain information, and Blockchain is applied to secure food traceability.

## Food chain interoperability

A pressing challenge facing FSCs is the need to coordinate information exchange across several types of commodities, transportation modes, and information systems. By analogy, a similar need was resolved in the healthcare industry through the implementation of Electronic Health Records (EHR) to provide access to an individual patient's records across all subdomains catering to the patient. The healthcare industry is presently working on enhancing EHR through the deployment of Blockchain to serve as a decentralized data repository for preserving data integrity, security, and ease of management (Shahnaz, Qamar, & Khalid, 2019). Closely resembling the role and function of the EHR in the healthcare industry, the creation of a Digital Food Record (DFR) is vital for FSCs to facilitate whole-chain traceability, interoperability, linking the different actors and data creators in the chain, and enhancing trust in the market on each product delivered.

FSC operators need access to business-critical data at an aggregated level to drive their business strategy and operational decisions, and many of the organizations operate at the global, international, or national levels. Data digitization and collaboration efforts of FSC organizations are essential to enable actionable decisions by the broader food industry. Currently, much of the data currently exist as siloed, disparate sources that are not easily accessible; including data related to trade (crop shortages/overages), market prices, import/export transaction data, or real-time data on pests, disease or weather patterns, and forecasts. With this in mind, and acknowledging the need for transparent and trusted data sharing, the Dutch horticulture and food domain created "HortiCube," an integrated platform to enable seamless sharing of data and enable semantic interoperability (Verhoosel, van Bekkum, & Verwaart, 2018). The platform provides "an application programming interface (API) that is based on the Open Data Protocol (OData). Via this interface, application developers can request three forms of information; data sources available, data contained in the source, and the data values from these data sources (Verhoosel et al., 2018, p. 102).

The US Food and Drug Administration is currently implementing the Food Safety Modernization Act (FSMA) with emphasis on the need for technological tools to accomplish interoperability and collaboration in their "New Era of Smarter Food Safety" (FDA, 2019). In order to enable traceability as envisioned in FSMA, a solution is required that incorporates multiple technologies, including IoT devices. Blockchain is envisioned as a platform of choice in accordance with its characteristic of immutability to prevent the corruption of data (Khan, 2018). Ecosystems suited for the application of Blockchain technology are those consisting of an increasing set of distributed nodes that need a standard approach and a cohesive plan to ensure interoperability. More precisely, FSCs comprised of various partners working collaboratively to meet the demands of various customer profiles, where collaboration necessitates an exchange of data (Mertins et al., 2012); furthermore, the data should be interchanged in real-time and verified to be originating from the designated source. Interoperability is a precursor of robust FSCs that can withstand market demands by providing small and medium enterprises with the necessary information to decide on the progress of any product within the supply chain and ensure the advancement of safe products to the end consumer. Blockchain technology enables an improved level of interoperability as FSC actors would be able to communicate real-time information (Bouzdine-Chameeva, Jaegler, & Tesson, 2019), coordinate functions, and synchronize data exchanges (Bajwa, Prewett, & Shavers, 2010; Behnke & Janssen, 2019). The potential interoperability provided by Blockchains can be realized through the implementation of GS1 standards. Specifically, the Electronic Product Code Information Standard (EPCIS), which can be used to ensure the documentation of all FSC events in an understandable form and the aggregation of food products into higher logistic units, business transactions, or other information related to the quantity of food products and their types (Xu, Weber, & Staples, 2019). A recent study by the Institute of Food Technologists found evidence that technology providers faced difficulty in collaborating to determine the origin or the recipients of a contaminated product (Bhatt & Zhang, 2013). Hence, the novel approach of Blockchain provides a specific emphasis on interoperability between disparate FSC systems, allowing technology providers to design robust platforms that ensure interoperable and end-to-end product traceability.

The use of IoT devices allow organizations within FSCs to send and receive data; however, the authenticity of the data still needs to be ascertained. A compounding factor is the technological complexity of FSCs (Ahtonen & Virolainen, 2009), due to the reliance on siloed systems that hamper collaboration and efficient flow of information. However, Blockchain architecture can accommodate interoperability standards at the variable periphery (the IoT devices) and other technologies used to connect FSC processes (Augustin, Sanguansri, Fox, Cobiac, & Cole, 2020). Blockchain is envisaged as a powerful tool (Ande, Adebisi, Hammoudeh, & Saleem, 2019) and an appropriate medium to store the data from IoT devices since it provides seamless authentication, security, protection against attacks, and ease of deployment among other potential advantages (Fernández-Caramés & Fraga-Lamas, 2018).

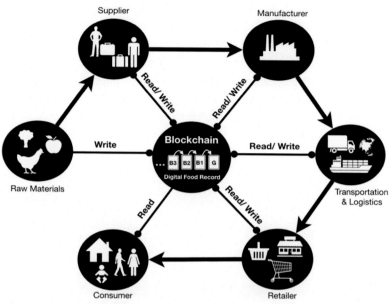

**FIGURE 17.5**

Blockchain: The FSC Interoperability Ecosystem

*Created by author.*

For FSC, Blockchain is seen as the foundational technology for the sharing and distribution (read and write) of data by the organizations comprising the ecosystem, as shown in Fig. 17.5. In this model, consumers can read data for any product and trace the entire path from the origin to the destination while relying upon the immutability of Blockchain to protect the data from any tampering. Supply chain data are stored as a DFR in the various blocks (e.g., B1, B2, B3) that comprise the Blockchain. The first block represented by G in Fig. 17.3 refers to the genesis block, which functions as a prototype for all the other blocks in the Blockchain.

## GS1, traceability, and Blockchain

GS1 ratified version 2.0 of the GS1 Global Traceability Standard (GS1, 2017b), documenting the business process and system requirements for full-chain traceability. The document is generic by design with supplemental, industry-specific documents developed separately. Of interest to FSCs are

- **GS1 Global Meat and Poultry Traceability Guideline** (legacy, developed for GS1 Global Traceability Standard 1.3.0) (GS1, 2015a)
- **GS1 Foundation for Fish, Seafood and Aquaculture Traceability Guideline** (GS1, 2019a)

- **Traceability for Fresh Fruits and Vegetables-Implementation Guide** (legacy, developed for GS1 Global Traceability Standard 1.3.0) (GS1, 2015b)
- **GS1 Global Traceability Compliance Criteria for Food Application Standard** (legacy, developed for GS1 Global Traceability Standard 1.3.0) (GS1, 2016b)

Together, these documents provide comprehensive guidance to FSCs on the implementation of a traceability framework. Figs. 17.6 and 17.7 below indicate a single and multiple company view of traceability data generation.

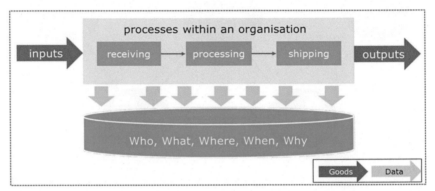

**FIGURE 17.6**

Generation of traceability data—a single company view.

*Source: (GS1, 2017a).*

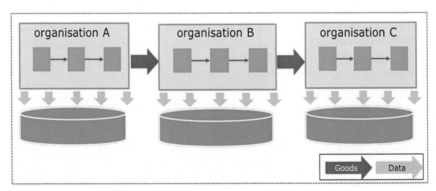

**FIGURE 17.7**

Generation of traceability data in a multiparty supply chain

*(GS1, 2017a)*

Underlying the GS1 traceability standard is the GS1 EPCIS (GS1, 2016a), which defines traceability as an ordered collection of events that comprise four key dimensions:

- **What**-the subject of the event, either a specific object (EPC) or a class of object (EPC class) and a quantity
- **When**-the time at which the event occurred
- **Where**-the location where the event took place
- **Why**-the business context of the event

The GS1 Global Traceability Standard adds a fifth dimension, "who," to identify the parties involved. This can be substantially different from the "where" dimension, as a single location (e.g., a third-party warehouse) may be associated with multiple, independent parties.

EPCIS is supplemented by the Core Business Vocabulary Standard (GS1, 2017a), which specifies the structure of vocabularies and specific values for the vocabulary elements to be utilized in conjunction with the GS1 EPCIS standard.

## Implementing EPCIS

EPCIS is a standard that defines the type and structure of events and a mechanism for querying the repository. Assuming that all parties publish to a common EPCIS repository (centralized approach) or that all parties make their repositories available (open approach), traceability is simply the process of querying events, analyzing them, and querying subsequent events until all relevant data are retrieved.

In practice, neither the centralized nor open approach is possible. In the centralized approach, multiple, competing repositories will naturally prevent a single, centralized repository from ever being realized. Even if such a model were to be supported in the short term by key players in the traceability ecosystem, as more and more players are added, the odds of one or more of them already having used a competing repository grows. In the open approach, not all parties will be willing to share all data with all others, especially competitors. Depending on the nature of the party querying the data or the nature of the query itself, the response may be no records, some records, or all records satisfying the query. For either approach, there is the question of data integrity: can the system prove that the traceability data have not been tampered with?

Blockchain is a potential solution to these problems. As a decentralized platform, Blockchain integration could provide EPCIS solution providers with a way of sharing data in a secure fashion. Furthermore, the sequential, immutable nature of the Blockchain platform either ensures that the data cannot be changed or provides a mechanism for verifying that it has not been tampered with.

The critical question is, what exactly gets stored on the Blockchain? The options discussed by GS1 in a white paper on a Blockchain (GS1, 2019b) are

- Fully formed, cryptographically signed plain text event data, which raises concerns about scalability, performance, and security if full events are written to a ledger;
- A cryptographic hash of the data that has little meaning by itself. This requires off-chain data exchange via a separate traceability application and a hash comparison to verify that data have not been altered since the hash was written to the ledger; and
- A cryptographic hash of the data and a pointer to off-chain data. This is the same as the above point with a pointer to the off-chain data source. Such an approach can enable the ledger to act as part of a discovery mechanism for parties who need to communicate and share data.

This then leads to the question of the accessibility of the data:

**Public**: Everyone sees all transactions;
**Private**: This includes a permission layer that makes transactions viewable to only approved parties.

## Blockchain integration challenges

Integrating EPCIS (or any other data sharing standard) with Blockchain often presents significant challenges:

In most cases, volumetric analysis can reveal sensitive business intelligence even without examining the data. For example, if company X is currently publishing 1000 records per day, and next year at the same time it is publishing only 800, it is reasonable to assume that company X's volume is down by 20% year over year.

Revealing the subject of an event (the "what" dimension) can reveal who is handling the expensive product, which may be used to plan its theft or diversion.

Publishing a record in plain text makes the data available to any party that has a copy of the ledger, but not all data should be available to all parties. For example, transformation events in EPCIS record inputs partially or fully consumed to produce one or more outputs. In the food industry, this is the very nature of a recipe, which is often a closely guarded trade secret. In order to mitigate this risk, the ledger would have to be firmly held by a limited number of parties that could enforce proper data access controls. Even if such a system were to be implemented correctly, it means that proprietary information would still be under the control of a third party, which is a risk that many food companies would not be willing to take.

Publishing a record in an encrypted form would solve the visibility issue, but in order to do so, the industry would have to agree on how to generate the keys for the encrypted data. One option is to use the event's subject (the "what" dimension) as the key. If the identifier for the subject is sufficiently randomized, this ensures that only parties that have encountered the identifier can actually decrypt the data;

while other parties could guess at possible values of the identifier, doing so at scale can be expensive and therefore self-limiting. There would also have to be a way to identify which data are relevant to the identifier, which would mean storing something like a hash of the identifier as a key. Only those parties that know the identifier (i.e., that have observed it at some point in its traceability journey) will be able to locate the data of interest and decrypt them.

Parties could publish a hash of the record along with the record's primary key. This could then be used to validate records to ensure that they have not been tampered with, but it means that any party that wishes to query the data would have to know ahead of time where the data reside. Once queried successfully, the record's primary key would be used to lookup the hash for comparison.

To enable discovery, data consisting of the event's subject (the "what" dimension) and a pointer to a repository could be published. In essence, this is a declaration that the repository has data related to the event's subject, and a query for records related to the event's subject is likely to be successful. To further secure the discovery, the event's subject could be hashed, and that could be used as the key. Volumetric analysis is still possible with this option.

To limit volumetric analysis, data consisting of the class level of the event's subject and a pointer to a repository could be published. This is essentially a declaration that objects of a specific type have events in the repository, but it does not explicitly say how many or what specific objects they refer to. It still reveals that the company using the repository is handling the product.

Over and above all of this is the requirement that all publications be to the same type of Blockchain ledger. There are currently no interoperability standards for Blockchains. The industry would, therefore, have to settle on one, which has the same issue as settling on a single EPCIS repository. Further technical research is required to determine the viability of the various options for publishing to the Blockchain.

## Discussion and conclusion

The standardization efforts in global FSCs have led to the need for best practice recommendations and common ways of managing logistics units in the food chain. The widespread use of GS1 standards reflects the tendency of food organizations to operate in an integrated manner with a universal language. This facilitates FSCs to structure and align with a cohesive approach to food traceability, empowering multidirectional information sharing, optimizing efficiencies, and added-value activities for FSC stakeholders. Moreover, the embeddedness of GS1 standards in global FSCs allows trading partners to work in an industry-regulated environment wherein food quality and food safety are of the utmost priority in delivering sustainable, authentic products to final consumers.

Today, the usage of GS1 standards is inevitable as they provide clear guidelines on how to manage and share event data across global FSCs (Figueroa, Añorga, & Arrizabalaga, 2019). This inevitability is further enhanced through the leadership of the global management board of GS1 (as of February 2020) that consists of senior executives from organizations such as Procter & Gamble, Nestle, Amazon, Google, J.M. Smucker, L'Oreal, Metro AG, Alibaba, and others. Similarly, the management board for the GS1 US organization includes senior executives from Walmart, Wegfern, Wendy's, Coca Cola, Target, Publix, Wegmans, Sysco, Massachusetts Institute of Technology, and others. The commitment of these organizations strongly supports the industry adoption of GS1 standards, and GS1 enabled Blockchain solutions as indicated by Walmart in their US-driven "fresh leafy greens" traceability initiative (Walmart, 2018). Moreover, many of these firms have announced Blockchain-related initiatives in their supply chains.

Walmart's traceability initiative reflects growing consumer concerns regarding food quality and safety and the recurring nature of product safety recalls. The combination of GS1 standards with Blockchain can provide immutable evidence of data provenance, enhance food traceability and rapid recall, and increase trust in the quality of food products. GS1 standards aid organizations in maintaining a unified view of the state of food while transitioning between processing stages across globalized and highly extended supply chains with multiple exchange parties. As such, the broad adoption of electronic traceability as identified by GS1 can endow the food industry with several capabilities, ranging from the optimization of trace-back procedures, the standardization of supply chain processes, the continuous improvement in food production activities, and the development of more efficient and holistic traceability systems.

The use of GS1 standards for the formation of interoperable and scalable food traceability systems can be reinforced with Blockchain technology. As envisioned by many food researchers, practitioners, and organizations, Blockchain technology represents a practical solution that has a positive impact on FSC collaborations and data sharing. Blockchain technology creates a more comprehensive and inclusive framework that promotes an unprecedented level of transparency and visibility of food products as they are exchanged among FSC partners. Combined with GS1 standards, Blockchain technology offers a more refined level of interoperability between exchange parties in global FSCs and facilitates a move away from the traditional or linear, stove-piped supply chains with limited data sharing.

By leveraging Blockchain, FSCs would be able to develop a management information platform that enables the active collection, transfer, storage, control, and sharing of food-related information among FSC exchange parties. The combination of Blockchain and GS1 standards can create a high level of trust because of the precision in data and information provenance, immutability, nonrepudiation, enhanced integrity, and deeper integration. The development of harmonized global FSCs gives rise to more efficient traceability systems that are capable of minimizing the impact of food safety incidents and lowering the costs and risks related to product recalls. Therefore, the integration of GS1 standards into a Blockchain can enhance the competitive advantage of FSCs.

In order to unlock the full potential from the functional components of a Blockchain and the integration of GS1 standards, several prerequisites need to be fulfilled. For example, a more uniformed and standardized model of data governance is necessary to facilitate the operations of FSCs in a globalized context. A balance between the conformance with diverse regulatory requirements and the FSC partners' requirements should be established in order to maintain a competitive position in the global market. The inter- and intraorganizational support for Blockchain implementations, including the agreement on what type of data should be shared and accessed, the establishment of clear lines of responsibilities and accountability, and the development of more organized and flexible FSCs should be considered prior to Blockchain adoption (Fosso Wamba et al., 2019).

In summary, a Blockchain is not a panacea, and non-Blockchain solutions are functioning adequately in many FSCs today. The business case or use case is crucially important when considering whether a Blockchain is required and whether its functionality adds value. Moreover, a Blockchain does not consider unethical behaviors and opportunism in global FSCs (bad character). Organizations need to consider other risk factors that could impact ex post transaction costs and reputation. Global FSC risk factors include slave labor, child labor, unsafe working conditions, animal welfare, environmental damage, deforestation and habitat loss, bribery and corruption, and various forms of opportunism such as quality cheating or falsification of laboratory or government records before they are added to a Blockchain. Product data governance and enhanced traceability can be addressed in global FSCs, but "bad character" is more difficult to detect and eliminate. Essentially, bad data and bad character are the two main enemies of trust in the food chain.

## Limitations of the study and further research

This study focused narrowly on existing research combining Blockchain, GS1 standards, and food. Due to the narrow scope of the research, we did not explore all technical aspects of the fast-evolving Blockchain technology, smart contracts, or cryptography.

Further research is needed to explore the risks associated with the integrity of data entered into a Blockchain, especially situations where bad actors may use a Blockchain to establish false trust with false data. In this regard, "immutable lies" are added to a Blockchain and create a false sense of trust. Because of this potential risk, and because errors occuring in the physical flow of goods within supply chains are common (e.g., damage, shortage, theft) as well as errors in data sharing and privacy, the notion of Blockchain "mutability" should be researched further (Rejeb et al., 2019, 2020).

Further technical research is encouraged to explore the relationship between the immutability features of a Blockchain and the mutability features of the EPCIS standard. In the latter, EPCIS permits corrections where the original, erroneous record is preserved, and the correction has a pointer to the original. Researchers should explore current EPCIS adoption challenges and whether EPCIS could provide Blockchain-to-Blockchain and Blockchain-to-legacy interoperability. The latter may mitigate the risks associated with FSC exchange partners being "forced" to adopt a single proprietary Blockchain platform or as a participant in multiple proprietary Blockchain platforms in order to trade with their business partners.

Researchers should explore if the latency of real-time data retrieval in Blockchain-based FSCs restricts consumer engagement in verifying credence claims in real time due to the complexity of retrieving block transaction history.

## Acknowledgment

The authors are thankful to Dr. Steven J. Simske, Dr. Subhasis Thakur, and Irene Woerner for their thoughtful commentary on this chapter.
Abderahman Rejeb, coauthor and Ph.D. candidate, is grateful to Professor László Imre Komlósi, Dr. Katalin Czakó, and Ms. Tihana Vasic for their valuable support.
Conflict of Interests
- No funding was received for this publication.
- John G. Keogh, the corresponding author, is a former executive at GS1 Canada and has not advised or worked with or for GS1 for more than 5 years.
- Kevin Dean is an independent technical consultant advising GS1.

## References

Ahtonen, A.-K., & Virolainen, V.-M. (2009). Supply strategy in the food industry — value net perspective. *International Journal of Logistics Research and Applications, 12*(4), 263–279. https://doi.org/10.1080/13675560903076107.

Ande, R., Adebisi, B., Hammoudeh, M., & Saleem, J. (2019). Internet of Things: Evolution and technologies from a security perspective. *Sustainable Cities and Society*, 101728. https://doi.org/10.1016/j.scs.2019.101728.

Augustin, M. A., Sanguansri, L., Fox, E. M., Cobiac, L., & Cole, M. B. (2020). Recovery of wasted fruit and vegetables for improving sustainable diets. *Trends in Food Science & Technology, 95*, 75–85. https://doi.org/10.1016/j.tifs.2019.11.010.

Autio, M., Autio, J., Kuismin, A., Ramsingh, B., Kylkilahti, E., & Valros, A. (2017). Bringing farm animal to the consumer's plate—the quest for food business to enhance transparency, labelling and consumer education. In N. Amos, & R. Sullivan (Eds.), *The business of farm animal welfare*. Greenleaf Publishing.

Bajwa, N., Prewett, K., & Shavers, C. L. (2010). Is your supply chain ready to embrace Blockchain? *Journal of Corporate Accounting & Finance*, 1–11. https://doi.org/10.1002/jcaf.22423.

Barnard, C., & O'Connor, N. (2017). Runners and riders: The horsemeat scandal, Eu law and multi-level enforcement. *The Cambridge Law Journal, 76*(1), 116–144. https://doi.org/10.1017/S000819731700006X.

Bartoletti, M., & Pompianu, L. (2017). An empirical analysis of smart contracts: Platforms, applications, and design patterns. In M. Brenner, K. Rohloff, J. Bonneau, A. Miller, P. Y. A. Ryan, V. Teague, et al. (Eds.), *Financial cryptography and data security* (pp. 494–509). Springer International Publishing. https://doi.org/10.1007/978-3-319-70278-0_31.

Behnke, K., & Janssen, M. F. W. H. A. (2019). Boundary conditions for traceability in food supply chains using Blockchain technology. *International Journal of Information Management*, 101969. https://doi.org/10.1016/j.ijinfomgt.2019.05.025.

Beulens, A. J. M., Broens, D.-F., Folstar, P., & Hofstede, G. J. (2005). Food safety and transparency in food chains and networks relationships and challenges. *Food Control, 16*(6), 481–486. https://doi.org/10.1016/j.foodcont.2003.10.010.

Bhatt, T., & Zhang, J. (2013). Food product tracing technology capabilities and interoperability. *Journal of Food Science, 78*(s2), B28–B33. https://doi.org/10.1111/1750-3841.12299.

BildtgÅrd, T. (2008). Trust in food in modern and late-modern societies. *Social Science Information, 47*(1), 99–128. https://doi.org/10.1177/0539018407085751.

Biswas, K., Muthukkumarasamy, V., & Tan, W. L. (2017). Blockchain based wine supply chain traceability system. *Future Technologies Conference*, 56–62.

Borras, S. M. (2020). Agrarian social movements: The absurdly difficult but not impossible agenda of defeating right-wing populism and exploring a socialist future. *Journal of Agrarian Change, 20*(1), 3–36. https://doi.org/10.1111/joac.12311.

Bosona, T., & Gebresenbet, G. (2013). Food traceability as an integral part of logistics management in food and agricultural supply chain. *Food Control, 33*(1), 32–48. https://doi.org/10.1016/j.foodcont.2013.02.004.

Bourlakis, M. A., & Weightman, P. W. H. (2008). *Food supply chain management.* Blackwell Publishing Ltd..

Bouzdine-Chameeva, T., Jaegler, A., & Tesson, P. (2019). Value co-creation in wine logistics: The case of dartess. *IEEE Engineering Management Review, 47*(1), 115–125. https://doi.org/10.1109/EMR.2019.2898631.

Buterin, V. (2014a). *A next-generation smart contract and decentralized application platform* (pp. 1–36) [Whitepaper] https://cryptorating.eu/whitepapers/Ethereum/Ethereum_white_paper.pdf.

Buterin, V. (2014b). *Proof of stake: How I learned to love weak subjectivity.* https://blog.ethereum.org/2014/11/25/proof-stake-learned-love-weak-subjectivity/.

Callon, M., Law, J., & Rip, A. (1986). How to study the force of science. In M. Callon, J. Law, & A. Rip (Eds.), *Mapping the dynamics of science and technology: Sociology of science in the real world* (pp. 3–15). UK: Palgrave Macmillan. https://doi.org/10.1007/978-1-349-07408-2_1.

CFIA. (2019, January 30). *Food fraud.* Reference material. Retrieved from https://inspection.gc.ca/food-safety-for-industry/information-for-consumers/food-safety-system/food-fraud/eng/1548444446366/1548444516192.

Chanchaichujit, J., Tan, A., Meng, F., & Eaimkhong, S. (2019). Blockchain technology in healthcare. In J. Chanchaichujit, A. Tan, F. Meng, & S. Eaimkhong (Eds.), *Healthcare 4.0: Next generation processes with the latest technologies* (pp. 37–62). Springer. https://doi.org/10.1007/978-981-13-8114-0_3.

Charlier, C., & Valceschini, E. (2008). Coordination for traceability in the food chain. A critical appraisal of European regulation. *European Journal of Law and Economics, 25*(1), 1–15.

Chemeltorit, P., Saavedra, Y., & Gema, J. (2018). *Food traceability in the domestic horticulture sector in Kenya: An overview.*

Cheng, M. J., & Simmons, J. E. L. (1994). Traceability in manufacturing systems. *International Journal of Operations & Production Management, 14*(10), 4–16. https://doi.org/10.1108/01443579410067199.

Cho, S., & Choi, G. (2019). Exploring latent factors influencing the adoption of a processed food traceability system in South Korea. *International Journal on Food System Dynamics, 10*(2), 162–175. https://doi.org/10.18461/ijfsd.v10i2.10.

Choi, T. Y., & Hong, Y. (2002). Unveiling the structure of supply networks: Case studies in Honda, Acura, and DaimlerChrysler. *Journal of Operations Management, 20*(5), 469–493. https://doi.org/10.1016/S0272-6963(02)00025-6.

Companik, E., Gravier, M., & Farris, M. (2018). Feasibility of warehouse drone adoption and implementation. *Journal of Transportation Management, 28*(2), 31–48. https://doi.org/10.22237/jotm/1541030640.

Cousins, P. D., Lawson, B., Petersen, K. J., & Fugate, B. (2019). Investigating green supply chain management practices and performance: The moderating roles of supply chain eco-centricity and traceability. *International Journal of Operations & Production Management, 39*(5), 767–786. https://doi.org/10.1108/IJOPM-11-2018-0676.

Dani, S. (2015). *Food supply chain management and logistics: From farm to fork*. Kogan Page Publishers.

Darby, M. R., & Karni, E. (1973). Free competition and the optimal amount of fraud. *The Journal of Law and Economics, 16*(1), 67–88. https://doi.org/10.1086/466756.

Dasaklis, T. K., Casino, F., & Patsakis, C. (2019). Defining granularity levels for supply chain traceability based on IoT and Blockchain. *Proceedings of the International Conference on Omni-Layer Intelligent Systems*, 184–190. https://doi.org/10.1145/3312614.3312652.

Donnelly, K. A.-M., Thakur, M., & Sakai, J. (2013). Following the mackerel — cost and benefits of improved information exchange in food supply chains. *Food Control, 33*(1), 25–31. https://doi.org/10.1016/j.foodcont.2013.01.021.

Dulleck, U., Kerschbamer, R., & Sutter, M. (2009). The economics of credence goods: An experimental investigation of the role of verifiability, liability, competition and reputation in credence goods markets. In R. Schob, M. Ahlert, L. Arnold, M. Lechner, R. Niemann, & O. Reimann (Eds.), *Proceedings of the annual conference of Verein Fur Socialpolitik 2009* (pp. 1–48). Verein Fur Socialpolitik. http://www.socialpolitik.ovgu.de/tagungsinformation/inhalt/programm_papers.print.

EthHub. (2020). *Ethereum proof of stake—EthHub*. https://docs.ethhub.io/ethereum-roadmap/ethereum-2.0/proof-of-stake/.

FDA. (2019, November 19). *New era of smarter food safety*. FDA. http://www.fda.gov/food/food-industry/new-era-smarter-food-safety.

Fernández-Caramés, T. M., & Fraga-Lamas, P. (2018). A review on the use of Blockchain for the Internet of Things. *IEEE Access, 6*, 32979–33001. https://doi.org/10.1109/ACCESS.2018.2842685.

Figueroa, S., Añorga, J., & Arrizabalaga, S. (2019). An attribute-based access control model in RFID systems based on Blockchain decentralized applications for healthcare environments. *Computers, 8*(3), 57. https://doi.org/10.3390/computers8030057.

Fosso Wamba, S., Kamdjoug, K., Robert, J., Bawack, R., & Keogh, J. (2019). Bitcoin, Blockchain, and FinTech: A systematic review and case studies in the supply chain. *Production Planning and Control, 31*(2−3), 115−142.

Frizzo-Barker, J., Chow-White, P. A., Adams, P. R., Mentanko, J., Ha, D., & Green, S. (2019). Blockchain as a disruptive technology for business: A systematic review. *International Journal of Information Management*, 102029. https://doi.org/10.1016/j.ijinfomgt.2019.10.014.

Giusti, R., Manerba, D., Bruno, G., & Tadei, R. (2019). Synchromodal logistics: An overview of critical success factors, enabling technologies, and open research issues. *Transportation Research Part E: Logistics and Transportation Review, 129*, 92−110. https://doi.org/10.1016/j.tre.2019.07.009.

Global Report: The Edelman Trust Barometer 2020. (2020, January 19). Edelman. Retrieved from https://www.edelman.com/sites/g/files/aatuss191/files/2020-01/2020%20Edelman%20Trust%20Barometer%20Global%20Report.pdf.https://www.edelman.com/trustbarometer.

Golan, E., Krissoff, B., Kuchler, F., Calvin, L., Nelson, K. E., & Price, G. K. (2004). *Traceability in the US food supply: Economic theory and industry studies (agricultural economics reports No. 33939*. United States Department of Agriculture, Economic Research Service. https://econpapers.repec.org/paper/agsuerser/33939.htm.

GS1. (2014). *Marsh holds place of honor in history of GS1 barcode* [Text]. Retrieved from https://www.gs1.org/articles/1606/marsh-holds-place-honor-history-gs1-barcode.

GS1. (2015a). *GS1 made easy—global meat and poultry traceability guideline companion document*. Retrieved from https://www.gs1.org/docs/traceability/GS1_Global_Meat_and_Poultry_Guideline_Companion_GS1_Made_Easy.pdf.

GS1. (2015b). *Traceability for fresh fruits and vegetables implementation Guide*. Retrieved from https://www.gs1.org/sites/default/files/docs/traceability/Global_Traceability_Implementation_Fresh_Fruit_Veg.pdf.

GS1. (2016a). *EPC information services (EPCIS) standard*. Retrieved from https://www.gs1.org/sites/default/files/docs/epc/EPCIS-Standard-1.2-r-2016-09-29.pdf.

GS1. (2016b). *GS1 global traceability compliance criteria for food application standard*. Retrieved from https://www.gs1.org/docs/traceability/GS1_Global_Traceability_Compliance_Criteria_For_Food_Application_Standard.pd.

GS1. (2017a). *Core business vocabulary standard*. Retrieved from https://www.gs1.org/sites/default/files/docs/epc/CBV-Standard-1-2-2-r-2017-10-12.pdf.

GS1. (2017b). *GS1 global traceability standard*. GS1. Retrieved from https://www.gs1.org/sites/default/files/docs/traceability/GS1_Global_Traceability_Standard_i2.pdf.

GS1. (2017c). *GS1 global traceability standard. Release 2.0. Ratified 2017 (GS1's framework for the design of interoperable traceability systems for supply chains)*. GS1.

GS1. (2019a). *GS1 foundation for fish, seafood and aquaculture traceability guideline*. Retrieved from https://www.gs1.org/sites/default/files/docs/traceability/GS1_Foundation_for_Fish_Seafood_Aquaculture_Traceability_Guideline.pdf.

GS1. (2019b). *Traceability and Blockchain*. Retrieved from https://www.gs1.org/sites/default/files/gs1_traceability_and_Blockchain_wp.pdf.

GS1. (2020). *How we got here* [Text]. Retrieved from https://www.gs1.org/about/how-we-got-here.

GS1 UK, The institute for Grocery Distribution, Cranfield School of Management (KTP project), & Value Chain Vision. (2009). *Data crunch report: The impact of bad data on profits and customer service in the UK grocery industry.* Retrieved from https://dspace.lib. cranfield.ac.uk/bitstream/handle/1826/4135/Data_crunch_report.pdf.?sequence=1.

Halaburda, H. (2018). *Blockchain revolution without the Blockchain.* https://doi.org/10.2139/ ssrn.3133313.

Helo, P., & Shamsuzzoha, A. H. M. (2020). Real-time supply chain—a Blockchain architecture for project deliveries. *Robotics and Computer-Integrated Manufacturing, 63,* 101909. https://doi.org/10.1016/j.rcim.2019.101909.

Hollands, T., Martindale, W., Swainson, M., & Keogh, J. G. (2018). Blockchain or bust for the food industry? *Food Science and Technology, 33*(4). Retrieved from https://www. fstjournal.org/features/32-4/Blockchain.

Hughes, L., Dwivedi, Y. K., Misra, S. K., Rana, N. P., Raghavan, V., & Akella, V. (2019). Blockchain research, practice and policy: Applications, benefits, limitations, emerging research themes and research agenda. *International Journal of Information Management, 49,* 114—129. https://doi.org/10.1016/j.ijinfomgt.2019.02.005.

Iansiti, M., & Lakhani, K. R. (2017). The truth about Blockchain. *Harvard Business Review, 95*(1), 118—127.

Iida, J., Watanabe, D., Nagata, K., & Matsuda, M. (2019). Sharing procedure status information on ocean containers across countries using port community systems with decentralized architecture. *Asian Transport Studies, 5*(4), 694—719. https://doi.org/10.11175/ eastsats.5.694.

Johnston, D. A., McCutcheon, D. M., Stuart, F. I., & Kerwood, H. (2004). Effects of supplier trust on performance of cooperative supplier relationships. *Journal of Operations Management, 22*(1), 23—38. https://doi.org/10.1016/j.jom.2003.12.001.

Kamath, R. (2017). Food traceability on Blockchain: Walmart's pork and mango pilots with IBM. *The Journal of the British Blockchain Association, 1*(1), 3712.

Kamble, S. S., Gunasekaran, A., Parekh, H., & Joshi, S. (2019). Modeling the internet of things adoption barriers in food retail supply chains. *Journal of Retailing and Consumer Services, 48,* 154—168. https://doi.org/10.1016/j.jretconser.2019.02.020.

Kano, Y., & Nakajima, T. (2018). A novel approach to solve a mining work centralization problem in Blockchain technologies. *International Journal of Pervasive Computing and Communications.* https://doi.org/10.1108/IJPCC-D-18-00005.

Kelepouris, T., Pramatari, K., & Doukidis, G. (2007). RFID-enabled traceability in the food supply chain. *Industrial Management & Data Systems, 107*(2), 183—200. https:// doi.org/10.1108/02635570710723804.

Keogh, J. G. (2018). *Blockchain, provenance, traceability & chain of custody.* https://www. linkedin.com/pulse/Blockchain-provenance-traceability-chain-custody-john-g-keogh/.

Khan, N. (2018). Fast: A MapReduce consensus for high performance Blockchains. In *Proceedings of the 1st workshop on Blockchain-enabled networked sensor systems* (pp. 1—6). https://doi.org/10.1145/3282278.3282279.

Kim, M., Hilton, B., Burks, Z., & Reyes, J. (2018). Integrating Blockchain, smart contract-tokens, and IoT to design a food traceability solution. In *2018 IEEE 9th annual information technology, electronics and mobile communication conference (IEMCON)* (pp. 335—340). https://doi.org/10.1109/IEMCON.2018.8615007.

Lacity, M. C. (2018). Addressing key challenges to making enterprise Blockchain applications a reality. *MIS Quarterly Executive, 17*(3), 201—222.

Lemieux, P. (2013). Who is Satoshi Nakamoto? *Regulation, 36*(3), 14—16.

Lemieux, V. L. (2016). Trusting records: Is Blockchain technology the answer? *Records Management Journal, 26*(2), 110–139. https://doi.org/10.1108/RMJ-12-2015-0042.

Liberati, A., Altman, D. G., Tetzlaff, J., Mulrow, C., Gøtzsche, P. C., Ioannidis, J. P., et al. (2009). The PRISMA statement for reporting systematic reviews and meta-analyses of studies that evaluate health care interventions: Explanation and elaboration. *Annals of Internal Medicine, 151*(4). W–65.

Lima, C. (2018). Developing open and interoperable DLT/Blockchain standards [standards]. *Computer, 51*(11), 106–111. https://doi.org/10.1109/MC.2018.2876184.

Mahalik, N., & Kim, K. (2016). 2—the role of information technology developments in food supply chain integration and monitoring. In C. E. Leadley (Ed.), *Innovation and future trends in food manufacturing and supply chain technologies* (pp. 21–37). Woodhead Publishing. https://doi.org/10.1016/B978-1-78242-447-5.00002-2.

Malhotra, A., Gosain, S., & El Sawy, O. A. (2007). Leveraging standard electronic business interfaces to enable adaptive supply chain partnerships. *Information Systems Research, 18*(3), 260–279. https://doi.org/10.1287/isre.1070.0132.

Manning, L. (2016). Food fraud: Policy and food chain. *Current Opinion in Food Science, 10*, 16–21. https://doi.org/10.1016/j.cofs.2016.07.001.

Manning, L., & Soon, J. M. (2016). Food safety, food fraud, and food defense: A fast evolving literature. *Journal of Food Science, 81*(4), R823–R834. https://doi.org/10.1111/1750-3841.13256.

Mertins, K., Jaekel, F.-W., & Deng, Q. (2012). Towards information customization and interoperability in food chains. In M. van Sinderen, P. Johnson, X. Xu, & G. Doumeingts (Eds.), *Enterprise interoperability* (pp. 92–103). Springer.

Moulding, R. (2019). *The promise of Blockchain and its impact on relationships between actors in the supply chain: A theory-based research framework.* Leeds University Business School [Master Thesis].

Nakamoto, S. (2008). *Bitcoin: A peer-to-peer electronic cash system.* https://doi.org/10.1007/s10838-008-9062-0. Retrieved from Www.Bitcoin.Org.

Nelson, P. (1970). Information and consumer behavior. *Journal of Political Economy, 78*(2), 311–329. https://doi.org/10.1086/259630.

New, S. (2010). The transparent supply chain. *Harvard Business Review, 88*, 1–5.

Olsen, P., & Borit, M. (2013). How to define traceability. *Trends in Food Science & Technology, 29*(2), 142–150. https://doi.org/10.1016/j.tifs.2012.10.003.

Olsen, P., & Borit, M. (2018). The components of a food traceability system. *Trends in Food Science & Technology, 77*, 143–149. https://doi.org/10.1016/j.tifs.2018.05.004.

O'Dwyer, K. J., & Malone, D. (2014). Bitcoin mining and its energy footprint. In *25th IET Irish signals & systems conference 2014 and 2014 China-Ireland international conference on information and communications technologies (ISSC 2014/CIICT 2014)* (pp. 280–285). https://doi.org/10.1049/cp.2014.0699.

Pan, X., Song, M., Ai, B., & Ming, Y. (2019). Blockchain technology and enterprise operational capabilities: An empirical test. *International Journal of Information Management.* https://doi.org/10.1016/j.ijinfomgt.2019.05.002.

Pigini, D., & Conti, M. (2017). NFC-based traceability in the food chain. *Sustainability, 9*(10), 1910. https://doi.org/10.3390/su9101910.

PTI. (2020). *The produce traceability initiative.* Retrieved from https://www.producetraceability.org/.

PWC. (2016). *Food fraud vulnerability assessment and mitigation: Are you doing enough to prevent food fraud?.* Retrieved from https://www.pwc.com/gx/en/services/food-supply-integrity-services/assets/pwc-food-fraud-vulnerability-assessment-and-mitigation-november.pdf.

Queiroz, M. M., Telles, R., & Bonilla, S. H. (2019). Blockchain and supply chain management integration: A systematic review of the literature. *Supply Chain Management: An International Journal*. https://doi.org/10.1108/SCM-03-2018-0143.

Ray, P., Harsh, H. O., Daniel, A., & Ray, A. (2019). Incorporating block chain technology in food supply chain. *International Journal of Management Studies, 1*(5), 115–124.

Rejeb, A., Keogh, J. G., & Treiblmaier, H. (2019). Leveraging the internet of things and Blockchain technology in supply chain management. *Future Internet, 11*(7), 161. https://doi.org/10.3390/fi11070161.

Rejeb, A., Keogh, J. G., & Treiblmaier, H. (2020). How Blockchain technology can benefit marketing: Six pending research areas. *Frontiers in Blockchain, 3*, 1–12. https://doi.org/10.3389/fbloc.2020.00003.

Rejeb, A., Sűle, E., & Keogh, J. G. (2018). Exploring new technologies in procurement. *Transport & Logistics: The International Journal, 18*(45), 76–86.

Richter, C., Kraus, S., & Bouncken, R. B. (2015). Virtual currencies like bitcoin as a paradigm shift in the field of transactions. *International Business & Economics Research Journal (IBER), 14*(4), 575–586. https://doi.org/10.19030/iber.v14i4.9350.

Roe, B., & Sheldon, I. (2007). Credence good labeling: The efficiency and distributional implications of several policy approaches. *American Journal of Agricultural Economics, 89*(4), 1020–1033. https://doi.org/10.1111/j.1467-8276.2007.01024.x.

Roth, A. V., Tsay, A. A., Pullman, M. E., & Gray, J. V. (2008). Unraveling the food supply chain: Strategic insights from China and the 2007 recalls. *Journal of Supply Chain Management, 44*(1), 22.

Sander, F., Semeijn, J., & Mahr, D. (2018). The acceptance of Blockchain technology in meat traceability and transparency. *British Food Journal*. https://doi.org/10.1108/BFJ-07-2017-0365.

dos Santos, R. B., Torrisi, N. M., Yamada, E. R. K., & Pantoni, R. P. (2019). IGR token-raw material and ingredient certification of recipe based foods using smart contracts. *Informatics, 6*(1), 11. https://doi.org/10.3390/informatics6010011.

Schaffers, H. (2018). The relevance of Blockchain for collaborative networked organizations. In L. M. Camarinha-Matos, H. Afsarmanesh, & Y. Rezgui (Eds.), *Collaborative networks of cognitive systems* (pp. 3–17). Springer International Publishing. https://doi.org/10.1007/978-3-319-99127-6_1.

Schiefer, G., & Deiters, J. (2013). *Transparency for sustainability in the food chain: Challenges and research needs EFFoST critical reviews #2*. Elsevier.

Shahnaz, A., Qamar, U., & Khalid, A. (2019). Using Blockchain for electronic health records. *IEEE Access, 7*, 147782–147795.

Skilton, P. F., & Robinson, J. L. (2009). Traceability and normal accident theory: How does supply network complexity influence the traceability of adverse events? *Journal of Supply Chain Management, 45*(3), 40–53. https://doi.org/10.1111/j.1745-493X.2009.03170.x.

Sousa, J., Bessani, A., & Vukolic, M. (2018). A Byzantine Fault-tolerant ordering service for the hyperledger fabric Blockchain platform. In *2018 48th annual IEEE/IFIP international conference on dependable systems and networks (DSN)* (pp. 51–58). https://doi.org/10.1109/DSN.2018.00018.

Staples, M., Chen, S., Falamaki, S., Ponomarev, A., Rimba, P., Tran, A. B., et al. (2017). *Risks and opportunities for systems using Blockchain and smart contracts. Data61*. Sydney: CSIRO.

Swan, M. (2015). *Blockchain blueprint for a new economy*. O'Reilly Media, Inc..

Sylim, P., Liu, F., Marcelo, A., & Fontelo, P. (2018). Blockchain technology for detecting falsified and substandard drugs in distribution: Pharmaceutical supply chain intervention. *JMIR Research Protocols, 7*(9), e10163. https://doi.org/10.2196/10163.

Szabo, N. (1996). Smart contracts: Building blocks for digital free markets. *Extropy Journal of Transhuman Thought, 16*, 1−10.

Szabo, N. (1997). Formalizing and securing relationships on public networks. *First Monday, 2*(9).

Tapscott, D., & Tapscott, A. (2017). *Realizing the potential of Blockchain A multistakeholder approach to the stewardship of Blockchain and cryptocurrencies*. Whitepaper, June, 46.

Tijan, E., Aksentijević, S., Ivanić, K., & Jardas, M. (2019). Blockchain technology implementation in logistics. *Sustainability, 11*(4), 1185. https://doi.org/10.3390/su11041185.

Toyoda, K., Takis Mathiopoulos, P., Sasase, I., & Ohtsuki, T. (2017). A novel blockchain-based product ownership management system (POMS) for anti-counterfeits in the post supply chain. *IEEE Access, 5*, 17465−17477. https://doi.org/10.1109/ACCESS.2017.2720760.

Tranfield, D., Denyer, D., & Smart, P. (2003). Towards a methodology for developing evidence-informed management knowledge by means of systematic review. *British Journal of Management, 14*(3), 207−222. https://doi.org/10.1111/1467-8551.00375.

UNFAO. (2018). *Food wastage footprint & climate change* [Press release]. Retrieved from http://www.fao.org/3/a-bb144e.pdf.

Vellema, S., Loorbach, D., & Van Notten, P. (2006). Strategic transparency between food chain and society: Cultural perspective images on the future of farmed salmon. *Production Planning & Control, 17*(6), 624−632. https://doi.org/10.1080/09537280600866884.

Verhoosel, J., van Bekkum, M., & Verwaart, T. (2018). Semantic interoperability for data analysis in the food supply chain. *International Journal on Food System Dynamics, 9*(1), 101−111. https://doi.org/10.18461/ijfsd.v9i1.917.

Voss, M. D., Closs, D. J., Calantone, R. J., Helferich, O. K., & Speier, C. (2009). The role of security in the food supplier selection decision. *Journal of Business Logistics, 30*(1), 127−155. https://doi.org/10.1002/j.2158-1592.2009.tb00102.x.

Walmart. (2018). *Fresh leafy greens new Walmart food traceability initiative questions and answers*. Retrieved from https://corporate.walmart.com/media-library/document/leafy-greens-food-safety-traceability-requirements-faq/_proxyDocument?id=00000166-0c8e-dc77-a7ff-4dff95cb0001.

Wang, Y., Dos Reis, J. C., Borggren, K. M., Salles, M. A. V., Medeiros, C. B., & Zhou, Y. (2019). *Modeling and building IoT data platforms with actor-oriented databases*. EDBT.

World Bank. (2018). *Food-borne illnesses cost US$ 110 billion per year in low- and middle-income countries* [Press release]. World Bank. Retrieved from https://www.worldbank.org/en/news/press-release/2018/10/23/food-borne-illnesses-cost-us-110-billion-per-year-in-low-and-middle-income-countries.

Xu, X., Weber, I., & Staples, M. (2019). Example use cases. In X. Xu, I. Weber, & M. Staples (Eds.), *Architecture for Blockchain applications* (pp. 61–79). Springer International Publishing. https://doi.org/10.1007/978-3-030-03035-3_4.

Yamoah, F. A., & Yawson, D. E. (2014). Assessing supermarket food shopper reaction to horsemeat scandal in the UK. *International Review of Management and Marketing, 4*(2), 98–107.

Yiannas, F. (2018). A New Era of food transparency powered by Blockchain. *Innovations: Technology, Governance, Globalization, 12*(1–2), 46–56. https://doi.org/10.1162/inov_a_00266.

Yoo, C. W., Parameswaran, S., & Kishore, R. (2015). Knowing about your food from the farm to the table: Using information systems that reduce information asymmetry and health risks in retail contexts. *Information & Management, 52*(6), 692–709. https://doi.org/10.1016/j.im.2015.06.003.

Yunfeng, H., Yueqi, H., Jiulin, S., & Qianli, Z. (2018). Current status and future development proposal for Chinese agricultural product quality and safety traceability. *Strategic Study of Chinese Academy of Engineering, 20*(2), 57–62. https://doi.org/10.15302/J-SSCAE-2018.02.009.

Zhong, R., Xu, X., & Wang, L. (2017). Food supply chain management: Systems, implementations, and future research. *Industrial Management & Data Systems, 117*(9), 2085–2114. https://doi.org/10.1108/IMDS-09-2016-0391.

# IT Data security

# Data security

# 18

**Vijay Laxmi, LPD, MSc**

*Security, Architecture & Engineering Director, Information Technology, Iron Mountain, Inc., Boston, MA, United States*

Digitization has become a necessity for the transformation and revitalization of every company, industry, and country that wishes to be relevant to the new digital economy. The food industry is no exception. With industrial automation and supply chain digitization, the agriculture market has seen an increase in production efficiency, quality improvements, and sustainability. Like any other industry, the food industry is also subject to regular monitoring, reporting, and compliance. The application of digital technology in food compliance is referred to as REGTECH.

In the recent few years, Blockchain, an emerging digital technology, has been a topic of research in agriculture and food supply chain. While stakeholders in the food industry-from farm to table-put more emphasis on food safety by leveraging digital technology, they also need to be aware of the security of the digital data generated and retained throughout the food journey. With digitization comes the risk of breaches in cybersecurity and data security. The frequency, volume, severity, and costs of data breach have increased since 2015. This section focuses on the aspects of digital data security in the context of the food industry.

This section is organized into five segments. The first one explores the role of digital data in all the five food-related contexts-quality, safety, authenticity, security/sustainability, and food defense-and how it has evolved. The second clarifies the word data security in this context. The third mentions laws, regulations, and framework in the food industry and data security. The fourth identifies common data security controls to address data security. The fifth highlights various methods to address these common data security issues, including Blockchain.

## Digital data in food industry

As food makes its journey from farm to the consumer, the data (digital or paper) associated with the food also go with it. For example, a farmer buys seeds and plants them to produce sellable goods. The farmer is a supplier, and the digital data include the place or the location from where the farmer bought the seeds. The farmer plants the seeds, manages the growth and harvest, and finally supplies the product to a producer. The producer accepts produce from various farmers or suppliers, processes (if needed), packages, and tags food products for the distributor. At every point in the process, data are generated and retained for various purposes. The producer site adds additional digital data, including the location of the farm, the time when produce was supplied, sell-by date, and shelf date. The distributor, on the other hand, selects optimal shipping routes, mode of transport, and the destination to maximize profit. Data collection at the distributor site may include the producer from which the product came, location, time, logistic company, and mode of transportation (by air, by water, or by road). The retailers, on the other hand, may add their own set of data such as price tag, sell-by date, and shelf date to the same product. The consumer buys the product by looking at the freshness, sell-by date, brand, and cost. On the retailer side, the digital data are related to the consumer who purchased the food, i.e., consumer credit card, loyalty card, phone number, and address. With the evolution of digitization in the food industry, digital data reside in various information systems, cash registers, and back-end supply chain databases. In addition to understanding the digital data journey in the food industry from the supply chain perspective, we need to clarify the role of digital data in terms of food contexts such as quality, safety, security/sustainability, authenticity, and defense.

*Food Quality* is associated with the quality of food, such as traceable sources of supply; external factors, such as flavor and texture; federal standards, such as safety and nutrition; and internal factors, such as chemical and physical. Digital data in the context of food quality include the source of the seed, the farm, the producer who packaged, the storage and transportation of food, and the temperature to keep food fresh and preserve its taste.

*Food Safety* refers to the process of handling, processing, and management of food to reduce the presence of food contaminants (biological, chemical, or physical), thus reducing the risk of consumers becoming infected by foodborne diseases resulting in illness and even death. Food safety, in terms of digital data, includes the inspection records of the production facility, distributor and retailer, and auditor information. The regulators play a significant role in verifying and validating digital data produced at and by the stakeholders in the food journey from the farm to the consumer table.

*Food Security* means availability and access to the food where people no longer starve. With an increase in world population and wealth in emerging countries, food security is a significant area to deal with. The international food security digital dataset includes country-level data such as annual yield, usage, and consumption.

*Food Sustainability* (a subset of food security) is a method of food production that protects the human and animal welfare environment and ensures future generations can do the same. Companies like Whole Foods, Mars, Nestle, and Dannon have already started moving toward food sustainability by bringing buyers and suppliers closer, understanding consumer preferences, reducing greenhouse gas emission, and continuing supporting farmers' cost of living standards. All this happens because of the disparate digital data being collected from various places to understand the real impact on the environment and living beings.

***Food Authenticity*** focuses on food identity and the criminal element of food fraud-another growing concern with the globalization of the good, especially when dealing with international spices, poultry, seafood, oil, and fats. Specific acts of concern include adulteration, tampering, overrun, theft, simulation, and counterfeiting. The digital data include the source, the testing results of food in question to validate if the composition of nutrients matches the required authentic layout. With additional impurities, the calculation to determine the composition becomes more complicated.

***Food Defense*** is a concern relating to the impact on consumers through any act characterized as "Economically Motivated Adulteration," "Corporate Sabotage," or "Food Bioterrorism." Though typically first identified as a failure in food safety or authenticity, the dishonesty and intent behind these actions are often difficult to determine and difficult to prosecute. After the "1984 Rajneeshee Incident" in The Dalles, Oregon (751 illnesses and 45 hospitalizations from *Salmonella enterica* Typhimurium) (Detwiler, 2016), a lengthy investigation found that the perpetrators' purpose was to incapacitate voters in order to influence the outcome of a local 1984 election in their favor, placing cult members, known as "Rajneeshees," into office. After the attacks on 9/11, the World Health Assembly, the decision-making body of the World Health Organization (WHO), adopted a 2002 resolution expressing serious concern about threats against civilian populations by deliberate use of agents disseminated via food. Later that year, WHO published "Terrorist Threats to Food"—a food safety/food terrorism document for national government policy-makers (WHO, 2002). Focusing on food, food ingredients, and water (in the forms of food ingredients and of bottled water), the document classifies food safety as an essential element of modern, global public health security.

## Data security in the food industry

Data travels within one company, company sites, and among many stakeholders within that industry and between states and countries. Some digital data reside at the individual stakeholder's site whether the stakeholder is a supplier, a producer, a distributor, or a retailer, and some digital data are sharable among one or other stakeholders. When the information system processes the data, then data are in the in-use stage, and when data travel within one site or many sites of the same stakeholder or between stakeholders, the data are in the in-transit stage. Sometimes data stay at one place for various purposes, and then the data are in the at-rest stage. In all three phases-in-use, in-transit, or at-rest-the security of the data is essential.

**Data security** means protection to retain confidentiality, integrity, availability, nonrepudiation, and authenticity to ensure data security. **Confidentiality** means protection from unauthorized access where only authorized users with relevant rights can access the specific information and not the whole data. **Integrity** means the data are not compromised or changed unknowingly or data have not been compromised by the unknown. **Availability** means data are available when needed by authorized persons. **Nonrepudiation** is another term that is frequently used with data security. Nonrepudiation says the author of the data cannot deny or dispute the authorship of the data. **Authenticity** is the establishment for a digital object to confirm indeed what it claims to be or what it is claimed to be.

Data at-rest requires assurances of three security principles-confidentiality, integrity, and availability-at the stakeholder, whether the stakeholder is a supplier, producer, distributor, or retailer. On the other hand, data in-transit needs four principles of data security-confidentiality, integrity, availability, and nonrepudiation. Data in-use demands all five components of data security-confidentiality, integrity, availability, nonrepudiation, and authenticity (see Table 1 below).

At the supplier site, data security requires information about seed location, crop nutrients, and the temperature and if they are safe and secure. If the information or data go in the wrong hands, then the unauthorized person can poison the seeds or change fertilizers' composition. This may create a situation of bioterrorism-a challenge to food defense, as well as to food safety and food authenticity. At the producer site, data security requires the protection of data from unauthorized changes in the packaging and storing of food. Changing the date of producing or sell-by date may affect food quality and food sustainability. The producer may be involved in creating the finished product from raw ingredients obtained from suppliers. Sometimes unauthorized modifications to food recipes that automated machines control can create a challenge to food quality. Distributors need to protect the food-related data from unauthorized access, nonrepudiation, and meddling with the integrity of the data. One can change the origin and destination data of food, divert the food to an unnecessary location, and hence violate food security and sustainability. These unauthorized changes can cause bioterrorism where food delivery to an emergency may not be delivered to the right place, keeping the needy people away from it. The retailer needs to protect data from changing the food quality if raw or processed, keeping customer personal data secure from unwanted data breaches.

The topic of data security becomes even more complicated in the case of precision agriculture. Precision agriculture uses a combination of sensors, embedded

**Table 1** Data alignment with security components at various stages in journey.

| Data security components | Data at-rest | Data in-transit | Data in-use |
|---|---|---|---|
| Confidentiality | X | X | X |
| Integrity | X | X | X |
| Availability | X | X | X |
| Nonrepudiation | — | X | X |
| Authenticity | — | — | X |

Table by author.

systems, and informed systems to maximize production by accounting for variability and uncertainties within agricultural systems. Tampering with any of these devices creates a threat to supply chain, food quality, food safety, and food authenticity.

With an increase in food safety and the nature of food supply chain awareness among consumers, traceability becomes an emerging issue. Any unknown change that impacts food or data associated with food traceability may affect food safety, authenticity, and defense.

## Laws, regulations, and framework in the food industry and data security

Countries and states apply different regulations to regulate food quality, food safety, food authenticity, food security, and food sustainability. In the United States, the laws are enforced by the FDA and the USDA. Similarly, digital data that travel with food are also regulated under various national data protection regulations.

To regulate food quality, the FDA has provisions within 21 C.F.R §110 (2011) pertaining to **Current Good Manufacturing Practices** (CGMPs) for food. CGMP regulates the quality of processed foods and dietary supplements by providing controls on food manufacturing methods, facilities, equipment, labeling, and packaging. The quality data of food is stored in digital format in the information systems at the producer site. The producer is responsible and accountable for maintaining the information for auditing purposes and ensures the integrity and availability of data-both at-rest and in-transit.

The purpose of the 2011 **FDA Food Safety Modernization Act ("FSMA")** (Pub.L. 111—353, 124 STAT 3885) is to transform the food safety system from reactive (i.e., responding to foodborne illness) to preventive. FSMA provides FDA authorities to protect the consumer and public health. Compliance with FSMA requires food stakeholders to comply with FDA food codes, data dashboards to show inspections, compliance actions recalls and reports, product tracing, supplier evaluation, food safety plans, and food defense plans. Digital information associated with all the above activities needs to be integrated with state or federal networks and requires data protection to maintain integrity and availability.

To regulate food security, FDA has developed the **Food Protection Plan** to protect the nation's food supply from both unintentional contamination and deliberate attack. There are rules on the food products that can be imported into the United States and exported from the United States. FDA posts various types of digital data such as food package database, the microbiological load of bagged, ready-to-eat produce, risk assessment data, adverse food, and events data. FDA also analyzes digital data to identify a potential threat and issues precautionary alerts. Digital data, in this case, although public, require a great precaution to maintain integrity and availability.

Food fraud is outlined in the FDA's **Prevention Control Rules** such as CGMP and risk-based controls for both human food and animals. Another global standard related to food fraud is **British Retail Consortium** (BRC), Version 8. The BRC defines standards to protect food authenticity and to prevent/reduce food fraud in three ways. One by having access to information and developing threats to the stakeholders in the supply chain that may create a risk of food fraud. Second, by performing a documented vulnerability assessment on all food raw materials. Third, by performing appropriate assurance and testing to reduce uncovered risks for raw materials. Vulnerabilities remediation and testing results are digital data, and tampering with any of this data will violate confidentiality, integrity, and availability.

The European Union's 2016 **General Data Protection Regulation** (GDPR) is a data protection law regulating European and non-European companies that serve European residents and became binding on May 25, 2018. The regulation secured the right to privacy across all digital communication. This new law has provided strong incentives for corporations to cooperate, not only for the safety of their customers but also to protect them from hefty fines, loss of reputation, and further regulatory inspection. While consumers and companies enjoy the benefits of speed, automation, integration, and connection, cyberattacks and data breaches have resulted in significant impacts on the individuals or users whose data are affected. This is also true for service providers whose reputations are also at stake. Because of compliance requirements, businesses must engage in the process of becoming fully GDPR-compliant. Hence, the GDPR seeks to clarify the responsibilities and liabilities of data-holding and data-processing companies. This regulation serves as the legal framework for digital security, establishing six fundamental principles and eight rights as described in Table 2 that follows.

Data protection and information security are two additional terms in the GDPR law. Under Article 78 and 83 of the GDPR, referring to the notion of privacy, the GDPR recommends addressing privacy needs in the design stage of a business. Before processing information, a company needs to assess the likelihood and

**Table 2** General data protection regulation (GDPR) principles and rights.

| GDPR principles (Article 5–11) | GDPR rights (Article 12–23) |
| --- | --- |
| Lawfulness, fairness, and transparency | Right to be informed |
| | Right of access to data and records |
| Purpose limitation | Right to rectification |
| Data minimization | Right to erasure—to "be forgotten" |
| Accuracy | Right to restrict processing |
| Storage limitation | Right to data portability |
| Integrity and confidentiality | Rights about automated decision-making and profiling |

*Table based on information from Laxmi, V. (2019). The impact of EU GDPR on Saudi Arabia's economy: A case study of tourism and logistics sectors,* ProQuest One Academic, *p. 21t.*

severity of risks. In the case of higher chances, data controllers must submit a **Data Protection Impact Assessment** to supervisory authorities during the project initiation phase of the system that will process and store covered information.

## Security controls to address data security

Violation of any of the underlying security principles-confidentiality, integrity, availability, nonrepudiation, and authenticity-affects data security. The standard data security issues and threats in the food industry are in the form of data breach, data manipulation, data corruption, and dissemination of confidential information in public.

A **data breach** can be stealing secret recipes, stealing employee's data and information, stealing manufacturing data or shipment locations, or unauthorized users gaining access to the digital data violating the confidentiality principle of data security. **Data manipulation** threat means unauthorized users are making unauthorized changes to the digital data breaking the integrity principle of data security. **Data corruption**, on the other hand, makes digital data unreadable or inaccessible and hinders the availability of data. **Dissemination of confidential information** can be damaging to customers and companies challenging the authenticity principle of data security.

To help protect data from the abovementioned threats, maintain security principles-confidentiality, integrity, availability, and nonrepudiation—and be compliant with various regulations, the US National Institute of Standards (NIST) has published the security control framework (NIST 800-53 Revision 4). The framework identifies the following key controls:

- **Access Control**: Defines who have access to digital data inside and outside the organization. How are users authorized, and what are they authorized for? For example, the supplier may want to control access to irrigation systems, or the producer may wish to limit the user's access to view or update supplier information or update the labeling or packaging. Access control allows authorized users to access specific data ensuring confidentiality. With proper access controls, chances of making unauthorized changes can be reduced, supporting data integrity.
- **Awareness and Training**: Defines the process to train users and employees on data security. Employees need to be aware of the data security risks and how these risks can impact an organization as a whole. Without proper training, users may make an unintentional change that may result in unauthorized data exposure, unauthorized data change, or poor system performance and hence violating data confidentiality, integrity, and availability principles.
- **Audit and Accountability**: Defines the process to log the trail of actions taken by the user-whether authorized or unauthorized. Regulators use audit trails to ensure compliance and data security. When incidents related to data security happen,

security professionals first review audit logs to identify and verify the attack. The attacker can be inside an employee or an outsider. If audit logs are in place, then the company can show nonrepudiation from an inside employee.

- **Configuration Management**: Defines the process to ensure any change in the system is restricted, monitored, and authorized. This process helps organizations in achieving integrity and availability principles.
- **Identification and Authentication**: Defines the process of authenticating and verifying the user to access digital information systems. This process addresses the confidentiality of the data as only verified users can access the confidential data.
- **Incident Response**: Defines the process of handling and responding to incidents- who is authorized to respond to the incidents, what actions to take, how to contain the incident, where to report, and how to remediate the incidents. Successful incident response systems support the availability principle.
- **Personnel Security**: Controls that are in place to ensure proper verification and background check of the users have taken place before employing them and providing access to the systems.
- **Physical Protection**: Refers to the controls that ensure data security from a physical access perspective. If the information system is in a nonsecure physical building, then the data are as secure as the security of the physical building.
- **Risk Assessment**: Controls in this category are related to the vulnerabilities assessment process that the company has in place to protect digital data. The majority of attacks exploit the vulnerability in systems. When the information systems are not running the latest patch, then the system is vulnerable to attacks, and a bad actor can manipulate the data or corrupt the data and could paralyze the company.
- **Security Assessment**: Refers to the effectiveness of security controls in place such as how the company measures and monitors its security controls. By doing a periodic assessment, the organization can determine the areas of potential weakness in protecting data.
- **System and Communication Protection**: Refers to the continuous monitoring of all data transfers, whether at-rest, in-use, or in-transit. Protecting the hardware and software from unwanted attackers is essential to protect data from being manipulated, corrupting, or stealing the data.
- **System and Information Integrity**: Refers to the controls that are in place to identify, detect, and remediate threats or risks in considerable time.

In theory, all these security controls make common sense; however, implementing these controls can be challenging because the data lie in disparate information systems across various teams within one organization. Interaction between different organizations is even more complicated, and achieving principles of data security—confidentiality, integrity, availability, and nonrepudiation-is even more strenuous. Technologies like cloud computing and Blockchain can help organizations in implementing these security controls if implemented correctly.

# Technologies to implement data security controls

When dealing with the complexities in the organization to ensure full visibility and data protection, implementing all security controls can be an expensive and lengthy process that requires skilled professionals, infrastructure, training, and continuous assessment. One way to reduce some of these complexities in the food industry is by migrating on-premise (physical environment) food quality management system or supply chain system to cloud-based. Cloud-based providers share security responsibility to ensure the infrastructure and data are secure, backed up, and can be available when needed. **Cloud computing** provides scalable, elastic, and on-demand storage and computing power, supporting the availability security principle. Cloud computing in the food industry allows companies in the food supply chain industry to collect and store data from various sources and analyze to gain insights about their assets, traceability of shipments, consumer choices, food trends, and proactive in reducing recalls incidents. Cloud-based providers have more on a stake on data security as one breach may bring more public damage to them.

While cloud computing addresses the availability pillar of data security, it is still the responsibility of the companies (producer, distributor, or retailer) to protect data confidentiality and integrity. Cloud computing may solve a problem for one company in the supply chain, but what about the other stakeholders in the supply chain who do not use cloud computing or the same provider? For example, a distributor in the food supply chain can take steps to protect the data and leverage cloud computing; however, the data before (i.e., at the producer side) and after (i.e., at the retailer side) are still prone to data manipulation, corruption, or nonavailability. In these disparate technology constrained environments, Blockchain technology can provide data protection by reducing chances of data manipulation, corruption, non-repudiation and supporting the integrity security principle.

**Blockchain** provides an immutable and tamper-resistant digital ledger implemented in a distributed manner and without a central authority. Blockchain enables a trusted group of users to record transactions in a shared ledger where no transaction can be changed once published under normal operation. For example, in the food industry, a supplier can upload data on antibacterial fodder that can be used by the producer. The producer adds information on required cuts, prepares meat, uploads the data such as weight, sell-by date, etc., and adds information for the distributor. The distributor on receiving notification selects an optimized shipping method and adds retailer information. The retailer has full details on where the food was initially produced, packaged, and distributed. The retailer adds information on the shelf and customer purchase information.

Blockchain technology is a data governance tool because it provides data management and distribution in accordance with data security principles and provides benefits compared with other contemporary solutions. Blockchain allows data sharing without the need for a central repository or authority and offers visibility as to who has accessed data. Once the transaction is submitted and approved by the trusted partners, then the transaction cannot be changed. Any change to the transaction is another transaction to the chain of transactions. Blockchain supports integrity and nonrepudiation principle of security. **Smart contracts**, based on Blockchain technology, can enable the data share among participants and reduce transaction costs. Smart contracts may include personal data such as name and address, which can be subjected to GDPR regulations in the European Union.

While complying with the security principles, Blockchain technology can be at odds with GDPR. First, Blockchain technology is based on the assumption that there is no central authority, but GDPR requires that there should exist at least one natural or legal person who is responsible for maintaining and preserving the personal data of the data subject. Second, Blockchain does not allow any change in the data, whereas GDPR provides data subjects the right of access or right to data portability and data erasure. Third, Blockchain keeps the data as long as the transaction is valid, which contradicts the data minimization principle of GDPR. There is no one technology or a service provider or a vendor that can solve the data security issues.

One has to assess the purpose and assess where and what technologies can be used. If one needs a shared consistent data store, or their transaction involves more than one entity to contribute data, requires once written transaction cannot be updated, allows only nonsensitive data to be stored, does not allow single party to control the data store, and ensures tamper proof log of all the transactions, then Blockchain is the appropriate technology.

## References

Detwiler, D. (2016, October 24). Death should not be on the Menu. *EC Nutrition, 5*(3), 1148–1149. Retrieved from https://www.ecronicon.com/ecnu/pdf/ECNU-05-0000158.pdf.

Laxmi, V. (2019). The impact of EU GDPR on Saudi Arabia's Economy: A case study of tourism and logistics sectors. *ProQuest One Academic*.

World Health Organization. (2002). "Terrorist threats to food: Guidance for establishing and strengthening prevention and response systems." Retrieved from https://apps.who.int/iris/handle/10665/42619.

# Legal issues concerning information, including data, in the agriculture and food industry

# 19

**David Mahoney, JD**
*Senior Corporate Counsel, Indigo Ag, Inc., Boston, MA, United States*

Agriculture and food production, taken collectively, serves as the most fundamentally important sector of industry due to its role in providing life-sustaining nutrition to the world's population. Advancements in the collection, analysis, and storage of large amounts of information, including data, hold promise in helping to maximize the efficiency and output of the process from farm to consumer. The types of legal protections required to protect such information will differ depending on the type of data collected and the manner of its use.

Information has always been valuable; however, technical improvements have fostered the increased commoditization of it and brought legal issues, such as those of security and privacy, to the forefront. In particular, legitimate concerns have arisen regarding the manner in which personal information is gathered and utilized by companies. As is often the case with any powerful tool, the extent to which it is utilized for the benefit, or conversely, the detriment, of the public at large, is dependent on the manner in which the user directs the use of such technology. This has partly resulted in the enactment of some new legislation to help create greater transparency and control for the personal information of individuals. As technology progresses, it is essential for laws and regulations to keep pace with new legal issues created as a result of the implementation of such advancements.

## The perennial value of information

In order to fully appreciate the importance of legal rights in information, we should consider the intrinsic value and inextricable relationship between people and information. Although the time period since the 1970s has often been described as the information age, its alternative characterization as the digital age seems more accurate, given the continuous importance of information throughout human history. Digitization enables the fast compilation, analysis, and rapid transfer of information that has transformed it into much more of a commodity during this era.

Building the Future of Food Safety Technology. https://doi.org/10.1016/B978-0-12-818956-6.00019-1

Information takes various forms. It is defined as including knowledge obtained from investigation, study or instruction, intelligence, facts, data, and information contained within sequences such as genetic sequences and computer code (Information, n.d.). Biological information, such as the genetic information contained within our DNA, is key to the continued existence of humans. Information obtained through experience, study, or testing allows for improvements in methods, as well as technology, and its conveyance to others benefits subsequent generations. Educational institutions are grounded in this straightforward premise.

The conveyance of information is especially important in the context of agriculture and food. For instance, knowledge of identifying edible and nontoxic foods has always been of critical importance. With the adoption of agrarian practices, information related to techniques for planting, cultivation, and harvesting, as well as the best varieties of seeds, has continued to be of key value to help maximize yields.

Failure of previous cultivation practices also generates data that enable subsequent improvements. For instance, the Irish Potato Famine (1845–49) highlighted the importance of crop diversity in order to minimize the risk of total crop loss due to stressors such as a disease infecting a single plant variety. Information gained as a result of the analysis of the Dust Bowl crisis in the Midwest of the United States (1930–36) resulted in critical changes such as cover crop rotation techniques and natural wind barriers to help mitigate the risk of massive topsoil loss in the future.

Thus, our present knowledge of agricultural practices and food derives from information gathered through the experience of previous generations. This process of continual learning can lead to critical advancements in techniques and technology, which can help us to progressively improve sustainable agricultural practices and food production in order to help feed the world in the most efficient and environmentally conducive manner possible. Greater access to functional data can help accelerate such beneficial improvements.

## Is the collection of data the latest gold rush?

The increasing commoditization of information does not necessarily mean that each individual portion of data is of greater value than in the past; rather, the latest technologies help make large amounts of information more useable such as efficiently identifying distinct patterns as well as predicting future trends. This has effectuated a rapid expansion in the collection and use of data across many industries. For instance, one report holds that in 2018, 11.9 billion dollars was spent in the United Sttaes on commercial information such as names, email addresses, IP addresses, home addresses, historical behaviors, preferences, and psychographic information ("The State of Data," 2018). In the same year, another 7.2 billion dollars was spent on technology to analyze such data, including artificial intelligence, which, taken collectively, represented an increase of 17.5% over the prior year ("The State of Data," 2018).

Some of the most well-known examples of data collection include that which is gathered through social media outlets as well as online service providers. The extensive level of detail obtained about users may be collected in an automated and seemingly undetectable manner. For instance, Google collects information from emails, photos, videos, and documents of users ("Google Privacy Policy," 2019).

The right type of data can be economically valuable to companies. For instance, information about the characteristics of users (such as preferences, habits, travel history, and friends) can help to predict possible future purchases of those individuals. Such acquisitions can include categories such as services, consumer electronics, cars, travel, clothing, and food purchases. For example, although Facebook asserts that it does not sell user data to outside entities, it collects data from users in order to offer advertisers the ability to specifically target ads to users who may be the most likely customers of those products (Facebook: Transparency, 2018).

What an individual may purchase in the near future with regard to food products is valuable to advertisers. It makes it possible to specifically target those groups of individuals who are most likely to choose a particular line of products. Customer loyalty programs offered by supermarkets collect user food purchase preferences for subsequent use and potential sale to other entities. Access to data was one of the significant benefits of Amazon.com, Inc.'s acquisition of Whole Foods Market, Inc. in 2017. Once acquired, Amazon replaced the loyalty program with Amazon Prime, thus integrating Whole Foods customer loyalty programs with Amazon Prime members. Amazon's access to the food shopping habits of Whole Foods customers provides Amazon the opportunity to target such shoppers with different types of products related to their purchasing habits as well as monitoring trends.

Apart from individual consumer interests for food products, data are increasingly important in the food and agriculture industry. Information related to food supply is valuable in maximizing the safety and efficiency of the food supply chain. Data related to the storage life, as well as the optimal temperature, can help ensure optimal condition of the food at the point of purchase or consumption by the consumer.

Data from agricultural practices helps demonstrate the effectiveness of new innovations or techniques. The harvest yield of a crop demonstrates success for that growing season in a specific region. Examples of other equally critical pieces of information include the growing conditions, various agricultural techniques utilized, climatic conditions, and the presence of any disease, insects, or other variables. In the event that producers of food products experience unusual or extreme climatic conditions, the ability to analyze such data is crucial to help ascertain the best possible methods and processes that can be implemented in order to maximize harvest yield. With the expansion of the world's population, these types of ongoing improvements and developments are especially critical.

Satellite image data can now be leveraged to help predict crop yields. Machine learning algorithms utilize the data gathered through satellite imagery and combine it with other relevant information, to enable more accurate harvest forecasts.

This type of innovation has the potential to provide more immediate insights to plant health and probable yield, particularly beneficial during growing seasons in which unexpected climatic events affect crop health.

Acquiring large volumes of data is not inherently valuable if there is no effective way to process or analyze it, nor if it lacks a specific purpose. However, if properly processed and analyzed to show meaningful trends or results, it can provide a commercially valuable benefit. Such value necessitates protection through legal measures such as contractual safeguards and proper IT infrastructures that provide for database protection systems. Also, depending on the jurisdiction, possession of personal information will result in the application of laws protecting such consumer information.

## With great information comes great responsibility

The type of information held by a company, as well its purpose and how it was obtained, will affect what legal obligations may apply. For valuable nonpublic information held by a business, a company will typically apply industry-standard safeguards. If information may constitute a trade secret, the company will need to apply reasonable levels of protection in order to maintain such status. For in-licensed data, the obligations of the holder will be subject to the terms of the license agreement. Depending on applicable law, possession of personal data of actual or potential customers gathered by the company will trigger different types of legal obligations.

- *Confidential Information*

Businesses will typically hold commercially valuable information as confidential and subject to standard safeguards, such as storing it within secured IT systems with proper access restrictions. Protecting it as confidential information requires ensuring that all individuals that have access to it are contractually obligated not to use or disclose the information beyond the restrictions set forth in such agreements. This is effectuated through the use of nondisclosure agreements commonly incorporated with employment agreements and also executed prior to extensive discussion with other business entities or individuals.

- *Trade Secrets*

Information that provides an economic benefit by not being disclosed to others may constitute a trade secret. For instance, this would include information that provides a competitive advantage to a company so long as it is not disclosed. In some instances, customer information may constitute a trade secret; however, decisions differ across various courts on this point. Trade secrets are required to be protected by reasonable measures. Thus, companies must treat it as confidential information and, depending on the circumstances, will often need to apply more stringent controls than other types of confidential information. For instance, disclosure should be limited only to those individuals that need to know the information for a specific business purpose.

Trade secret law was historically governed only by state law; however, the enactment of the Defend Trade Secrets Act of 2016, 18 U.S.C Sec. 1836 ("DTSA"), now allows the option for an action of trade secret misappropriation to be taken in federal court if the trade secret is used in or intended for use in interstate or foreign commerce. With regard to state trade secret laws, the Uniform Trade Secrets Act ("UTSA") has been adopted, in some form, by every state except New York. Although, as of this publication, New York currently has Bill SB 2468 pending for adoption of the UTSA (SB 2468, 2019). There are still variations among the state trade secret laws due to different versions of the UTSA and differences in the manner of what UTSA language was adopted. There are a number of differences between the DTSA and the UTSA as well. For instance, the DTSA applies the trade secret definition under 18 U.S.C Sec 1839 that is slightly more detailed than under the UTSA and its definition includes all forms of financial, business, technical, and economic information as well as information related to methods, techniques, and processes among others listed.

- *In-licensed Data*

Some data may be in-licensed by a company from another entity. The legal obligations that apply to the licensee will be dependent on the license terms. It will likely specify the type of law that applies. The license will specify the type of license as well as the permitted uses of the data by the licensee. It should also specify the types of standards that may be required with regard to restricting access to the data.

- *Personal Information*

If the information collected is personal information, specific obligations must be followed pursuant to any applicable privacy laws. The privacy laws impose a number of obligations on companies, including to clearly identify the basis for which the company is collecting information, the type of information that is being collected, and the manner in which it is being collected. Individuals may also possess the right to request the deletion of the collected personal information. To the extent that companies deal directly with consumers, misrepresentations about the use of consumer information may result in enforcement from agencies such as the Federal Trade Commission (FTC). These aspects are covered in further detail below.

- *Rights to Personal Information*

The recognition of people holding rights to their personal information predates the enactment of the GDPR by the EU or the California Consumer Privacy Act ("CCPA") by the State of California. The GDPR refers to an individual's information as "personal data" and the CCPA refers to it as "personal information." These laws seek to uphold those concepts of rights to personal information in the face of modern technology that enables the silent gathering and analysis of large volumes of personal data through a growing number of sources. While differences exist between these latest privacy protection laws, there are common fundamental concepts underlying them described below.

I would describe the three key tenets espoused by these privacy laws as disclosure, control, and accountability. Disclosure is provided to the individual through the provision of clear and specific information about how a company may gather, use, and transfer a person's information. With this insight, an individual is better able to understand the type and manner of use of their personal information so that they are better able to make an informed decision regarding their consent for its use. Control manifests from the ability of individuals to have their personal information deleted. Accountability on the part of companies is established in clear penalties provided for companies that fail to abide by these laws.

## Protection of personal data in the European Union

The GDPR came into effect on May 25, 2018, in the European Union. This regulation creates requirements that allow for greater transparency of how and why companies gather personal information of individuals that use their products or services. Companies are required to disclose how the information is collected; the categories of information collected; how it is utilized; the legal basis for processing it; when the company may disclose it; if it may be transferred internationally; how a person can contact the company to receive a copy of their information or have it corrected and/or deleted; how long the information is retained; and a listing of the rights of the user.

The GDPR does not apply to information in which an individual is no longer identifiable, referred to as anonymous information. One of the most important rights is empowering the customer to have their information deleted, although there are a few narrow exceptions for this obligation. This right to have personal information deleted is also known as the "right to be forgotten." If the data are processed by a business performing services for the company that collected the information, it is necessary to have a contract in place that ensures that such processing is performed in accordance with the provisions of GDPR. The European Commission provides standard contractual clauses for the international transfers of information under the GDPR to processors. Depending on the type of violation, the maximum administrative fines under Article 83 of the GDPR may be 10 million Euro (or 2% of total worldwide revenue of the previous fiscal year) or up to 20 million Euro (or 4% total worldwide revenue of the previous fiscal year) for more severe fines.

However, GDPR was not the first law in the European Union that addressed the protection of personal information. While GDPR provides a comprehensive set of regulations for the protection of personal data, it was preceded by Directive 95/46/EC from October 24, 1995, that addressed the processing and use of personal data. This directive was the basis for the action taken under case C-131/12,

*Google Spain SL, Google Inc. v. AEPD, Mario Costeja Gonzalez*, 2014, ECLI:EU:C: 2014:317. The court in that case held that Google was required to remove links to third-party web pages that contained information related to a person who justifiably objected to such use. This case set an important ruling on the protection of personal information prior to the implementation of the GDPR.

In the 2019 decision of the case of C-507/17, *Google LLC v. Commission nationale de l'informatique et des libertes* (CNIL), 2019, ECLI:EU:C:2019:772, the court ruled that the protection for the personal information of the EU individual, under Article 17(1) of the GDPR, does not extend to requiring a search engine provider to remove links to web pages containing personal information for versions of the service beyond the European Union. Practically, this means that the "right to be forgotten" did not apply to versions of the service outside of the EU Member States. This case provided valuable guidance with regard to a specific example of the "right to be forgotten" under the GDPR.

## Protection of personal data in the United States

At the state level, California is the first state in the United States to have enacted an extensive privacy law applicable for all California residents. At the federal level, there is no single, all-inclusive law in the United States that provides for protection of personal information across all areas. Rather, an individual's right to privacy of personal information is currently protected under various existing laws within specific areas. Some of those specific laws are not relevant for the purposes of this discussion, such as HIPAA (Pub.L. 104-191, 110 Stat. 1936), DPPA, FCRA, or the Financial Services Modernization Act.

## California leads the way for comprehensive privacy protection in the United States

The CCPA provides a comprehensive privacy law to protect the personal information of all individuals that is the first of its kind in the United States. It came into effect on January 1, 2020. Its enactment stemmed from the efforts of a California real estate developer who had deep concerns about the manner in which personal information was being gathered and utilized by businesses such as Google.

The CCPA has many similarities to the protection provided under the GDPR, such as the requirement to identify the categories of personal information collected, the purposes for its use, the purposes for which it will be utilized, and how a person can contact the company to receive access to their information or have it deleted. There are also some narrow exceptions with regard to deletion of information. In some instances, the CCPA builds upon aspects of the GDPR. For example, the definition of personal information found in the CCPA provides greater detail than that set forth under GDPR. The CCPA definition also provides numerous examples as well as identifying information that is specifically excluded. The CCPA allows the individual to specifically prevent a service provider from reselling that information to any third parties. A company may not provide a different level of service if an individual exercises their rights under the CCPA. If a company discloses or sells the personal information of an individual, there are additional disclosure obligations.

Companies that meet the definition of business under the CCPA and interact with California residents need to ensure that their online privacy policies meet the CCPA disclosure requirements. The CCPA does not constrain the ability of a business to use data that does not identify consumers, specifically referred to as deidentified or aggregated consumer information. A business that experiences a data breach due to not utilizing reasonable security measures can be liable directly to consumers for damages from $100 to $700 dollars per incident or actual damages, if greater in amount. The intentional breach of the requirements can result in a penalty up to $7500 per violation.

## Current Status of federal protection in the United States

An individual's right to privacy has been recognized by the US Supreme Court in ruling that there is an implied constitutional right of privacy based upon the collective interpretation of certain amendments of the US Constitution (*Griswold v. Connecticut*, 381 U.S 479, 1965). The Court's ability to adapt its application of privacy rights in light of new data collection technology is evident in their 2018 decision in *Carpenter v. United States*, 138 S. Ct. 2206, 2220, involving an individual's reasonable expectation of privacy of location information involuntarily documented in cellphone records. The Court considered the automatic collection of the data, as compared to voluntary submission, and also highlighted that the Court has not automatically applied prior legal decisions "when confronting new concerns wrought by digital technology." While these privacy rights address governmental access to personal information rather than business use, it provides the basis of recognition of privacy rights, and the *Carpenter* case demonstrates the importance of courts upholding fundamental privacy rights in the face of the potentially intrusive new data gathering capabilities.

In the United States, the Data Privacy Act of 1974, 5 U.S.C § 552a, as amended, addresses practices relating to the collection, use, and disclosure of the personal information of individuals that is maintained by federal agencies. However, the purpose of this law puts limitations on the use of individuals' personal information by the government. Information gathered by businesses does not fall within the scope of the Data Privacy Act.

The Children's Online Privacy Act of 1998, P.L. 105-277 (COPA) was the first legislation in the United States at the federal level that specifically focused on online service providers and placed restrictions regarding the collection of personal information by companies of children under 13 years of age. COPA requires that an online service directed to children that is collecting information must obtain parental consent and identify the type of information collected, how it is used, and how the business may disclose it. Companies that do not direct their online services to children and do not intend to collect information from children will include such a statement, to that effect, in their privacy policy.

Currently, the US FTC protects some instances of consumer personal information matters on the basis of its power to prevent unfair or deceptive acts or practices that affect commerce, as provided under the FTC Act of 1914, 15 U.S.C, Ch, 5. §5. The FTC has brought actions in 2019, such as FTC *and People of the State of New York* versus *Google LLC and YouTube* LLC, 2019, Civil Action Number 1:19-cv-02642, for allegations that Google and its subsidiary YouTube illegally collected personal information in violation of COPA. Google agreed to settle in the amount of 170 million dollars.

The aggregation of vast volumes of data has increased the impact of data breaches such as that which occurred with the Facebook-Cambridge Analytica data scandal in 2018. The issue revealed a functionality in Facebook that allowed third-party apps to access the personal information not only of those individuals who utilized that app but also the information of their friends in Facebook who did not explicitly consent to use of the app. The ability of such apps to access the information of friends was alleged to be due to the lack of safeguards put into place by Facebook. Through the efforts of the US FTC and the US Department of Justice (DOJ), an action was brought against Facebook (*United States of America v. Facebook*, 2019, Case No. 19-cv-2184) for its failure to adequately protect the privacy and confidentiality of the personal information of its users as required under an FTC Commission Order issued in 2012. Facebook was also alleged to have engaged in deceptive practices in violation of the FTC Act by requesting users to submit personal information in order to take advantage of security measures but did not disclose that the information would be utilized for advertising. In 2019, Facebook agreed to settle with the DOJ and the FTC in the amount of $5 billion in addition to agreeing to implement changes to its privacy practices.

Ultimately, a comprehensive federal law protecting personal information would be beneficial for the consumer as well as companies. For the same reason that it is advantageous for the laws governing food, drug, and medical device requirements to exist at the federal level, a comprehensive federal law could provide a consistent set of requirements to be followed across the country. Otherwise, a system of potentially inconsistent state laws could create extremely burdensome efforts for companies seeking compliance across the United States.

## Protection of personal data in Brazil

Brazil's new consolidated privacy law (that is scheduled to come into effect in August of 2020, as of the writing of this publication) is known as the Lei Geral de Proteção de Dados Pessoais (LGPD) or translated as the General Data Privacy

Law. However, this will not be the first time that Brazil addresses this issue as there are currently 40 regulations at the federal level that protect personal data. The LGPD will have a number of features that are similar to that of GDPR such as the rights of individuals to direct the deletion of their personal data.

## To the future of agriculture and food

The agriculture and food industry has the potential to achieve further important gains by leveraging advances in the collection, processing, and analysis of various types of information. While greater access to data may not provide a single "magic bullet" solution, it promises to help augment improvements for a more efficient and sustainable food supply. Companies need to be diligent in preparing for the different types of legal obligations that may be triggered based upon the type of information collected and utilized. With regard to personal information, the enactment of privacy laws such as the GDPR and the CCPA demonstrates updated legislation addressing the different types of legal concerns that often arise through the implementation of new technology. Balance is ideal not only in nature but also in the legal realm. With the appropriate laws that enable functional and responsible practices, the improved capabilities promise to benefit industry as well as the public.

## References

ECLI:EU:C. *C-131/12, Google Spain SL, Google Inc. v. AEPD, Mario Costeja Gonzalez, 2014* (2014 (p. 317).

ECLI:EU:C. *C-507/17, Google LLC v. Commission nationale de l'informatique et des libertes (CNIL), 2019* (2019 (p. 772).

*Carpenter v. United States, 138 S. Ct. 2206, 2220.*

*Griswold v Connecticut, 381 U.S. 479.*(1965).

*Facebook: Transparency and use of consumer data: Hearing before the House Committee on Energy and Commerce, house of representatives, 115th cong. 95.*(2018) (testimony of Mark Zuckerberg).

*Federal trade commission and people of the state of New York vs. Google LLC and YouTube LLC.*(2019). Civil Action Number 1:19-cv-02642.

Google Privacy Policy. (2019, December 19). *Google. Effective 2019.* Retrieved 2020, January 1, from https://policies.google.com/privacy?hl=en-US.

Information. (n.d.). *Dictionary.* Merriam Webster Online, Retrieved 2019, December 26, from https://www.merriam-webster.com/dictionary/information.

SB 2468. (2019, January 25). *An ACT to amend the general business law and the civil practice law and rules, in relation to the uniform trade secrets act.* Retrieved from https://legislation.nysenate.gov/pdf/bills/2019/S2468.

*The Children's Online Privacy Act of 1998, P.L. 105-277 (COPA).*

*The Data Privacy Act of 1974, 5 U.S.C. § 552a.*

*The Defend Trade Secrets Act of 2016, 18 U.S.C. Sec. 1836.*

*The Federal Trade Commission Act of 1914, 15 U.S.C., Ch, 5. §5.*

*The Health Insurance Portability and Accountability Act of 1996 (HIPAA). (Pub.L. 104-191, 110 Stat. 1936).*

The State of Data 2018. (2018). *The Winterberry group.* Retrieved from https://www. winterberrygroup.com/our-insights/state-data-2018.

*United States of America v. Facebook* .(2019). Case No. 19-cv-2184.

# Implementing blockchain and regulatory technology (REGTECH)

# Implementing future food safety technologies

# 20

## Darin Detwiler, LP.D

*Assistant Dean and Associate Teaching Professor, Northeastern University, Founder and CEO of Detwiler Consulting Group, LLC., Boston, MA, United States*

Until recently, most food safety has focused on food production, manufacturing, and supply chain. Massive amounts of brain power, capital, and technology have poured into this segment of food's journey to the family table. Agriculture is still seen, however, as "one of the last traditional industries" that is embracing advanced technologies-including monitoring tools, centralized digital platforms, data analytics, and precision agriculture (Lynch, 2018). While these technologies offer hope for resiliency and sustainability, the FDA's "New Era of Smarter Food Safety" sees technology as a means for traceability and transparency. When viewed across the entire food spectrum, food safety is a continuous process from farm to fork where critical milestones, checkpoints, and (far too many) assumptions are made along the way.

Data collected annually by the US Department of Commerce since 1992 revealed in March 2015 that sales at restaurants and bars had surpassed those at grocery stores (Jamrisko, 2015). Essentially, this reflects US consumers' changing eating habits as we are now spending more money dining out or eating foods prepared outside the home than buying groceries to prepare food in the home. That stated, restaurants and retail locations-that "last mile"-are where food safety is arguably the most perilous. This actually reflects the last 100 feet of food's journey that is most likely to cause consumers to become ill, hospitalized, or worse.

Some experts hold that the future of technology in the food industry is, perhaps, most visible in restaurants and retail locations-often referred to as the "last mile" of food's journey. Here, consumers can easily find evidence of technologies' impact on marketing, ordering, and delivery options, whereas those in the industry are using new technologies for sourcing, inventory, management, and even automation (Avant, 2017).

At the same time, others see retail food safety as not having received the attention it deserves as the baseline, protective element of the $6 Trillion food consumed each year at the Retail and Food Service level in the United States (Conway, 2020). All of the work and investment in protecting the food we consume is lost the minute food products land at the loading dock of the food establishment-if the food is not stored, prepared, and served properly. The FDA recognizes the importance of this "last mile" and has created the biannual, voluntary, model Food Code that provides guidance on Food-borne Illness Risk Factors and Public Health Interventions as well as Good Retail Practices to help mitigate these risks (FDA, 2019).

However well intended, this food code is often insufficient due to the lack of enforceability, poor training, and a dearth of technology solutions designed specifically for the regulatory authorities and owner/operators who are supposed to keep the public safe.

It is important to note that some states may have updated to the 2017 Food Code in recent months, while many still operate under adopted versions from 2013 and even older versions dating as far back as 1995. However, these wide-ranging and inconsistent regulatory requirements provide significant challenges for multistate retailers and restaurant chains that operate in numerous jurisdictions because they must comply with each iteration of the Food Code throughout the 3000 US regulatory jurisdictions (FDA, 2018; Weeda, 2017).

The greatest challenges that retailers that operate in numerous jurisdictions face when attempting to comply with the various Food Code editions include

**(1)** inconsistent health inspection standards;
**(2)** inconsistent training requirements; and
**(3)** inconsistent jurisdictional authority.

Each of these inconsistencies create tremendous barriers for retailers and restaurants to protect public health to the best of their abilities. Due to the lack of one single version of the Food Code, consumers must worry whether the zip code they are eating food in will place them at a higher risk of contracting foodborne illness.

The need in this "last mile" exists, then, for a digitized, mobile platform for the entire inspection process so inspectors have all of the tools they need in the field, exactly when they need them. This technology solution would also need to allow users to select the applicable version of the FDA Food Code for the jurisdiction of concern. Few examples exist of a technology such as this-including one created by a leading, national food safety consulting firm in Boston.

Many perspectives and responsibilities must be considered when evaluating new food safety technologies.

- Maslow's Hierarchy of Needs (1943) reminds us that food and water are human's most basic, physiological needs. Second to that is safety and well-being-not only the safety of consumers, but also, as the COVID-19 pandemic has revealed, that of employees—especially in slaughterhouses and meat packing plants.
- Archie Carroll's Pyramid of Corporate Social Responsibility holds that economic, legal, ethical, and philanthropic responsibilities are also at play (Carroll, 2016).
- Comparing the two allows one to consider that ethical and philanthropic responsibilities (higher in the CSR pyramid) related to food safety (at the bottom of Maslow's hierarchy) are increasingly impacting companies' economic and legal concerns.

- Economically speaking, discussions of the ROI on investing in such technology have often come with the criticism that cost/benefit analyses must take into consideration the long-term benefits not only for the company's profit and reputation but also for consumers' well-being.
- Legally speaking, a company being sued for causing the illness or death of a consumer due to failures in food safety will have a hard time making the argument that investing in proven food safety technologies was not necessary.

## References

Avant, M. (2017, October). 5 technology trends to know: A rundown of what's new and what's next in technology as it relates to five aspects of running a restaurant business. *QSR Magazine*. Retrieved from https://www.qsrmagazine.com/technology/5-technology-trends-know.

Carroll, A. (2016). "Carroll's pyramid of CSR: Taking another look. *International Journal of Corporate Social Responsibility, 1*, 3. https://doi.org/10.1186/s40991-016-0004-6.

Conway, J. (2020, February 21). *Total retail and food services sales in the U.S. 1992-2018*. Statista. Retrieved from https://www.statista.com/statistics/197569/annual-retail-and-food-services-sales/.

FDA. (2018, October 26). *Retail food protection*. Retrieved from https://www.fda.gov/Food/GuidanceRegulation/RetailFoodProtection/ucm2006807.htm.

FDA. (2019, December 11). *FDA food code*. Retrieved from https://www.fda.gov/food/retail-food-protection/fda-food-code.

Jamrisko, M. (2015, April 14). *Americans' spending on dining out just overtook grocery sales for the first time ever*. Bloomberg News. Retrieved from https://www.bloomberg.com/news/articles/2015-04-14/americans-spending-on-dining-out-just-overtook-grocery-sales-for-the-first-time-ever.

Lynch, S. (2018, December 4). *The 7 technologies that will make farming smarter—and more productive*. Fast Company. Retrieved from https://www.fastcompany.com/90272045/the-7-technologies-that-will-make-farming-smarter-and-more-productive.

Maslow, A. (1943). A theory of human motivation. *Psychological Review, 50*, 370–396. Retrieved from https://psychclassics.yorku.ca/Maslow/motivation.htm.

Weeda, J. (2017, October 12). *FDA report on food code adoption*. Retrieved from https://www.ofwlaw.com/2017/10/12/fda-report-food-code-adoption/.

# Quality assurance: considerations for the future of food safety technology

# 21

**David Shelep**

*Microbiologist and Consultant, Paramount Sciences, Los Angeles, CA, United States*

The FDA Food Safety Modernization Act (FSMA) was signed into law by President Obama on January 4, 2011, to better protect public health by strengthening the food safety system. It enables FDA to focus more on preventing food safety problems rather than relying primarily on reacting to problems after they occur.

While there had been many companies very active in the areas of food safety for years, often companies had operated such that food safety was a hindrance to business or productivity. After years of well-known recalls and many illnesses and deaths, FSMA has driven the food industry to diligently concentrate on further providing safe products. In the past, there were not any "Directors of Food Safety" within organizations, however post-FSMA, that or similar titles are commonly seen. There are more and more conferences, workshops, products, and services all geared toward food safety matters. This is a clear indication of change.

Another significant change is with the quality assurance departments. In the past quality assurance roles within organizations often reported into the operations team of a food company. This could create conflict within an organization. It is becoming more common to have the food safety interest of an organization's report to the legal team, a C-level person or similar position outside of manufacturing operations that can drive the interest of food safety above all before any products are released to the public. This gives those whose primary focus was more technical in the past a greater business focus in their responsibilities.

As a microbiologist who was trained in the bench-level technical aspects of my field, I was given little training on what the discovery of a pathogen or environmental contaminant truly meant to the business and what my role would be to resolve the problem. What did it truly cost our organization, how did it affect customer or employee safety, etc.? This is a welcomed change and it is further empowering quality professionals to think beyond the laboratory bench and into their significance within an organization.

Building the Future of Food Safety Technology. https://doi.org/10.1016/B978-0-12-818956-6.00021-X

Manufacturers now proactively practice recall readiness, mock regulatory inspections, perform diligent supplier audits, and use other measures to produce a safe product. Product testing remains an important part of food safety; however, testing of the final product is too limited at times and can miss potential problems.

One of the biggest changes has been the building of robust environmental monitoring (EM) programs. The food industry's approaches to EM are now mirroring what the pharmaceutical industry has undertaken for years. It just makes sense that a way to prevent contamination is to discover a potential problem in the manufacturing area before it can get into a product.

Robust EM programs have allowed organizations to better understand their manufacturing environments and be able to react to problems faster. This is the basis and goal of any EM program. Organizations are undertaking thorough sampling and as they have greater understanding of where problems may occur, modifying their programs to better respond.

While the industry is getting up-to-speed (in regard to revealing contaminations), responses and decontamination approaches often seem to be less developed and, at times, very disorganized. These companies' reactions to situations are characterized by the "Henny Penny, the sky is falling" approach rather than an "all hands-on deck, everyone is prepared and has a specific function" approach.

Once cleaning procedures have been conducted, in aligning with the "Era of Smarter Food Safety" there are three ways in which I recommend advancing an organization.

## Develop a strategic sanitation program

In developing your strategic sanitation program (SSP), completely map out all the options you have available to control or eliminate contaminations. Understand then where each method fits into your processes and which contaminants and to what level of kill they offer. It is also imperative to understand the effect each has on your equipment, staff, budget, timelines, etc.

Simply mapping out all options in a table is helpful. (In this example, generic terms are shown under usual application conditions, however, list all options in detail.)

Developing the SSP and this table gives each member of the team the ability to visually see when each method can and should be used. In addition, consider where each method can be used. Will a chemical be used on a specific processing equipment, a drain, spiral freezer, full facility, etc.? What equipment needs to be avoided due to corrosion or other incompatibilities?

The goal of the SSP is

- To be focused as a team in the approaches undertaken.
- Not use methods unnecessary or ineffective (i.e., using a sporicidal chemical when you have only bacterial contamination).

| Method | What it *kills* | Level of kill | Timeline considerations | Implementation considerations | Safety on equipment | Safety for staff | Initial price | Cost to the organization |
|---|---|---|---|---|---|---|---|---|
| UV-C | Sterilant (bacterial, viruses, yeast, mold, spores) | 3–6 log | Fast, exposure can be managed easily | Direct kill where light is exposed, not around corners, etc., simple equipment | Yes | Yes | Medium priced equipment | Over time very low |
| Foam A | Disinfectant (no spores) | 3–4 log | Fast | Misses nooks and crannies, no complex equipment | Yes | Yes, also can bring in service | Inexpensive | High, can be ineffective |
| Foam B | Sterilant (bacterial, viruses, yeast, mold, spores) | 5–6 log | Slow, requires long exposure | Misses nooks and crannies, complex to mix or use proper concentration | Can be corrosive | Need PPE in implementation, also can bring in service | Inexpensive | Medium, unless destroys equipment |
| Powder | Sterilant (bacterial, viruses, yeast, mold, spores) | 5 log | Slow, requires long exposure | Misses nooks and crannies, no complex equipment | Yes | Need to be careful with dispersing | Medium | Low |
| Spray | Disinfectant (no spores) | 4–5 log | Fast | Gets just about everywhere it is applied, easy to mix or use proper concentration | Can be corrosive | Need to be careful with dispersing | Inexpensive | High if ineffective and destroys equipment |
| Gas A | Sterilant (bacterial, viruses, yeast, mold, spores) | 5–6 log | Slow, requires long exposure, set up complex | Gets everywhere—nooks and crannies, but not great for whole facility | Yes | Generally little training or risk if used properly, PPE as backup, also can bring in service | High priced equipment, supplies inexpensive | Over time very low as complete sterilant |
| Gas B | Sterilant (bacterial, viruses, yeast, mold, spores) | 5–6+ log | Fast, exposure can be managed easily | Gets everywhere—nooks and crannies, great for whole facility, complex equipment | Yes | Generally little training or risk if used properly, PPE as backup, also can bring in service | High priced equipment or service, supplies inexpensive | Over time very low as complete sterilant and owning equipment |

Table by author.

- Use less resources both in labor and chemicals to not waste money.
- Solve the problem faster and return to producing a safe product with greater ease.

## Practice mock contamination events and resulting decontamination plans

Organizations practice mock recalls and mock regulatory inspections with their teams. This gives them the ability to plan how to react, determine if they have proper documentation in place, and make changes in their approaches.

There is complete logic in developing the same in regard to contaminations. If there was an immediate call to the food safety leader within your organization that a *Listeria* isolate was found in a critical area, what would happen? Are teams ready and in place (along with the SSP above) to easily handle the situation? Does everyone within the organization fully understand their role in food safety and how a contamination affects their work? A simulated event such as this would reveal areas of expertise or problem areas that need to be addressed. If you asked a line worker or a human resources professional what a *Listeria* means to them and the organization, how would they respond?

Consider flight crews on commercial airlines. While we see them as ambassadors of service, they are fully trained (and retrained, and retrained) on safety. Ninety-nine percent of the time their jobs are routine, but should an event occur, they know their roles and they are trained to play them and promptly do so. This is for safety and swift resolution of the event. Or, consider the Emergency Department in your local hospital. Staff deal with a lot of routine and mundane times, but when a significant event occurs, a major trauma arrives, each member goes into action and knows their role. Again, for safety and swift resolution of that event (or in this case a patient trauma).

The teams involved in your organization would go beyond those generally involved in mock recalls or regulatory inspections. Besides the food safety and operations teams, consider involving

- **Purchasing**—they care about the spend, is it done wisely ...
- **Materials Management**—they know supplies, inventory, orders/back orders ...
- **Sanitation**—consider many members from this team and those that work different shifts
- **Human Resources**—they know limits on hours staff can work, what is available and costs to the organization with overtime
- **Maintenance**—they know what equipment is easily cleanable and what is not and time needed to get back to functioning if disassembly needs be performed
- **Environmental Health and Safety**—if intimately involved developing the SSP, they need to be on this team and fully prepared with any documentation, permits, employee protective equipment needed, etc.

During an event, it is not the time to put the team into place, it must be established beforehand and ready at any time to step into action. Practicing a mock contamination event and the decontamination plans is wise.

## Elevate the sanitation teams within the organization

I urge the food industry to look at their sanitation and decontamination staff and how they fit within the organization. Could their reporting structure be changed to give them more significance and therefore that of food safety as it relates to sanitation? Are their titles and pay or compensation congruent with their work? Many would initially say yes; however, if the question was asked "are their titles and pay or compensation congruent with their role in regards to food safety in an era of new food safety"?

While there are some training programs and even university attention to sanitation, the industry as a whole must elevate and compensate these teams based on their critical role in sanitation and food safety.

This may require significant training staff in understanding of each of the available methods developed in your SSP, but the organization would gain much more strategic approach in routinely controlling their environments and then reacting to problems when they occur. Staff fully understanding why they do something and why they do it will follow procedures better, gain more ownership of the processes, and be more efficient in their duties.

If the sanitation and decontamination teams are the weakest link or a constraint in regard to food safety, change it. Compensate them and elevate them.

The future of food safety is all about being proactive and less and less reactive. Considering these approaches mentioned may require some to adapt to completely new business models. While for others, simple modifications will be made. Either way, under FSMA the expectations are high to make the food supply where the FDA maintains responsibility, the safest in the world.

# Regulatory compliance: executive level considerations for food safety technology

# 22

**Jennifer Crandall**

*Founder and CEO, Safe Food En Route, LLC., Independence, KY, United States*

A key to understand what type of food safety technology needs to be in place is by what types of food safety programs need to be managed and the associated data that go along with those programs. Most food manufacturing and food facilities have a single person or department designated to manage the food safety and quality programs. The person in charge manages the programs to meet requirements set by legal authorities, customer requirements, and expectations for any certifications the facility chooses for branding purposes to follow (such as SQF, BRC, etc.). The person is usually in charge of other programs as well including Kosher, Halal, Organic, Non-GMO, Gluten-free, and many other branding type decisions that need managed appropriately as well. A great deal of responsibility falls upon this department and/or person and it is often difficult for a facility to justify all the expense that might go into managing it all.

The Quality Department is often the department that oversees all related programs. As such, these teams work with an insurmountable amount of data and paperwork to prove that the company understands what they are doing and that they are doing what they say they are doing. These programs include, but are not limited to, the following programs provided below.

## HACCP/Food safety plans

Depending on the sector of the food industry, Hazard Analysis Critical Control Points (HACCP) and/or Current Good Manufacturing Practices (CGMPs), Hazard Analysis and Risk-Based Preventive Control for Human Food and/or Animal Feed Safety plans might be a regulatory requirement. Let us quickly dive into what these programs cover and what type of data might need to be managed with them.

Per the International HACCP Alliance (n.d.), "HACCP is a process control system that identifies where hazards might occur in the food production process and puts into place stringent actions to take to prevent the hazards from occurring. By strictly monitoring and controlling each step of the process, there is less chance

Building the Future of Food Safety Technology. https://doi.org/10.1016/B978-0-12-818956-6.00022-1

for hazards to occur." In layman's terms, an HACCP plan is a risk-based assessment conducted on all foreseeable hazards associated with the production of the product being sold for consumption from the facility in question and making sure there are controls in place to prevent the hazards from getting to the consumer. The plan includes listing all raw materials, processing steps, evaluating, and demonstrating into practice policies, procedures, and documented processes verifying the hazard is controlled and is backed by science. HACCP plans have seven principles that include paperwork surrounding each one:

1. **Conduct hazard analysis**: each step is listed in a process flow diagram and each raw material used in the process of each different type of product including food and packaging and the associated hazards with each of those points in the process.
2. **Identify the critical control points (CCPs)**-in general, this is the last point that the hazard can be controlled prior to leaving the facility and going to the next user (manufacturing, packaging, distributing, etc.) or customer.
3. **Establish critical limits**-critical limits are established to manage the CCPs and make sure that the facility is not allowing product to pass the point in the process flow without meeting those limits.
4. **Establish CCP monitoring requirements**-this includes identifying what it will take to meet those critical limits through a processing step such as cooking to a specified temperature for a specified amount of time. There are several ways to manage the CCP and would be used and monitored in the process.
5. **Establish effective recordkeeping**-recordkeeping includes how the records are maintained to prove that the facility managed the hazard appropriately and that it was within the critical limits specified. Using the cooking time/temperature example above, a digital thermometer recording the time the temperature was met and how long before it dropped below the required temperature. Knowing the relationship of the time and temperature during each batch product will prove that the facility met the appropriate CCP monitoring requirement and stayed within the critical limits.
6. **Establish procedures for verifications**-this step includes someone making sure that the CCP critical limit was met. This is different than a validation process where there is scientific evidence proving that the CCP is appropriate for the hazard identified. The verification means that someone made sure that the process worked the way it was supposed to. Using the same time/temp cook example from above, this might include someone reviewing the charts to make sure that the calibration was done properly on the temperature gauge and that the time/temp was met and if it was not that appropriate corrective actions were taken to ensure that only safe product went to the consumer.
7. **Recordkeeping**-it did not happen if it was not recorded. Though this is very cliché, this is the reality. Everything must be documented and proven.

Usually the HACCP plan also contains prerequisite programs including GMPs and Sanitation Standard Operating Procedures (SSOPs), which control the operational conditions within a food establishment and promote environmental conditions that are favorable to produce safe food. According to Cornell University's Dairy Extension services (Cornell, 2020) and the FDA's 2015 Grade "A" Pasteurized Milk Ordinance (PMO) (FDA, 2015), prerequisite programs may include things like

1. Water, steam, and ice safety (proven possibly by periodic lab testing or water charts from public water supply).
2. Condition and cleanliness of food-contact surfaces (proven possibly by preoperational check off sheets).
3. Prevention of cross contamination (proven possibly by sanitation records).
4. Maintenance of hand-washing, hand-sanitizing, and toilet facilities (proven possibly by daily paperwork).
5. Protection from adulteration (proven possibly by lab results).
6. Proper labeling, storage, and use of toxic compounds (proven possibly by daily paperwork and regularly reviewing raw material specifications).
7. Control of employee health conditions (proven possibly by training documents).
8. Exclusion of pests (proven possibly by pest management paperwork).
9. Additional programs might include several other aspects from calibrations, temperature controls, receiving, training, recall, etc.

As you can imagine, there would be ways to prove all this through various types of paperwork collected and managed on a daily basis in the facilities.

CGMP, Hazard Analysis and Risk-Based Preventive Controls for Human Food, and/or Animal Feed Food Safety Plans are now required by the 2011 FDA Food Safety Modernization Act ("FSMA") (Pub.L. 111−353, 124 STAT 3885), for specific types of manufacturers of food. According to Illinois Institute of Technology's Food Safety Preventive Controls Alliance (FSPCA):

> The Current Good Manufacturing Practice, Hazard Analysis, and Risk-based Preventive Controls for Human Food regulation (referred to as the Preventive Controls for Human Food regulation) is intended to ensure safe manufacturing/processing, packing and holding of food products for human consumption in the United States

**FSPCA, 2020**

One way that some experts think about Preventive Controls for both Human Food and Animal Feed is like HACCP on steroids. The biggest difference in the programs, in my opinion, reminded me of Simon Sinek's book, *Start With Why: How Great Leaders Inspire Everyone to Take Action* and his description of the Japanese automaker measuring every step of the process to ensure that a car door fits at the end of the assembly line (Sinek, 2009). This is the same as Preventive Controls rules where the hazards are evaluated, controlled, and have critical limits defined with appropriate documented corrective actions to take when metrics are not met, whereas HACCP is like the American automaker in his story hammering the door into place after it gets to the end of the line as it only measures and documents the last possible critical step the hazard can be controlled and performs corrective actions at defined critical control point only. There are other differences regarding Preventive Controls rules including different hazard categories to assess and basic requirements for specific prerequisite type programs and many more documents that must be managed by the facilities to prove that they are saying what they are doing. All of this can be considered for managing electronically.

## Food safety audit certifications/audits/regulatory inspections

The principles and standards of HACCP are internationally recognized and a key component of many food safety audit requirements including those of GFSI (Global Food Safety Initiative) benchmarked audit schemes, such as BRC, SQF, FSSC 22000, IFS, Global GAP, PrimusGFS, and many more. These core principles are foundational of a good food safety program and audit companies build the requirements into their guidance documents to provide the framework for facilities to meet internationally recognized standards. Though GFSI has gained recognition over the past 20+ years, there are also third-party food safety audits that are conducted that cover these areas as well. Though they do not scrutinize the hazards assessment as much as GFSI benchmarked audit schemes, they still ensure that the companies have an HACCP plan in place. Also, third-party food safety audits cover a lot of the GMP (Good Manufacturing Practices) that are now required for many facilities to meet FSMA requirements. And a key to all of this is that these types of audits review that facilities have procedures, policies, and appropriate documentation that ties into each major food safety element required by whatever authority reviewing their programs (regulatory or third-party food safety audits and even customer audits).

## Other related programs to manage

Other key areas for managing a lot of food safety data management are supplier programs, supply chain programs, product development programs, recall and traceability programs, and branding decisions such as Kosher, Halal, Organic, and Gluten-free programs. These are all tied together by documentation and data management.

## Foundation of food safety programs takeaway

The quality assurance managers at a facility must manage all these programs and keep track of policies, procedures, SOPs (Standard Operating Procedures), and operational documentation and keep those records for a specific amount of time determined by whatever authority is overseeing the program. Keep in mind that some paperwork is required to be managed and kept for up to 5 years.

## Improving programs through the era of smarter technology

Though technology has been used in the food industry for a while, most of the technology that has been available has been centered around other parts of the business, such as inventory management or purchase order writing. For the past 20 years, the regulatory, food safety, and quality assurance sections of the industry have been attempting to create solutions that are built onto systems that manage these other types of business-related functions. In my experience, in retail environments and in manufacturing, trying to build on to a software system designed for a completely different reason creates a recipe for large expenses and, oftentimes, systems that do not fully manage the additional feature sufficiently.

With FDA's focus on improving programs through the Era of Smarter Technology, the time is coming where companies will be mandated to review their programs and determine what makes sense to manage with technology. According to the FDA's 2019 statements related to their "New Era of Smarter Food Safety" (FDA, 2019), things to consider will include tech-enabled traceability and foodborne outbreak responses, smarter tools, and approaches for prevention, adapting to new business models and retail food safety modernization and improving the food safety culture. As these things are considered, a great importance should be placed on including supplier compliance management programs, raw material management, lot number and traceability programs, and real-time processing, storage conditions, and in-line recording devices. The following are suggestions of things to consider in each category.

## Tech-enabled traceability and foodborne outbreak response

While myriad conferences and publications focus on Blockchain, this platform is not alone. Tangle is the other name to describe the Internet of Things Applications' directed acyclic graph (DAG)—a data integration and transaction settlement layer that acts as a string of individual transactions which are interconnected to one another and stored in a decentralized network node of the participants. Essentially, the Tangle platform replaces Blockchain with DAG to store its ledger (Arogyalo-kesh, 2020).

The FDA is asking that when looking at technologies, the food industry looks at data streams, and processes that will greatly reduce the length of time needed to track and trace the origin of a contaminated food and respond to public health risks.

Blockchain and the emerging Tangle platform will be technologies to keep an eye on and use to a company's advantage while developing programs to meet FDA's future requirements.

A frequently discussed Walmart traceability exercise with some large companies provides an example of how managing data with Blockchain reduced the amount of time to trace a product back to its origin from days to seconds ("Case Study", 2018). To be able to track data this way would be a huge advantage to the industry and to consumers as well. A real-world risk to consider, however, would be that the relationship from product to retailer is usually not a one-to-one basis where the product is managed and handled by one company. EVERYONE in the supply chain would have to be engaged. But keep in mind that a one-to-one relationship is not normal. Normally, a product is sourced from multiple sources and sold to multiple customers; therefore, the traceability must be done with that in mind where it is a many-to-many relationship.

Another example of how the Blockchain/Tangle technologies can be used is with the sharing of data. Suppliers are constantly asked to provide data to their customers—including supplier compliance programs, third-party food safety audits, certifications, product data, specifications, and branding certifications (such as Organic, Kosher, and Halal). Often, retailers ask for various software platforms to be used for uploading these data to them from the supply chain. The data are then integrated into other internal programs that might need supplemental data from the vendors. With Blockchain and Tangle technologies, these data can be encrypted and shared with permission-based encryptions to allow vendors to share the data once instead of having to upload the data multiple times to multiple customer programs and multiple software platforms. If the software systems that the vendor is using to manage these programs had this technology built into the software, they could utilize internal systems to share data with customer systems with the click of a button. Although this might be a utopian point of view, the possibilities are endless to be able to incorporate programs related to supplier management, raw material management, lot number, and traceability programs.

## Smarter tools and approaches for prevention

Another great use for the Blockchain and Tangle technologies is with the real-time data recording devices. Examples of this might include in-line thermometers, in-line pressure gauges, satellite recording thermometers used in transit of refrigerated or frozen goods, storage conditions digitally recorded with remote alarm systems, in-line pH meters, and many other types of tools to monitor the real life conditions of raw materials, storage environments, finished products, and processing controls. These types of tools, according to the FDA's documents on its "New Era of Smarter Food Safety," can be used to enhance the "use of new knowledge from traceback, data streams and tools for rapidly analyzing data" (FDA, 2019). The FDA is looking to the industry to start using these data in a more revolutionary type way, such as using it for predictive analytics and artificial intelligence built in for trending data in ways to assist in preventing public harm.

Some of this type of technology is already in existence and self-corrects when critical limits are not met. An example would be a dairy high temperature short time (HTST) pasteurization unit. Most dairies in the United States are required to have a diversion procedure in place where the HTST unit automatically diverts milk back to the raw tank when the temperature and/or pressure does meet required limits that are substandard according to the FDA requirements for pasteurizing milk. The HTST has digitally controlled recording devices that cause automatically diversion when those limits are not met and the operator and the regulatory authorities test the unit on a regular basis to ensure that it is working properly (FDA, n.d.). These are the types of real-time technologies that can be put into place throughout the supply chain to assist with management of safe foods. These are also areas where the data are automatically captured and monitored in some type of recording device.

## Adapting to new business models and retail food safety modernization

The FDA's "New Era of Smarter Food Safety" includes an expressed desire of the administration to advance "the safety of both new business models, such as e-commerce and home delivery of foods, and traditional business models, such as retail food establishments" (FDA, 2019). As these technologies are rapidly being developed, there are some obstacles suppliers should consider.

- Large company legacy systems do not always connect to each other and ask for same data.
- Often retail systems require subscriptions to be paid by suppliers.
- Retailer data silos—new technology is not always integrated across all departments.
- One-time sharing is not always possible.
- Global Trade Item Number (GTIN) technology (the GS1 developed identifier for trade items) adopted by retailers is NOT consistent among all retailers.
- Information is as good as the quality of the data (if fields are not required, then gaps will persist).

## Food safety culture

The FDA wants to promote and recognize "the role of food safety culture on farms and in facilities" (FDA, 2019). The goal is to ensure that companies are doing their best to improve the thought patterns around influencing employees and overall companies to have better food safety programs and be able to "demonstrate" their commitment to the work. The intent is to also strengthen this culture to homes and educate consumers on safe food handling practices.

All parts of the supply chain must be engaged in making sure programs are embraced and utilized. GFSI certification audit programs and regulatory compliance audits cover leadership commitment by leadership demonstrating (not just on paper) that they support and prioritize food safety.

Examples of leadership commitment include, but are not limited to, the following:

- Incentivized programs around quality and food safety metrics
- QA/food safety management teams in higher positions or equivalent positions to operations management
- Resources allocated to prioritizing food safety—education, training, programs, policies, meetings
- Ongoing investment into programs, software, technology, consulting, expand departments, etc.

The less obvious benefits to these programs and this smarter era of technology can include many areas:

- Supplier/product approval processes
- Supplier/product management
- PM programs
- Real-time monitoring
- Less paper
- Policy and document management centralization
- Reduced labor
- Automatic logging devices = less human error
- Linked information—easily onboarded and deboarded
- Free up management time/reduced labor

## Things to consider when purchasing solutions

Before considering purchase of solutions to meet the future requirements of FDA with smarter food safety management, a good first step would be to review several options, as multiple decisions will need to be made along the way. Many important decisions to be made center around how a company wants to use technology. Below are several dimensions of questions to ask prior to reviewing technology.

**A.** Questions to ask regarding the volume of data to manage:
  **1.** How many suppliers and documents associated with onboarding and maintenance of supplier programs?
  **2.** How many raw materials and documents associated with onboarding and maintenance of information?

3. How many products/formulations and documents associated?
4. How many documents for all policies, programs, procedures?
5. How much daily paperwork is managed at the facility?

**B.** Questions to ask regarding the need for automation:

1. Do documents expire? What types of documents are they? Do you need to maintain documents based on their expirations? Do you need copies of the audit reports, certifications, policies, etc.?
2. Do you need email alerts/notifications? Do you need automatic reminders?
3. Do you need reporting features? Do you need dashboard management?
4. Is it easy to connect documents to different parts of the supply chain? For example, PO numbers to Bills of Lading to Lot codes to manufacturing data to customers (one step backwards, one step forward).

**C.** Questions to ask regarding the robust level for data management you need:

1. Do you need to maintain version control of policies, procedures, and/or operational paperwork for audit guidance documents and references?
2. Do you need to create HACCP or Food Safety Plans from scratch, or do you have it already created and just need a place to store it?
3. Do you need a document repository for centralization purposes? Would this be beneficial to your audit preparedness?
4. Do you need to store GFSI/third-party audit reports for your suppliers? Do you need to monitor their expiration dates?
5. Do you need to review regulatory audits?
6. Do you need a place to store all daily paperwork? Do you need an electronic system to manage the daily paperwork instead of using paper? This could apply to processing records, production paperwork, sanitation records, preventative maintenance, in-house pest management programs, allergen management programs, internal and external lab paperwork.
7. Do you need version control for product development/formulas? How to manage scale-up trials and tweaking of formulas?
8. Do you need Nutritional calculating software? Do you need to store current product specifications for raw materials and finished products?
9. How to manage current label versions?
10. How to manage shelf-life testing?
11. Do you have HACCP Challenge/Validation studies to monitor and conduct periodically?
12. Do you need a dashboard for quick reporting and/or a reports feature and searchability in the documents? Are the documents and words easy to search?
13. How do you track employee training on each program? Is it connected to the documents or is it in a separate file? How do you handle it when someone is absent from training the day of training for the entire crew? How do you document it?

**D.** Questions to ask around Blockchain/Tangle readiness:
1. How is privacy, permissions managed for internal and external purposes?
2. How much individual attention will you get with the software providers to ensure that you can correct any concerns you might have?
3. Is there capability for easy sharing (one click vs. multiple uploads)? Can you upload sets of documents once instead of multiple times for multiple customers/participants? Is there capability for one-time share subscriptions?
4. What type of remote accessibility (cloud) and backup options are there?
5. Are there any space restraints? How do you manage backups? Can you go 100% paper free?
6. What kind of maneuverability will you have with the system? Can you integrate it to other systems such as SAP, Inventory, and other food safety and quality management systems, etc.? Is it customizable, configurable? Are there data feeds you can tap into such as FDA Dashboard information? What are the sources to those?
7. Is there a traceability method to manage and connect all the documents and supply chain paperwork that might go together?
8. Can other departments benefit potentially?

Keep in mind that, though affordability might mean you cannot please everyone, consider everyone before finalizing project scope. Document management is document management. If the software solutions are not designed 100% for one purpose or another, there is potential to modify a system to be able to manage many compliance-related documents as they typically need managed the same way with expirations and resubmissions by the customer, the supplier, or someone else within the supply chain. Departments to discuss this with are the following at minimum:

1. Legal/Contract compliance management
2. Sustainability programs
3. Ethical compliance
4. Supplier diversity programs
5. Transportation programs
6. Sourcing teams
7. Human resources

## Summary

In summary, I want to send a note to the entities that might be considering these types of programs for data management. In my experience with working at a retailer that owned manufacturing facilities as well and had a corporate department dedicated to managing policies, procedures, regulatory compliance, food safety, and quality programs and product development, plus my experience in working at manufacturing facilities, I have had a pretty good vantage point of some of the pitfalls and ways to manage these types of programs. My below suggestions are advice to each entity to consider how to develop technology that assists with programs and maximize how your programs can all work together for your best interest.

## Note to Growers:

Depending on your size, managing paperwork in an electronic format might seem way too advanced and overwhelming. Also depending on your size, the regulations might not apply to you the same way that they do to everyone else. But, if you are planning to grow your operation to a larger scaled size, it is good to develop your programs earlier and consider going electronic as quickly as possible. Because the FSMA Produce Safety rule was implemented for growers larger than $25,000/year in sales, it is a good idea to create programs with the document management portion of that rule in mind. It is also good to review any GAP (Good Agricultural Practices) requirements as well as many retailers and food service companies require these types of programs as a minimum standard. These types of programs include, but are not limited to, documents related to the following:

1. Worker health, hygiene, and training
2. Soil amendments
3. Wildlife and domesticated animals, surrounding land use
4. Agricultural water: production and postharvest
5. Postharvest handling and sanitation
6. Traceability programs
7. HACCP/food safety plans

   Consider incorporating these into a document management program using software and use live feeds for temperature control and water controls where possible. You can also consider using electronic management of field harvest and pest management. The soil amendment and pesticide applications also are great to be managed electronically. All these types of live data feeds are good to have centralized and easily accessible along with policies and procedures and the proof of training surrounding these types of programs on file. Having these data easily accessible to auditors and regulatory authorities, not to mention your customers, helps those processes go smoother and make you appear more organized and more in order. Taking food safety programs seriously and proving what you say you are doing will take your facility far and take you to the level that retailers and food service companies expect in their supply chain. Not to mention, it is the right thing to do for public health and safety.

## Note to Manufacturers:

I highly recommend that you review how you want to use technology and to look for the most robust system you can find for internal purposes. Food safety management is not just the Quality Assurance department either—this is a full company effort. Work together to find solutions that work across the entire company. And know that thinking strategically often means stepping outside of the four walls of your facility. You may want to consider hiring consulting companies to assist with this process or shutting down for a few days and working together to solve multiple problems together. This is difficult to do in the manufacturing world, but it is critical to develop this strategically instead of reactively. Also, it is good to divide your programs into categories when selecting software programs. The three main dimensions I suggest considering are as follows:

1. **Supplier management and monitoring**—most of the regulations require that you have some type of supplier approval program, supplier management program, and some type of monitoring program in place. Consider how to do this and how to maintain an approved supplier list and, if possible, a way to monitor them and keep it all connected. This is a combination of

monitoring their history with regulatory agencies in all areas they sell into globally as well as monitoring their history with your company and their food safety audit history. This program cannot just be one of those areas. It needs to consider all of them.

2. **Policy/Procedure/Guidance document management and version control**—how do you manage all the versions of documents in place in the facility? How are old versions kept out of the use? This is critical to ensure that old versions of formulas, of raw materials, etc., are not used in the facility if a new version is developed. Do not forget managing the training of your teams in this system as well. You need to have all of that on file and quickly accessible and it's in your best interest to have it managed together. Centralized data make your life so much easier. Also, do not forget documents like your kosher, halal, organic, and natural management and fair trade, sustainability programs, and anything related. These are all relevant to being managed this way.

3. **Live data management**—how do you manage all documents used to measure and monitor your processes from start to finish? Consider supplier approvals and purchase systems connections, supplier maintenance, receiving, traceability data, storage and inventory management, process controls, and shipping records. Also, consider what you can gather electronically and connect the dots inside the system with your preventive controls programs, allergen management, sanitation, operational paperwork, lab results, and temperature monitoring systems. These are mere examples of how you can connect it all together.

## Note to Retailers:

When considering technology solutions, it is wise to consider the experience of everyone involved and not one party solely. The easier that it is for the entities providing the information, the more success your program will have in the long run. In my experience, the most data needed usually are from the supplier base. The suppliers should not be the forgotten entity in the development process and should be considered when developing automation and easy management. The documents they need to provide are large and usually require a lot of back and forth between your teams and them to get the right information to evaluate their programs. Consider all processes that ask for the documentation as well and try to connect those dots, such as bidding and approval processes versus supplier maintenance processes. Look at ways you can automate that as much as possible and ways that you can make it a one-stop shop. If possible, collaborate with other retailers, so that the experience is easy, and they can comply easily to all programs. Though the suppliers do have to pay a "cost of doing business" with companies, per say, it is not necessary to make it so difficult that they never fully comply. This only puts strain on your internal teams and not necessarily the supplier themselves. The internal teams are the ones that must manage the aftermath and the back and forth and it puts you at risk of not complying fully to the regulatory requirements you have in place. Another responsible way of managing this program is to use the automatic features as much as possible, such as automatic email reminders and reports when documents expire.

You will have obstacles with your legacy systems, and that is understandable. Look for ways to piece things together and have integration instead. Yes, software development usually means expensive, so I recommend prioritizing the main user in the process and automate as much as possible to them. Too often, priorities are only focused on the internal teams and the external users are the ones that might have better ways to upload information and do it faster. This is especially true for the larger companies that are engaged. They already have methods to manage this all and sometimes want everyone to comply to their standards, but the suppliers must hire full time people to upload documents to each customer system because there are so many different systems to upload information, thus adding unnecessary cost to the supply chain. The earlier you get engaged with the

Blockchain/Tangle technology to help define that, the better it will be. But do not forget the little guys. They are the core of your business and they may not have access to all of the technology conversations you have been involved in.

## Final word

Anything that is required for the GFSI type audits and/or third-party audits and/or regulatory requirements are good to consider for managing in a smarter and technological way. The more digitalized you are and the easier it is to manage the data, the better off you will be. Think strategically with how you manage it, think how you can automate, and think how you can protect your data, yet provide it easily and quickly to those companies. That will help you land the customer faster. Speed and efficiencies are always respected if it represents the reality of your programs. However, you cannot speed up baking a cake, so be sure to check all the ingredients and go through the appropriate steps to have your cake and eat it too.

## References

Arogyalokesh. (2020). *Tangle technology.* Mindmajix Technologies, Inc. Blog. Retrieved from https://mindmajix.com/tangle-technology.

*Case Study: How Walmart brought unprecedented transparency to the food supply chain with Hyperledger Fabric.* (2018). The Linux Foundation. Retrieved from https://www.hyperledger.org/resources/publications/walmart-case-study.

FDA. (n.d.). *HTST pasteurization of milk.* Retrieved from https://www.accessdata.fda.gov/orau/pasteurization/PAS_03_summary.htm.

FDA. (2015). *Grade "A" pasteurized milk ordinance.* Retrieved from https://www.fda.gov/media/99451/download.

FDA. (2019, November 19). *New era of smarter food safety.* Retrieved from https://www.fda.gov/food/food-industry/new-era-smarter-food-safety.

FSPCA. (2020). *Preventive controls for human food.* Illinois Institute of Technology. Retrieved from https://www.ifsh.iit.edu/fspca/fspca-preventive-controls-human-food.

International HACCP Alliance. (n.d.). *HACCP questions and answers.* Retrieved from http://haccpalliance.org/alliance/haccpqa.html.

Prerequisite Programs. (2020). *Cornell university college of agriculture and life science, dairy extension.* Retrieved from https://dairyextension.foodscience.cornell.edu/resources/food-safety/food-safety-planhaccp/prerequisite-programs/.

Sinek, S. (2009). *Start with why: How great leaders Inspire everyone to take action.* N.Y.: Penguin.

# Index

Printed in the United States
By Bookmasters